When Doctors Kill

Joshua A. Perper · Stephen J. Cina

When Doctors Kill

Who, Why, and How

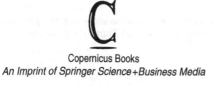

Copernicus Books
An Imprint of Springer Science+Business Media

Joshua A. Perper, M.D., LL.B, M.Sc.
Fort Lauderdale, Florida
USA
perperj@bellsouth.net

Stephen J. Cina, M.D.
Fort Lauderdale, Florida
USA
cinasj@pol.net

Cover design: Dr. Edward J. Perper, Animation MD

Published in the United States by Copernicus Books,
an imprint of Springer Science+Business Media.

Copernicus Books
Springer Science+Business Media
233 Spring Street
New York, NY 10013
www.springer.com

Library of Congress Control Number: 2010923613

Manufactured in the United States of America.
Printed on acid-free paper.

The opinions expressed herein solely represent the views of the authors and do not reflect the opinions of Broward County government, the Office of the Medical Examiner and Trauma Services, or any organizations to which the authors belong.

ISBN 978-1-4419-1368-5   ISBN 978-1-4419-1369-2 (eBook)

From Dr. Joshua A. Perper
To my greatly missed and beloved wife,
Sheila, who made me a better compassionate
physician and man.

From Dr. Stephen J. Cina
To Ali, Kyle, Tucker, and Bella,
Most doctors don't kill people. As a matter
of fact, why don't one of you go to med
school?—Dad

Preface

It would come as no surprise that many readers may be shocked and intrigued by the title of our book. Some (especially our medical colleagues) may wonder why it is even worthwhile to raise the issue of killing by doctors. Killing is clearly antithetical to the Art and Science of Medicine, which is geared toward easing pain and suffering and to saving lives rather than smothering them. Doctors should be a source of comfort rather than a cause for alarm. Nevertheless, although they often don't want to admit it, doctors are people too. Physicians have the same genetic library of both endearing qualities and character defects as the rest of us but their vocation places them in a position to intimately interject themselves into the lives of other people. In most cases, fortunately, the positive traits are dominant and doctors do more good than harm.

While physicists and mathematicians paved the road to the stars and deciphered the mysteries of the atom, they simultaneously unleashed destructive powers that may one day bring about the annihilation of our planet. Concurrently, doctors and allied scientists have delved into the deep secrets of the body and mind, mastering the anatomy and physiology of the human body, even mapping the very molecules that make us who we are. But make no mistake, a person is not simply an elegant biological machine to be marveled at then dissected. A person has a soul or, if you prefer, an innate uniqueness that can never be perfectly replicated. When a human being has been reduced to a compilation of tissues, cells, lab tests, radiological images, neuroses, and infirmities, it is easy to dehumanize a person. Ultimately, when an individual has been reduced to a cluster of symptoms, a list of billable diagnoses, a curiosity, an experiment, a pawn, or an inconsequential plaything, physicians may kill.

Doctors take lives for a variety of reasons, many of which are shared by other members of society. They may kill for financial gain or out of jealousy. They may maim and dismember in search of sexual gratification. They may torture to impose their will on another helpless human being simply because they have the opportunity to do so. They may kill just to prove they can get away with it. Or they may just become addicted to death and pain. Physician killers, however, also have been involved in murder for reasons not shared by the average Joe. Sometimes doctors have killed out of real or perceived "Acts of Mercy." They have murdered thousands in the name of advancing science and medicine. They have been recruited by despots to twist their life-saving skills into tools of control, intimidation, and unspeakable horror.

They have focused their intellect on ruling countries with an iron fist instead of a comforting touch. Further, some doctors have been active participants in terrorism holding key roles in al-Qaeda and several Palestinian organizations. Simply put, when the Hippocratic Oath states, "above all do no harm to anyone," they have claimed an exemption.

To understand "Bad" it is important to first understand "Good." Physicians have served as healers prior to written history. Textbooks of medicine date back thousands of years and physicians have been featured in myths, plays and novels for centuries. In most cases, doctors have been portrayed as benevolent healers. Most advanced civilizations have developed codes of behavior for their physicians, ethical standards imparted to them above and beyond those to which an average person would be held. The first two chapters of the book present the background against which Medicine came into being and the forces that molded the social, psychological and professional profile of healers. We acknowledge that this part of the book has more of an academic coloration to it and some readers may skip to the "juicier" chapters.

We will continue with profiles of infamous serial killer physicians throughout the world. Some "practiced" over a hundred years ago, others in recent decades. It will become self-evident that evil doctors are spread throughout the world – no place is immune. Murderous physicians have employed all of the scientific tools available to them in their killing sprees. It is highly likely that several are still honing their craft as you sit here reading. It is only a matter of time until we see the first genetic homicides, murder by means of chromosomal manipulation.

Physicians have actively and passively participated in the taking of thousands of innocent lives. Physician-scientists have engaged in medical experimentation on captives, prisoners of war, children, the aged, inmates, the mentally challenged, and their own military personnel. They have been instrumental in genocide as witnessed by their activities during the Holocaust of World War II. In addition to Nazi experimentation, Japanese physicians of the same era committed innumerable atrocities. America is guilty as well, particularly in developing means of breaking the human mind. To be fair, doctors don't only experiment on helpless victims; many have staked their careers and lives on self-experimentation.

Physicians have been involved in politics for decades, often behind the scenes but occasionally as active participants. They have also ruled as malevolent dictators, been the targets of extermination, and most recently contributed to the horrors of international and domestic terrorism. These creative minds invented such atrocities as "suicide bombers" and "skyjackings." What a waste of their talent, choosing to kill thousands rather than curing hundreds.

We will share our thoughts on some of the ethical issues facing physicians today. It can be hard to draw the line between compassionate patient care and murder. Is "Mercy Killing" all that merciful? Is euthanasia ethical and, if so, how does it differ from the philosophy promulgated by the Nazi regime? When does malpractice cross the line into murder? There are many gray areas between Medicine and Law. We cannot hope to resolve these but we hope that we can at least get you thinking.

We will end with current fashions and trends. Complementary medicine and alternative therapies have brought relief to many patients. They have also resulted in disability, suffering, and death. Bear in mind, just because something is natural doesn't always mean it's good for you – cocaine and heroin come from plants, you know. We will take a look at how doctors are portrayed in fiction and attempt to answer why medical professionals are so prominently featured on television and in movies. How exactly did Dr. Kildare morph into Hannibal "the Cannibal" Lecter? We will finish up with the timely topic of the potentially unhealthy, master/pet relationships characteristic of celebrities and their personal physicians.

The authors of this book have been doctors for over 60 years. As forensic pathologists, we see death every day and have investigated hundreds and hundreds of murders. You will be relieved to know that most people are not killed by physicians. Quite the contrary, every day we see evidence of the heroic efforts made by healthcare providers to save lives. By and large, doctors are good people.

This book contains accounts of horrible atrocities, but it is not a horror story. It features descriptions of graphic murders committed by healers, but it is not pulp fiction. It follows the rise of tyrants and the torture of their subjects, but it does not make a political statement. It brings to light the risks patients face today given the wide array of treatment options, but it is not an exposé. All we hope to do is to accurately relay the circumstances of when, how, and why doctors kill.

Acknowledgments

From Dr. Perper

My thanks to my sons Ed and Harry and to my daughter Blanca (Perper) Greenstein for loving and constant support. Without their moral support this book would have never been written.

From Dr. Cina

I would be greatly remiss if I failed to thank my lovely wife, Julie, for her tireless critical review of this manuscript and putting up with our countless revisions. She has ensured its readability by reviewing our chapters on innumerable plane flights, often blocking the view of interested co-passengers attempting to peer over her shoulder.

Contents

Section 3   In the Name of Science

Section 4   Politics and Medicine

Section 5   What Now?

Section 1
Ethics and the Physician

Chapter 1
In the Beginning

I am the Lord your physician!

– Exodus 15:26

From the dawn of history, humankind has been awed by the power of healing. To restore the rosy color of health to skin bleached by illness and misery; to quiet a bone-rattling, hacking cough; to morph the gasps of suffocation into refreshing breath; to quench the fires of burning fever; and to return a soul on the threshold of another world back to life, certainly appeared to be mighty magic. And to many, it still does. Therefore, it is no wonder that from the earliest times man has believed that the power to heal is, in truth, a Godly power that only supernatural beings can possess.

Many early polytheistic religions have anthropomorphic Gods of Healing or Medicine. According to the more than 6,000 year-old Hindu mythology, Brahma, the creator of the Universe, was the first to make a compilation of Ayurvedic texts of medicine and surgery – secrets of healing known only to Gods. The name "Ayurvedic" is derived from the title of the ancient Veda writings which espouses this method of healing. Ayurvedic medicine is the Indian traditional medicine that forms the basis of Tibetan healing practices. It includes the use of various herbal medicines and cures as well as a holistic approach to health. Another major Hindu deity, Lord Vishnu, is also believed to be associated with medicine. He ordered the "churning of the ocean of milk" from which Dhanvantari, the God of Medicine, was said to have been born.

In Egyptian mythology, the Goddess Isis (1,500 BC) was considered the "Divinity of Medicine" and her name was invoked against all kind of diseases. Imhotep, the first recorded celebrity physician (who incidentally also designed the first pyramid of Sakara for King Zoser of the third dynasty (cca. 2800 BC)), was considered a demigod a hundred years after his death. By 525 BC this pre-Renaissance, "Renaissance man" was elevated to the status of God of Healing. His mythical prowess extended beyond Egypt. Even the rival Greeks worshipped him as a God.

This is not to say that the Greeks were devoid of their own deities with respect to medicine. Apollo was considered the earliest God of Medicine and it was he who taught the healing arts to the centaur Chiron. Asclepius, the most famous of the Greek physicians and a pupil of Chiron, cured many patients of a variety of ailments around 130–40 BC. The myth of Asclepius is particularly interesting because it highlights both the benefits and risks associated with the magical art of

J.A. Perper and S.J. Cina, *When Doctors Kill: Who, Why, and How*,
DOI 10.1007/978-1-4419-1369-2_1, © Springer Science+Business Media, LLC 2010

healing. It also foretells the hubris that continues to afflict many physicians to this day. Asclepius was said to be Apollo's offspring from his union with Coronis, the daughter of the king of the Lapiths. While she was pregnant by Apollo, however, Coronis fell in love with a mortal. Enraged that Coronis preferred a mortal to a God (not unlike preferring a ditch digger to a neurosurgeon – if you ask a neurosurgeon), Apollo sent his twin sister Artemis to kill and burn Coronis. Before the body was totally consumed by fire, Apollo rescued the infant child from the flames and took him to Chiron who raised him. Athena, the Goddess of wisdom, also helped Asclepius by giving him two samples of the magical blood of the Gorgon Medusa, one containing blood from her right veins that could heal sickness and even reverse death and the other from her left veins, which was a lethal poison. Asclepius became a great healer but his ego took over. He had the audacity to resurrect Hyppolytus, the son of Theseus, as well as other warriors clearly stepping over the line that separated Man from God. An angry Zeus smote him with a thunderbolt, perhaps as a warning to other healers that Nature has borders that cannot be crossed. Nonetheless, the Gods and men alike eventually recognized his profound skills and he was eventually deified.

In Buddhism, Buddha as a Healer is portrayed as the Lapis Lazuli Buddha with his hand extended, palm outward in a generous gesture, holding a magical fruit that can heal any disease. Buddhist teachings claim that merely seeing an image or a statue of the Medicine Buddha or hearing or saying His name is greatly beneficial to physical and mental health. Tibetan Buddhist leaders such a Lama Tashi Namgyal, the founder of the Victoria Buddhist Dharma Center believe that "If one meditates on the Medicine Buddha, one will eventually attain enlightenment, but in the meantime one will experience an increase in healing powers both for oneself and others and a decrease in physical and mental illness and suffering." Perhaps this approach has been worked into the new Healthcare Reform Law (it may be necessary as there may not be many doctors around in a few years).

In Judaism God is also seen as the ultimate healer. In the Torah (the Old Testament) God states about himself: "I am the Lord your physician" (Exod. 15:26). In Genesis, the tale of the patriarch Abraham and his wife Sarah positions God as both causing illness as a punishment and curing it upon repentance. The story relates that God (Yahweh) directed Abraham and Sarah to migrate and settle in Gerar (the southern Negev area of the Land of Israel). Sarah was very beautiful and when Abraham introduced Sarah to the local king, Avimelech, he presented her as his sister. King Avimelech was struck by her beauty and took her into his harem. God was angered at this indiscretion and struck Avimelech and his servants with impotence. Clearly, the Lord knows how to hurt a man. Avimelech then had a dream in which God told him the reason for his illness and that Sarah was Abraham's wife. Avimelech promptly returned Sarah to Abraham and confronted Abraham in righteous indignation. Upon the return of his wife, the bible notes: "… Abraham prayed unto God: and God healed Abimelech, and his wife, and his maidservants; and they conceived children." (Genesis 20:17). In essence, the Lord provided Viagra for the soul. Later, God promised the people, "If you obey God … keeping all His decrees, I will not strike you with any of the sicknesses that I brought on Egypt. I am God, your Physician" (Ex. 15:26). The prophets also acknowledged God as a Healer and Jeremiah stated: "Heal us, and we will be healed" (from the blessing for healing, Jeremiah 17:14). Throughout the Torah, God is imbued with great healing powers. It is no wonder that it is written, "The Lord giveth, the Lord taketh away" when it comes to health, wealth, and life itself.

In biblical times and many centuries later, even to this very day for some, illness was accepted as God's punishment for the sins of an individual or of a community of people against the ultimate healer, God. Historically, there have been five recognized sources of illness. Infirmities may be caused by:

1. God for his own purposes;
2. Intermediaries of God;
3. Evil spirits, devils or Satan;
4. The stars and;
5. Sins.

It was also believed that there were four means of healing by the Spirit of God:

1. Faith and prayer;
2. Exorcism;
3. Virtuous living and;
4. Magical means.

Two thousand years ago Ben Sira, a Jewish sage, portrayed the ideal Jewish physician as an instrument of God and wrote, "From God the physician gets wisdom… God brings forth medicines from the earth. With them the physician soothes pain and the pharmacist makes a remedy". This position clearly states that man may practice medicine for the good of his fellow man, as his skills are a gift from God. A contrarian view from other sages, such as Ibn Ezra, a great Biblical commentator, opined that God's permission for man to heal was restricted. God had provided man with "a sign that permission has been granted to physicians to heal blows and wounds that are externally visible. But, all internal illnesses are in God's hand to heal". Ibn Ezra argued that biblical passages permitting limited healing by man, namely the ability to treat injuries, but that God acts as the (sole) healer of all disease. This viewpoint implies an extremely limited role for physicians (essentially validating only emergency room physicians and trauma surgeons). Seeking care from a physician for a non-traumatic condition would equate with a lack of faith in God's ability to cure an illness.

Ibn Ezra's position is supported by the biblical story relating to the healing of Asa (King of Judah in 928 BC) when he became ill. The Bible records that when the king became sick, "he did not seek out God, but only doctors" (Chronicles II 16). The implication is that the king committed a grave error when he only sought out doctors and did not pray for healing from God. Most current Judeo-Christian believers assert that healing is a partnership between God and a man. While God is the ultimate healer, He delegates part of His role to humankind and asks the physician to practice medicine for the good of man. The Jewish approach to illness and medicine requires the righteous man to recognize the preeminent role of God in healing, while seeking out appropriate medical care. God gives man the power to heal but only if it is His Will that the patient be healed.

The Christian scriptures recurrently depict Jesus Christ as a Healer both metaphorically and factually. The Gospels and subsequent books record the many healings done by Jesus going "throughout Galilee, teaching in their synagogues, preaching the good news of the kingdom, and healing every disease and sickness among the people." (Matthew 4:23). The healing done through the "Holy Spirit" through Jesus was accomplished by either verbal command, thought, gesture, and/or by laying his hands on the diseased body part of the ill person. His cures included relief from severe pain, fever, bleeding, dysentery, paralysis, leprosy, blindness, deafness, demonic possession, restoration of withered limbs, and re-attachment of a severed ear. Jesus also resurrected an older man and a young girl, the ultimate form of healing. At the end of his earthly life, the New Testament tells us that he resurrected himself (exemplifying the adage "physician heal thyself"). In several instances, Christ's physical healing coincided with spiritual healing of the afflicted, truly "chicken soup for the soul."

In Islam, God is seen as the ultimate Physician and Healer. The Quran calls itself a book of healing: "We have sent down in the Quran that which is healing and a mercy to those who believe" (Quran 17:82). According to Moslem believers, Allah laid down in the Quran three types of healing:

1. Faith in Allah, not only as Creator but also as the Sustainer and the Protector. This faith can be demonstrated by the performance of obligatory prayers, fasting, charity and pilgrimage to Mecca;
2. Compliance with health practices including the consumption of honey, olives, fruit, lean meat, and the avoidance of alcohol, pork, excessive eating, sexual promiscuity and sex during menstruation and;
3. Direct healing by Quaranic prayers and recitations.

Many Islamists strongly believe that the very recital of Allah's name or specific passages from the Quaran are therapeutic. Further, some modern Islamic physicians have claimed that sound waves produced during Quaranic recitations generate electrical stimuli that activate various physiological centers in the brain and body in a most beneficial manner. The Quran's recitations must be done in loud voice following the instructions of Muhammad who stated "The comparison between a silent reader and a recitor is like a bottle of perfume when it is closed and when it is opened."

To this very day, many religious people see in God the ultimate and sole healing power. Human healers are, at best, a tool of Providence and, at worst, a superfluous intrusion into the healing process. Many Christian Scientists dispense altogether with physicians and modern medical care and proclaim that healing may and should be achieved only by the power of prayer. Jehovah's Witnesses adamantly refuse blood transfusions even if they are potentially life-saving because of their interpretation of passages in both the Old and New Testament. The overriding principle seems to be that God will heal believers without transfusions if it is His Will.

Whereas this philosophy renders physicians useless, worse things have been said about doctors. For example, although the Talmud generally portrays physicians in a favorable light, it also states that even the best of physicians are headed for Gahenna (Hell). An argument can be made that while Hell is clearly the proper destination for poorly skilled physicians who inadvertently or intentionally kill, even good physicians should head there because they are under the mistaken belief that they have cured the patient when, in fact, God was the healer. This arrogance may be punishable by eternal damnation in the eyes of some zealots. While physicians of today may not face the prospect of Hell, they are constantly menaced by the specter of court and malpractice litigation.

Humankind has I long recognized that the power of healing is only one side of the magical medical coin and that the other side is the power to cause harm. Apollo, the God of Archery as well as Medicine, was said to be a bringer of death-dealing plagues. The Old Testament mentions that God punished the Israelites with a plague that killed thousands because they returned to idolatry while Moses was communing with the Lord and receiving the Ten Commandments. He also infested their camp with poisonous snakes. Job also suffered greatly due to the direct intervention of God. If one accepts the monotheistic premise that God is the Creator of everything that exists, then it is logical to infer that He also created disease, pain and suffering. This jibes with God's promise of death to Adam and his descendents upon expulsion from the Garden of Eden. It follows then that if doctors have been blessed with the power to heal, they should also have the power to kill.

Since physicians have been imbued with the divine power of healing, these fallible humans are held to a very high, if not impossible, ethical and professional standard of perfection. Though physicians may have the near supernatural power to bring back patients from the brink of death, they also have the capacity, by failure of hands or unsound judgment, to cause great harm and death either intentionally (very rarely so) or in a failed, good faith effort. It is interesting to note that the Codex of Law, devised more than 4,000 years ago by the wise King Hammurabi of Babylon, included statutes which liberated the practice of medicine from the chains of magical practices and witchcraft. In so doing, it also set clear penalties for physicians that harmed or killed patients. The Code in keeping with Hammurabi's philosophy of lex talionis ("an eye for an eye") decreed: "If a physician makes a large incision with a bronze lancet (the operating knife), and causes the man's death, or opens an abscess with a bronze lancet, and destroys the man's eyes, they shall cut off his fingers." It is doubtful whether a great number of pre-medical students would knock on the portals of our institutes of high learning if such penalties were in effect today.

Chapter 2
Perfect Intentions, Imperfect People

May no strange thoughts divert my attention at the bedside of the sick, or disturb my mind in its silent labors, for great and sacred are the thoughtful deliberations required to preserve the lives and health of Thy creature.

– Daily Prayer of Maimonides

It is a trite fact of life that the old Latin maxim "Human erare est" (It is human to err) has lost none of its truth. For centuries, however, healers have sworn to err as little as possible in the performance of their art. As medical practice became more organized and education more uniform, most societies developed ethical and professional codes to provide their physicians rules to live and work by. It seems reasonable to assume that most young doctors would gladly swear to uphold a set of guidelines in lieu of having their fingers lopped off for a mistake.

One of the earliest and best known of the medical codes of ethics is the Hippocratic Oath. The Oath is generally recognized as the brainchild of the fifth century BC Greek physician Hippocrates, a contemporary of both Plato and the historian Herodotus. Legend has it that Hippocrates belonged to a noble family that claimed to trace its roots directly to the mythical Aesclepius, son of Apollo. The Oath requires the physician entering the profession to honor his teachers; to give patients proper diet and cause them no harm; to refrain from giving drugs that may induce abortion or any drugs that may harm the patient; to restrict the practice of surgery exclusively to skilled surgeons; to refrain from any harmful activities; to avoid sex with anyone in the patient's household (still a very good idea); and to keep confidential the general and medical information about a patient. Twenty-five hundred years later Congress enacted the Health Insurance Portability and Accountability Act (HIPAA) and formalized the ancient concept of patient confidentiality. Hippocrates was way ahead of his time. In several seminal works, he began to lay the foundations of modern medical ethics. In *Epidemics* he states that that the first commandment of the medical profession is "To do no harm" ("Primum non nocere"). In *Aphorism* he wisely notes, "Life is short, and the Art long; the occasion fleeting; experience fallacious, and judgment difficult. The physician must not only be prepared to do what is right himself, but also to make the patient, the

J.A. Perper and S.J. Cina, *When Doctors Kill: Who, Why, and How*, DOI 10.1007/978-1-4419-1369-2_2, © Springer Science+Business Media, LLC 2010 attendants, and externals cooperate." Taken literally, the modern day physician must behave ethically and ensure that insurance companies, legislators, attorneys, and noncompliant patients do the same. No problem.

The Hippocratic Oath, now well established as the cornerstone of the medical ethics edifice, took centuries to catch on in European medical schools. The first major institution of medical learning to include it in the curriculum was the University of Wittenberg in Germany in 1508. In 1804, the Oath was first incorporated into commencement exercises at a medical school graduation in Montpellier, France. This custom spread sporadically on both sides of the Atlantic during the nineteenth century and early 1900s but relatively few American physicians formally took the Oath. According to a survey conducted for the Association of American Medical Colleges in 1928, only 19% of the medical schools in North America included the Oath in their commencement exercises. It was only after the Second World War that it became much more frequently utilized. Today most medical schools in United States administer some type of professional oath to the 16,000 men and women entering the field each year. In many schools, the Oath has been revised to compensate for changes in the practice of medicine and fluctuations in societal values. Many medical schools administer an Oath that has deleted references to Greek deities, statements advocating obligatory teaching of medicine to physicians' sons, and the prohibition for general practitioners to perform surgery, abortion and euthanasia. In fact, according to a 1993 survey of 150 U.S. and Canadian medical schools only 14% of modern oaths prohibit euthanasia, 11% preserve the covenant with a deity, and 8% forbid abortion. Interestingly only a mere 3% forbid sexual contact with patients. It is safe to say that Western society has a more liberal attitude than the Greeks with respect to medicine; rumor has it that the ancient Greeks had their less conservative sides as well.

The Hippocratic Oath and its various permutations are not the only codes of ethical behavior available to novice physicians. The Oath of Asaph, also known as the Oath of Asaph and Yohanan, is a code of conduct for Hebrew physicians dating back to the sixth century AD. Maimonides, a great Jewish philosopher, rabbi, and renowned physician of the twelfth century also devised an Oath and Prayer that is still used in a number of medical schools. Ali ibn Sahl Rabban al-Tabari, the chief Muslim physician in the ninth century AD, described the Islamic code of medical ethics in his book *Firdous al-Hikmah* stressing the desirable character traits of the physician and the physician's obligations towards his patients, community, and colleagues. The modern Oath of the Muslim Physician was adopted at the first International Conference on Islamic Medicine held in Kuwait in January 1981. This Oath requires the physician to protect human life in all of its stages, respect the body of the patient, pursue knowledge, and live in faith in piety and charity. In 1997, the Islamic Medical Association of North America adopted a somewhat different oath that included the Quranic verse stating: "Whoever killeth a human being, not in liew [sic] of another human being nor because of mischief on earth, it is as if he hath killed all mankind. And if he saveth a human life, he hath saved the life of all mankind." Strict interpretation of this verse suggests that the physician would be in great trouble if he killed a patient unless it was through an act of mischief or in lieu of killing another person. In reality, physicians can also get in a lot of trouble by killing people through acts of mischief.

Just as some cultures pre-date the Greeks, some ethical codes existed for centuries prior to the Hippocratic Oath. The oath of the Hindu physician, also known as the Vaidya's Oath, was an oath taken by Hindu practitioners dating back to the fifteenth century BC. This ethicoreligious code requires physicians not to eat meat, drink, or commit adultery. Further, the Vaidya's Oath commands physicians not to harm their patients and to be solely devoted to their care, even if this put their lives in danger. A Chinese Hippocratic-like oath was devised by a famous traditional Chinese doctor, Sun Simiao (581–682 AD), of the Sui and Tang Dynasties. The code is included in Simiao's book *"On the Absolute Sincerity of Great Physicians"* which is still required reading for many Chinese physicians. The Seventeen Rules of Enjuin, for students of the Japanese Ri-school of medicine in the sixteenth century, emphasized that physicians should love their patients and that they should work together as a family. Physicians were also instructed to respect their patients by maintaining confidentiality of their medical records. This commitment to patient confidentiality stated in both the Rules of the Enjuin and the Hippocratic Oath is alive and well today.

The Declaration of Geneva was adopted by the General Assembly of the World Medical Association in 1948 and it was subsequently amended in 1968, 1984, 1994, 2005 and 2006. It was created to remind physicians that their calling and primary professional mission was to provide service to humanity. The first draft was largely prompted by the painful recollection of medical crimes recently committed in Nazi Germany. It was intended to modernize and adapt the moral directives of the Hippocratic Oath to the realities of modern medicine. The Declaration of Geneva, as currently amended, states:

At the time of being admitted as a member of the medical profession:

- I solemnly pledge to consecrate my life to the service of humanity
- I will give to my teachers the respect and gratitude that is their due
- I will practice my profession with conscience and dignity
- The health of my patient will be my first consideration
- I will respect the secrets that are confided in me, even after the patient has died
- I will maintain by all the means in my power, the honor and the noble traditions of the medical profession
- My colleagues will be my sisters and brothers
- I will not permit considerations of age, disease or disability, creed, ethnic origin, gender, nationality, political affiliation, race, sexual orientation, social standing or any other factor to intervene between my duty and my patient
- I will maintain the utmost respect for human life
- I will not use my medical knowledge to violate human rights and civil liberties, even under threat
- I make these promises solemnly, freely and upon my honor

The amendments to the Declaration have been criticized on the grounds that they are intruding on the inviolability of human life. Hippocrates made "health and life" the doctor's "first consideration" whereas the amended Declaration removes the words "and life." The original Oath demanded respect for human life "from the time of its conception" whereas the Geneva Declaration replaced this with "from its beginning" in 1984 prior to deleting it entirely in 2005. These changes have been criticized as departing from the Hippocratic tradition and as a deviation from the post-Nuremberg concern of respect for human life.

Not to be confused with the Geneva Declaration, the Geneva Convention governs the behavior of military members, including physicians, in wartime. Anyone familiar with the altruistic behavior of Hawkeye Pierce and the other doctors of "*M.A.S.H.*" can tell you that a military physician should impartially treat both his own troops and the enemy based solely on the severity of the wounds and accepted field triage standards. He is allowed to carry and fire a gun, but only in self-defense or to protect his patients. If a physician is captured, the Convention states that the doctor is to be treated as a non-combatant and should be "detained" rather than "imprisoned." In return for humane treatment, he is obligated not to attempt to escape and to treat both his comrades and injured enemy soldiers to the best of his ability. These ideas are great in concept, however many physicians and countries don't play by this set of rules. Red Cross-labeled vehicles and tents may become military targets. Hospitals may be bombed and patients are murdered in their beds. Captured physicians may be tortured or killed. And up to 25% of U.S. military physicians have admitted that they would not provide the same level of care to enemy soldiers as they would to their own countrymen. Perfect intentions, imperfect people.

Most every culture created deities with healing powers early in its evolution. As humans were invested with the power to heal (in essence, the power to turn death into life) it is no surprise that each society eventually developed a code of ethics to govern their healers. All of the codes have a similar theme – physicians are to behave as honorable, good, respectable, and compassionate men and women – and more. They are to value all life, do no harm, and to put their patients above themselves. It is easy to say an Oath; it is harder to live by it. In the 1990s, medical schools experienced a resurgence of students' interest in taking the traditional Hippocratic Oath. Some older professors, however, were initially reluctant to administer the Oath to these graduating doctors. Some were convinced that these young physicians were not capable of understanding and reaching the high ethical standards inherent in the Oath. Although most eventually relented and swore in these neophytes, we wonder whether they might have been right after all. Would our teachers be proud of the way in which twenty-first century physicians practice medicine? Would Hippocrates?

Section 2
When Doctors Kill

Chapter 3
The Alpha Killers: Three Prolific Murderous Doctors

> Doctors are the same as lawyers; the only difference
> is that lawyers merely rob you, whereas doctors rob you
> and kill you too.
>
> – Anton Chekhov

Doctors are supposed to heal people, not kill them. Murders by physicians always arouse a great deal of public interest and invariably instigate a media frenzy. Physicians enjoy a high level of trust and respect as essential providers of life-saving medical care. The doctor is, or at least has been, viewed as a father figure by society – a source of security, safety, and comfort. When a member of the medical profession violates this important public trust, society at large experiences a psychological shock similar to that occurring when a high-ranking military officer or a respected political leader commits treason.

It has been pointed out that because of their close contact with a relatively large number of patients and their unchallenged mandate to recommend treatments with many potentially toxic or lethal side effects, physicians may injure or kill many people if they choose to do so. A physician's knowledge of human behavior, anatomy, and physiology coupled with a familiarity with drugs, poisons, and sharp instruments may certainly facilitate serial murders by evil or mentally disturbed practitioners. A physician, even if psychologically impaired, may put on a façade of normalcy and assume the guise of a model citizen. Internally, however, there may be an unquenchable desire to inflict pain, subjugate wills, and, ultimately, to choose between life and death for his victims. For every Dr. Jekyll there is a potential Mr. Hyde. Some studies have shown that among serial murderers a significant number are doctors. Researchers such as psychiatrist Dr. Herbert G. Kinnel have argued that medicine has given rise to more serial killers than all the other professions put together because the medical profession seems to attract some people with a pathological interest in the power over life and death. This infatuation can lead to horrific crimes.

Serial killings by medical professionals are always good for at least a few headlines. Depending on what else is happening in the world, the stories may stay in the public eye for days to weeks. If Nancy Grace dislikes the suspect, he can be on the air for months before fading back into obscurity. But one-hit wonders are a dime a dozen.

J.A. Perper and S.J. Cina, *When Doctors Kill: Who, Why, and How*,
DOI 10.1007/978-1-4419-1369-2_3, © Springer Science+Business Media, LLC 2010

It takes either a large series of victims or a cluster of cases with particularly grue-some features to permanently etch the murders and murderer into the collective mind. The Jack the Ripper slayings are a case in point.

Saucy Jack (MD?)

The most famous series of killings possibly committed by a medical professional were those of Jack the Ripper. This pseudonym was given to an unknown serial killer, or killers, active in the Whitechapel area of London beginning around April 1888 and perhaps lasting until February 1891. The sobriquet was plucked from a letter sent by someone who claimed to be the murderer to the Central News Agency. A total of five women were definitely killed by the Ripper, all East End prostitutes, but the total number of victims may have reached 11. The five "confirmed kills" were murdered over an interval of 10 weeks between August and November 1888.

Mary Ann "Polly" Nichols, a married 42 year-old woman with five children, was the first widely acknowledged victim. She was found by two men on their way to work at 3:40 in the morning on Friday, August 31, 1888. She was lying on her back with her clothing in disarray, still quite warm. Her throat had been slashed twice with the second cut almost separating the head from the body. According to Doctor Henry Llewellyn who examined the body, she had also suffered a very deep wound on her lower abdomen "running in a jagged manner" together with "several other incisions running across the abdomen" and "three or four similar cuts" on her right side "all of which had been caused by a knife which had been used violently and downwards."

Over the preceding 2 months two other prostitutes had been killed but their deaths had not been initially linked to each other by either the police or the media. With the murder of Mary Nichols, however, the newspapers claimed that a serial killer was running amuck in the city. On September 1, 1888, *The Star* reported, "Have we a murderous maniac loose in East London? It looks as if we had. Nothing so appalling, so devilish, so inhuman – or, rather non-human – as the three Whitechapel crimes have ever happened outside the pages of Poe or De Quincey. The unraveled mystery of "The Whitechapel Murders" would make a page of detective romance as ghastly as The Murders in the Rue Morgue (a mystery novel of Edgar Alan about a gruesome murder committed by a monstrous (sic) ape). The hellish violence and malignity of the crime, which we described yesterday, resemble in almost every particular the two other deeds of darkness, which preceded it. Rational motive there appears to be none. The murderer must be a Man Monster, and when Sir Charles (The Lord Mayor) has done quarrelling with his detective service he will perhaps help the citizens of East London to catch him." *The Star* went on to say that, "There is a terribly significant similarity between this ghastly crime and the two mysterious murders of women which have occurred in the same district within the last three months. In each case the victim has been a woman of abandoned character, each crime has been committed in the dark hours of the morning, and more important still as pointing to one man, and that man a maniac, being the culprit, each murder has been accompanied by hideous mutilation."

It is possible that these three crimes were linked, but there are some inconsistencies in the killer's *modus operandi*. The first alleged victim, Emma Elizabeth Smith, survived for 2 days and related that she was beaten, robbed and raped by a gang of three or four young men who also shoved a blunt object into her vagina resulting in severe lacerations and hemorrhage. The second supposed victim, a middle-aged prostitute by the name of Martha Tabram, had a total of 39 stab wounds mostly in the areas of her breasts, belly, and groin. She had been sexually assaulted but her throat was not cut and she was not disemboweled. Clearly these were cruel and sadistic crimes but, despite the assertions of the columnist, critical analysis of these cases suggests that at least the first murder was likely not committed by the Ripper. The mechanism of injury in this case was blunt force rather than cutting, the latter being a hallmark of the Ripper killings. Martha Tabram, on the other hand, may well have been killed by the Ripper and may represent the primitive efforts of a serial killer who was honing an evolving craft.

The killings triggered a growing sense of fear amongst the inhabitants of the East End fueled, no doubt, by the sensational press coverage. *The Daily Telegraph* noted that, "At the present moment the nerves of the Metropolis are stirred and thrilled by the appalling Whitechapel murder; while in the immediate neighbourhood (sic) of the scene of the tragedy nervousness has been aggravated to the proportions of a panic." The murder also prompted the local Whitechapel police, headed by Detective Inspector Edmund Reid, to call for assistance from Scotland Yard who dispatched Detective Inspector Frederick Abberline to oversee the investigation. Additional manpower was mustered and deployed to police London's East End.

The second victim, Annie Chapman, aged 47, was discovered by John Davis at about 6:00 AM on September 8. A Spitalfields Market porter, he went downstairs after having had a cup of tea and discovered her in the rear yard of 29 Hanbury Street. Annie's throat had also been savagely cut and her body mutilated with her uterus and portions of her bladder removed in a manner which suggested that her attacker had anatomical knowledge. The organs could not be located and had presumably been taken away as trophies. She had been partially disemboweled with her intestines placed above her right shoulder but still connected with the body by shards of skin and tissue. Her stomach had been partially removed and placed on her left shoulder along with some skin fragments and her rings had been torn from her fingers. The only possible clue was a leather-apron soaked in water found nearby. Dr. George Bagster Phillips MBBS, MRCS, the Police Surgeon for the Metropolitan Division which covered London's Whitechapel district stated at the subsequent inquest:

> The left arm was placed across the left breast. The legs were drawn up, the feet resting on the ground, and the knees turned outwards. The face was swollen and turned on the right side. The tongue protruded between the front teeth, but not beyond the lips. The tongue was evidently much swollen. The front teeth were perfect as far as the first molar, top and bottom

and very fine teeth they were. The body was terribly mutilated... the stiffness of the limbs was not marked, but was evidently commencing. He noticed that the throat was dissevered deeply; that the incision through the skin were jagged and reached right round the neck...On the wooden paling between the yard in question and the next, smears of blood, corresponding to where the head of the deceased lay, were to be seen. These were about 14 inches from the ground, and immediately above the part where the blood from the neck lay.

The doctor stated that the instrument used on the throat and abdomen was the same. It must have been a very sharp knife with a thin narrow blade at least 6–8 in. in length, probably longer. The cuts could have been done by the type of instrument "a medical man" might use for postmortem purposes, but not a routine surgical instrument. Blades used by the slaughter men might have caused them but knives used by those in the leather trade would not be long enough, in his opinion, to have inflicted these wounds. He felt there were indications that the killer knew anatomy. He went on to surmise that deceased had been dead at least 2 hours prior to his arrival on scene, probably more, and that she had entered the yard alive. His observations could easily have earned him a starring role in *CSI: London*.

Only half an hour before the discovery of her body, Annie had been seen by a park keeper's wife in the company of a somewhat shabbily but respectably dressed man in his forties wearing a deerstalker (the kind of cap worn by Sherlock Holmes). On Sunday, 2 days after the crime, the police arrested a Polish Jew named John Pizer. He was promptly nicknamed "Leather Apron" due to the evidence (later proven unrelated to the murder) at the scene but he had unshakable alibis. After his release the killings continued and the hysteria grew resulting in a wave of anti-Semitism. Several members of the local Jewish community were beaten because of a widespread belief that a God-fearing, Christian Englishman simply could not have committed such a crime.

On September 27 a letter written in red ink was received by the Central News Agency addressed "Dear Boss." The author took credit for the murders and signed his name as "Jack the Ripper." Though some detectives at Scotland Yard believed the letter was a publicity stunt, its authenticity was somewhat validated a few days later. Elizabeth Stride, known as Long Liz, was the third certain victim. It appears she was attacked while walking home from a local bar. She was discovered by Louis Diemschutz when he turned his pony and carriage into the yard behind 40 Berner Street at 1:00 AM Sunday September 30. Liz had deep slashes to her neck but she was not disemboweled. From the position of the corpse it was presumed that the murderer had intended to mutilate her but was apparently was disturbed by the arrival of the cart. An examination of the body established that she had only been dead for some 15–30 minutes prior to discovery. The fourth victim Catherine Eddowes, aged 46, was found inside London at Mitre Square by P.C. Watkins less than an hour after Elizabeth Stride had taken her ill-fated walk. She was lying on her back in a pool of blood having been savagely stabbed and cut. Her throat was slit, her face disfigured with her nose partially cut off, and her abdomen was flayed open. Like Annie Chapman, some of her internal organs had been removed and taken, most notably her uterus and left kidney. Trust us, these organs are not easy to get to unless you know your anatomy and know where to look. Her stomach was cut open and most of her intestines had been ripped out. According to the police she "looked like a pig in a butcher's shop." Her right ear had also been partially amputated in partial fulfillment of the prophecy of the "Dear Boss" letter: "The next job I do I shall clip lady's (sic) ears off and send to the police officers just for jolly." The Ripper had time to complete his morbid fantasy in this case.

A postcard to the press on October 1 described the "double event" of September 30 and referred to the "Dear Boss" letter which had not been published. In this note, the killer referred to himself as "Saucy Jack." This was followed by a letter beginning with the greeting "From Hell" to Mr. George Lusk, Chairman of the Whitechapel Vigilance Committee. This note, signed by Jack the Ripper, was accompanied by ½ of a human kidney. Other letters of dubious authenticity were received by Mr. Lusk and other agencies.

The fifth and possibly the last victim was 25 year-old Mary Jane Kelly. She was murdered in her home at 4:00 AM on Friday November 9. This was the killer's most savage and gruesome attack. Kelly, unlike all the other victims, had been killed indoors affording the killer more time to commit his unspeakable crime. Resultantly, the defilement of her body was far more extensive than previously seen. Most of the flesh had been stripped from her body with her internal organs placed around the room. Her face was mutilated beyond recognition. And her heart had been removed as a personal trophy. The widespread and sensational coverage in the media fueled the public's panic and placed intense pressure on London's police and Scotland Yard. Fear was not, of course, the only emotion the murder inspired. Morbid curiosity was also rampant with the murder sites becoming tourist attractions. *The Telegraph* reported that the "house and the mortuary were besieged by people" and that a good trade had been established in charging a penny a time to view the "blood stained spot in the yard." Others made a living by selling waxwork tableaus that reconstructed the murder scenes. As cold as this sounds, we currently behave no differently. Wax was replaced by film then television then DVDs to meet the demands of the marketplace. Then the Internet came along allowing us to watch suicides and murders in real time.

In their attempts to catch the killer, the police used bloodhounds and dispatched undercover police officers dressed as prostitutes. The efficacy of this ploy is questionable since most London police officers were men. The Lord Mayor of London announced a reward of 500 pounds for information leading to the arrest of the perpetrator. On October 13, 1888, the police conducted a thorough house-to-house search of the entire Whitechapel area but found nothing. There was mounting dissatisfaction with the investigation, especially amongst local businessmen who found that the murders frightened customers away. Local prostitutes, whose business had plunged precipitously, were badly in need of a financial bailout. Then, abruptly, the prototypical "Ripper" murders stopped.

Though the murderer was never found there were a number of suspects, the most famous being the eldest son of King Edward VII, Prince Albert Victor, the Duke of Clarence. This theory makes for a great story but the prince's involvement is unlikely. Similarly, Queen Victoria's doctor, Sir William Gull, has been accused of the crimes and portrayed as the killer in fictional renditions of the murders but the facts militate against his involvement. The most legitimate suspects appear to be a Polish barber/surgeon, George Chapman (real name Severin Klosowski), who had poisoned three of his wives and Montague John Druitt. Druitt, a lawyer, was the son of a doctor and had some familiarity with his father's work. He committed suicide in December 1888, very close to the time the murders stopped. Other possibilities include "Dr" Francis Tumblety, a misogynistic quack doctor connected to the deaths of some of his patients; Aaron Kosminski, a Polish Jew who later died in an insane asylum; Sir John Williams, a friend of Queen Victoria and the obstetrician to her daughter, Princess Beatrice; a midwife ("Jill the Ripper"); John Pizer ("Leather Apron"); and Dr. Thomas Neill Cream (who we will discuss shortly). Obviously the medical community is over-represented in this short list.

It is rather difficult to understand why the Jack the Ripper murders raised such persistent, worldwide interest and prompted the creation of so many books and movies. The savagery of the attacks and the public's panic and anger over the butchery explains the initial interest, but it doesn't explain why "Ripperologists" busy themselves with the case over 100 years later. Over the past century, there have been many serial killers who murdered tens and, possibly, hundreds of victims compared to the paltry 5–11 victims killed by Jack the Ripper. The Ripper stabbings, slashings, and mutilations were certainly cruel but even more horrible manners of homicide have been reported. In the Ripper cases, all of the victims were prostitutes (or "sex-workers" as we call them today) who are known to be at risk for violent death and do not usually elicit much sympathy or public interest. Perhaps our infatuation with this serial killer resides in the mystery itself. This prolific killer could vanish into thin air and blend into society without arising any suspicion. He could be your barber, your lawyer, your midwife, your doctor. To date more than 200 works of non-fiction have been published about Jack the Ripper making him one of the most written about criminals of the past century. In 2006, Jack the Ripper was selected by the BBC History Magazine and its readers as the worst Briton in history. Now that is impressive!

In looking at this case through the binoculars of modern criminology one easily recognizes some of the typical characteristics of serial killers in general and medical murderers in specific including:

- Assault techniques and mutilation indicative of anatomical knowledge;
- Features of "missionary type" serial murderers claiming to "punish sinning whores" and cleanse the world of their polluting presence;
- Gradual progression in the viciousness of the attacks as the homicidal fantasy is refined and perfected;
- Ritualistic arrangements of disemboweled organs implying ultimate control and unreserved power combined with underlying sadistic sexuality;
- Removal of physical "mementos" designed to objectify the murderer's ownership of the victim and to provide a record of the killing to facilitate re-enactment of the homicidal fantasy. Removal of the heart of one of the victims is also clearly symbolic as the heart symbolizes both love and bravery. In removing the heart of the victim the murderer stole her very living essence; by taking her uterus, he stripped the victim of fertility, and;
- Feeling a need to communicate with the police with taunting letters and boasting of invulnerability.

Was Jack the Ripper a physician? Possibly, but maybe not. His contemporary, Dr. Thomas Neill Cream was.

Dr. Thomas Neill Cream: The Misogynistic Serial Killer

Either biology or God or both have bound man and woman together in an everlasting partnership, an indivisible link forged by love and passion. Without the company of a fertile woman, the last man on earth would die lonely (and very tense) mourning the end of humankind. If this irrevocable bond is maintained, our species is virtually assured of its future. Haters of women, misogynists, subvert the fundamental union of man and woman as colleagues, friends, lovers, and soulmates. Some misogynists abuse women in the workplace or harass them in bars. Others poison them.

Dr. Thomas Neill Cream hated women, especially lower-class women and prostitutes, and he killed seven of them in the late 1800s. He was born in Glasgow, Scotland on May 27, 1850, the first of eight children of William and Mary Cream. In 1854, the Creams migrated to the frontier of Wolfe's Cove, Quebec, Canada where his father found a job with the province's top shipbuilding and lumber firm. He came to own an independent lumber company and all of his children except Thomas entered into the family business. Thomas never displayed much interest in lumber choosing instead to spend his time reading books and teaching Sunday school. He was resolute to be a doctor from an early age. In September 1872, Thomas left the Cream Lumber Mill to start his medical studies at the well-known and respected McGill University in Montreal. Throughout his college years, he appeared to be a somewhat stiff-collared dandy, very much self-conscious of his attire. According to the records of McGill University, Cream was a thoroughly average student with an intense interest in drugs. He wrote his doctoral thesis on the topic of chloroform, an anesthetic which is poisonous when used in high doses. He earned his degree of Doctor of Medicine and Master of Surgery in 1876. Following graduation, Cream apparently set fire to his lodgings in order to collect $350 in insurance money. In retrospect, it appeared that the arson was a harbinger of much more severe crimes.

In 1876, as a full-fledged doctor, Cream prepared to leave town and take advantage of better professional opportunities in England. However, when he was just about to leave he was confronted by an angry family led by the shotgun-toting father of a young woman named Flora Brooks (whom Cream had seduced and then abandoned). Flora had recently been very ill, and while being examined by her family doctor, she admitted that she had an abortion performed by Cream. Holding him at gunpoint, the irate father forced Cream to return to town and marry his daughter. The morning after the wedding, Flora woke up to find that Cream had fled to London, leaving a note promising he would keep in touch, a promise that he kept (unfortunately for her). Shortly after Cream's departure, Flora once again became severely ill. When her doctor asked her if she had taken any medications for her illness, she mentioned taking some pills her husband had sent her. Flora mysteriously died in 1877, less than 1 year after the nuptials. Dr. Phelan, her personal physician was highly suspicious that the "medication" send by the estranged husband was responsible for her death.

In order to obtain British medical certification, Cream studied and worked at the famous St. Thomas' Hospital in South London, the hallowed grounds where Dr. Thomas Lister and Florence Nightingale had healed the sick. Lister was the innovative surgeon whose espousal of aseptic procedures during childbirth saved thousands of women from succumbing to puerperal fever and Nightingale was the renowned mother of modern nursing. When Cream arrived, England was at the waning end of the industrial revolution, bringing on one hand prosperity and a better life for the middle class but creating hellish slums rampant with poverty, prostitution and disease in the larger cities. Cream, a mustached, handsome young man accustomed to a rather rustic Canadian environment was dazzled by London's vibrancy and sophistication. He plunged enthusiastically into the vivacious nightlife frequenting the bars, music halls and vaudeville theaters while seeking the company of both affluent society women and prostitutes working under the Waterloo Bridge. His voracious sexual appetite ranged from filet mignon to week-old hamburger. This frantic social life, however, allowed him little time for studies and he failed to pass the medical examinations required to obtain his license to practice. Following this devastating failure Cream moved to Edinburgh, Scotland where he successfully completed his studies at the Royal College of Physicians and Surgeons prior to returning to Canada.

Cream developed a thriving medical practice in Ontario, addressing common ailments by day and performing abortions on the side. However, in 1879 Dr. Cream ran afoul of the Canadian police. A young, pregnant woman, Kate Gardener, was found dead in a shed behind Cream's office and it was determined that she died of chloroform poisoning. Cream was arrested and under questioning, he confirmed that Gardener had requested an abortifacient from him but claimed that he had refused. He suggested that Gardener must have committed suicide. However, in view of the fact that there was no chloroform container at the scene and that the victim's face and body were badly scratched, the investigating Coroner's Jury issued a verdict of homicide. Cream was the obvious prime suspect but somehow he persuaded the Coroner that he had only tried to help the dying girl and successfully avoided murder charges. As soon as he was set free, with his reputation as a physician now in tatters, Cream moved to Chicago and set up a practice not far from the city's red-light district.

Police quickly suspected him of performing abortions, which were strictly forbidden both morally and legally in the 1880s. The police also knew that women who used the services of non-physician abortionists often died because of bleeding or infections so they tended not to pursue physicians who performed safe abortions. Cream, who may become addicted to cocaine and morphine, narrowly escaped homicide charges when two prostitutes died after receiving abortions from him. One simply bled to death and the other was given "anti-pregnancy pills" later discovered to be strychnine (effective, to be sure, but deadly). Police were suspicious of Cream, but they could not positively link him with the crimes. Ironically, Cream's downfall in Chicago occurred after he poisoned not a woman but a man. Around the time that he killed the two prostitutes, Cream was selling an elixir supposedly effective in the treatment of epilepsy. One of his patients, Daniel Stott, was very pleased with the medication and would often send his wife to Cream's office for the pills. Cream started an affair with the Stott's wife, and as the husband became bothersome and suspicious, Cream added strychnine to Stott's medication. The patient obligingly died in June 1881. Cream would probably have got away with this murder had it not been for his unusual compulsive and meddling behavior. He wrote to the Coroner accusing the pharmacist of poisoning Stott with strychnine. Having drawn attention to a possible crime, the body was exhumed and the poison detected. However it was Cream, not the pharmacist, who stood trial for murder. He was found guilty and sentenced to life imprisonment at Illinois State Penitentiary. After serving only 10 years of his life sentence, he was set free in 1891 after he bribed Illinois politicians to grant him a pardon. It is hard to believe that such a thing could happen in Chicago.

After his release, he hurriedly returned to London. He visited his old haunts, such as Waterloo Bridge, and took residence in South London near St. Thomas' Hospital. He posed as a resident doctor from the hospital, signing his name "Thomas Neill, MD." In October 1891, Ellen Donworth, a prostitute, was seen walking in the company of a rather elegant gentleman in a top hat. Soon thereafter she was found slumped in her bed, apparently drunk, but experiencing periodic, agonizing convulsions. Between the painful spasms, she was able to tell witnesses that a tall, dark, cross-eyed man had given her something to drink. She died in agony on the way to hospital of what was later shown to be strychnine poisoning. Just 2 days later Cream killed again, this time another prostitute, Matilda Clover, who had her death incorrectly attributed to alcoholism. The following April, Cream carried out his first double murder. After accompanying two prostitutes to their house, Alice Marsh and Emma Shrivell, he left them to die in excruciating pain. Autopsies revealed lethal doses of strychnine in both women's stomachs. Strychnine, commonly used as a rat poison, produces some of the most painful symptoms of any poison. Within less than half an hour the victim starts to experience very painful and continuous muscular spasms and convulsions, starting at the neck and spreading over the entire body. The convulsions progress, increasing in intensity and frequency, until the backbone arches like a bow. In some instances, the spine may snap. Death comes from asphyxia caused by paralysis of the neural pathways that control breathing or by cardiac arrest due to exhaustion from the convulsions. The subjects usually die after 2–4 hours of unbearable pain. Allegedly, at the point of death the body becomes rigid immediately, even in the middle of a convulsion, resulting in instantaneous rigor mortis. Of all of the poisons available to Dr. Cream, strychnine was a particularly sadistic choice.

Lou Harvey, a smart, Piccadilly prostitute did not fall for Cream's deadly "medical treatments." After accosting her, Cream succeeded in convincing her to meet him later that evening for dinner and a night at the theater. Before they parted at the Charring Cross Embankment near the Thames River, "Dr. Neill" gave her some pills which he guaranteed would greatly improve her rather pale complexion caused by the unhealthy London air. With the deeds of Jack the Ripper still reverberating in her mind, the streetwise Ms. Harvey was suspicious of Cream and she tossed the pills into the Thames once he was out of sight. Nevertheless, she showed up at the appointed place and time later that evening to meet Cream but he never appeared as he likely assumed she was already dead. It was only after two more prostitutes were found dead from strychnine poisoning that Scotland Yard realized they were dealing with a serial murderer. It is very possible that Cream would have avoided detection if his own meddling did not once again bring him to the attention of the authorities. After committing his crimes, Dr. Cream wrote a blackmailing letter to Dr. Joseph Harper, the father of a medical student in the same rooming-house where he lived, saying he had evidence that his son had committed the murders. Signing his name "W. H. Murray," Cream said he would destroy the evidence if the father paid him 1,500 pounds. The father sent the letter to his son in the belief it was from an insane person (a very good guess). The son immediately turned it over to Scotland Yard who just happened to be following up on a complaint from Cream that he was being followed and was concerned about his safety. Ordinarily, Scotland Yard ignored such reports since it received so many of them but something about Cream alerted them to follow up in this case. A series of events then transpired which trapped Cream in a web of irrefutable evidence.

A constable who had been on patrol in the neighborhood where the two women (Marsh and Shrivell) were murdered recognized Cream as the man whom he had seen leaving the house where one of the murders had taken place. Dr. Cream also began to discuss the murders in great detail with an acquaintance, John Haynes, a retired New York detective. As a former detective, Haynes was obviously very interested in these conversations and was quite surprised to hear how much this new friend knew about the murders. After the men had supper one night, Cream actually took Haynes on a tour of the murder sites and talked at length about each of the victims, including Lou Harvey. When Haynes asked Cream how he knew so much about the murders, Cream claimed he had just been following the cases closely in the newspapers. So had Haynes, but he did not recall any mention in the newspapers of a victim named Lou Harvey. Whoops! Haynes contacted a friend of his at Scotland Yard, Inspector Patrick, and the Cream investigation began in earnest. His prior convictions were uncovered, a handwriting analyst confirmed that Cream had written the accusatory letters to Dr. Harper, and the passport identifying him as Thomas Neill proved to be a forgery. Police were trailing Cream round the clock while trying to solve the mystery of his missing victim, Lou Harvey. Finally, to their surprise and great relief they found her to be alive and well and willing to cooperate fully with the police.

With mounting evidence against him, Cream was arrested on June 3, 1892. Further investigation turned up two more murders in the U.S. during a visit by Cream. The doctor confided in someone that he "used strychnine in connection with the prevention of childbirth" of the women he had had relations with. His medical reasoning is quite sound; it cannot be denied that childbirth can be prevented by the murder of the mother. Throughout his incarceration and during the beginning of his inquest, Cream maintained unfazed that he was an innocent man. He betrayed no emotion and remained composed with a stoic expression on his face, according to many historical accounts. It was not until the bailiff introduced Lou Harvey to the courtroom that Cream appeared suddenly surprised and apprehensive. After Harvey testified about her encounter with "the doctor" and his pills, Cream was found guilty of murdering four women. He was sentenced to death by hanging.

On November 16, 1892, crowds gathered outside of Newgate Prison calling for Cream's death. One Canadian newspaper wrote, "Probably no criminal was ever executed in London who had a less pitying mob awaiting his execution." According to legend, right before the trapdoor released Cream to his death, he supposedly shouted, "I am Jack..." and then was cut off as his neck cracked in the noose. This, of course, implies that Cream was confessing to being Jack the Ripper, although this seems rather implausible because he was jailed in Illinois when the Ripper murders took place. Some researches, however, including the late Canadian writer Donald Bell noted that Dr. Cream and Jack the Ripper shared several similar traits an overlapping modus operandi. In support of his theory, Bell argued that:

– Both chose prostitutes as victims;
– Both wrote letters to authorities boasting about their evil deeds;
– Both were very cruel and merciless in their choice of "weapons" and;
– Their victims, as though intoxicated, nearly never cried out in fear.

Although Cream was apparently in jail at the time when Jack the Ripper murders occurred, Bell points out that prisoners sometimes paid substitutes (men willing to serve a prison sentence for a fee) to serve in jail in their stead. Considering the widespread corruption in Chicago during the 1880s, this was a very attractive arrangement for a man of financial means. A handwriting expert, Derek Davis, corroborated Bell's assumption by reporting that he found similarities between Cream's handwriting and the writing in Jack's letter. Nevertheless, to this very day the identity of the Ripper remains shrouded in secrecy.

The serial murders of Dr. Cream epitomize the characteristics of the sadistic serial killer who enjoys both the suffering of his victims, their powerlessness, and their deaths. His crimes imbue him with a sense of superiority which convinces him he is immune from detection and smarter than the police investigators who he taunts. As is often the case with these types of killers, they are brought down by their own inflated egos. Cream was a misogynist and it was his "mission" to rid society of trashy, perverted women. Yet he also loved the company of his victims and actively sought out their favors. He made his rounds among the prostitutes, slept with them, and then murdered them. A rather incongruous behavior for the self-designed "missioner of virtue."

Dr. Harold Frederick Shipman: The Champion Serial Killer

The scary image of the mad scientist or the psychopathic doctor is, for horror-loving readers and viewers, a great crowd pleaser. The titillation and fear experienced from the safe haven of a comfortable armchair, a plush theater seat, or a couch in a dark living room is intoxicating and, for some, truly addicting. However, the thought that those imaginary creatures can step into real life and threaten our existence is more frightening than any fiction. Physicians deal with us at times when we are very vulnerable, not just physically but emotionally as well. Disease, injury, and the ravages of aging disable many of us to some extent. We look up to the doctor as a figure of wisdom and compassion. The thought that this helping hand can turn into the claws of a monster preying on patients is truly terrifying. Nevertheless, such monsters have existed and likely still practice in the medical profession.

Dr. Harold Frederick Shipman, the champion of serial murder, was born the middle child of a working-class family on June 14, 1946, in Nottingham, England, the old prowling grounds of Robin Hood. Out of the three siblings, Harold (or rather Fred or Freddy as he was commonly called) was clearly the favorite child of his mother Vera, a rather domineering woman. From an early age, she fostered a sense of uniqueness and superiority that engendered in him both arrogance and aloofness while isolating him from other children. In 1963, when he was 16, his beloved mother was stricken with cancer and Shipman devoted a great portion of his free time to being with her. Over several months, he watched her being progressively consumed by the disease often writhing in great pain that could only be miraculously dampened by injections of morphine. Ultimately he watched his mother die peacefully at age 43, after a large morphine injection. His mother's death greatly affected young Shipman and likely prompted him to choose medicine as a career. After a bumpy start, he was admitted to Leeds University Medical School at age 19 and graduated after 5 years of study. As a student, he did not make any lasting impression on his peers except that he appeared to be a loner, somewhat haughty and patronizing (an attitude not completely foreign to some physicians of our present era). He met his future wife, Primrose Oxtoby, after her father rented him a room and they were married when she was 17 (and 5 months pregnant with his child). Primrose had a family background similar to Shipman's as her mother had also been very controlling. From Leeds, Shipman moved to Pontefract where he was employed for 12 months as a house officer at the Pontefract General Infirmary before being fully registered with the General Medical Council in August 1971. Thereafter, he continued to work at the same hospital as a senior house officer gaining a diploma in child health in 1972 and a diploma in obstetrics and gynecology in 1974.

By 1974, he was a father of two and had joined a lucrative medical practice in Todmorden, West Yorkshire. He conducted himself appropriately with his peers and his patients. The senior physicians were pleased with his work, but he clearly antagonized the office staff. He was arrogant, overbearing, aggressive and cantankerous, and displayed a belittling behavior to his support staff, deeming assistants "stupid" if they did not comply exactly with his wishes. Then unexpectedly Shipman started to experience unexplained blackouts that he claimed were due to epilepsy. In 1975, his medical colleagues found out that he had ordered large amounts of Pethidine, a pain-killing narcotic, for the office using fake prescriptions. When confronted with the incriminating evidence of his likely narcotic addiction, Shipman asked for a second chance. When this was denied he stormed out of the meeting in a violent rage. Shipman refused to resign from the group but eventually was forced to leave and shortly thereafter entered a rehab clinic. Protracted disciplinary proceedings concluded 2 years later, and he was found guilty of multiple violations of national drugs laws as well as fraudulent behavior and forgery of prescriptions. Surprisingly this resulted only in a small fine of about $1,000. The BBC reported that the senior partner at the Todmorden practice, Dr. Michael Grieve, explained the light sentence by saying: "If Fred hadn't at that point gone straight into hospital, perhaps his sentence would have been more than just a fine. I think it's perhaps the fact that he put his hands up and said 'I need treatment' and went into hospital, and then the sick-doctor routine takes over." Shipman paid his fine and worked 2 years as a clinical medical officer before resuming general practice in 1977 at the Donneybrook Medical Centre in the North of England.

By that time, he was the father of four. In the Donneybrook group, Shipman earned a reputation as a hardworking and dedicated doctor who enjoyed the trust of patients and colleagues alike. He remained on staff there for 15 years before going into solo practice in 1992. Despite his solid reputation with the group by 1985 a disturbing trend emerged among his clientele. Allen Massey, the local undertaker, noticed that Dr. Shipman's patients seemed to be dying at an unusually high rate and in a very uniform pattern – most were fully clothed and sitting up or reclining on a chair. There was no evidence that the person had been severely ill at the time of death and Dr. Shipman was present at many of the deaths. The undertaker approached Shipman directly about his concerns, but was apparently reassured that there was nothing to worry about and that the practice's books, always available for inspection, backed up his story.

Suspicions resurfaced in 1998 when a medical colleague, Dr. Susan Booth, complained to the local Coroner who in turn contacted the police. A covert investigation followed, but Shipman was cleared since his patients' records detailed diagnoses and treatments consistent with the causes of death listed by him on the death certificates. Later, a more thorough investigation revealed that Shipman had altered and forged the medical records of his patients to corroborate their alleged causes of death.

The majority of Shipman's killings were carried out in a rather monotonous fashion. The doctor's routine was to make a house call to patients on a weekday afternoon and inject them with morphine or heroin. The patient was then found dead either in the doctor's presence or within 30 minutes of his departure. The mechanism of death was described as syncope or collapse and the cause of death certified by Shipman was a heart condition, a stroke or old age. The families were advised by Shipman that the manner of death was natural, no autopsy was necessary, and prompt cremation of the body was recommended. Shipman's killing spree was brought to an end largely because he altered his discrete methods.

While most of his murders did not involve monetary manipulations, for some reason he decided he would not only kill one of his patients but would act as her sole beneficiary as well. Kathleen Grundy, a well-known former mayor of Hyde and a highly active and wealthy 81 year-old widow, was found dead in her home on June 24, 1998 following a brief visit by Shipman. Shipman told her daughter that Grundy had died of natural causes and that an autopsy was not required. Shipman recommended cremation and had already signed the cremation authorization but the daughter firmly objected and Kathleen was buried in a funeral attended by hundreds of people. Unbeknownst to Dr. Shipman, the daughter was an attorney. She had always handled her mother's affairs, so she was quite shocked when informed of the existence of a second will leaving her mother's estate, valued at 386,000-pound sterling, to Dr. Shipman. Upon examination of the recently "signed" will, the daughter became convinced the document was a cheap forgery, as it was badly worded, badly typed, and totally out of character for her mother who was a very tidy and meticulous person. Furthermore, her mother's signature appeared to be forged. Believing that Shipman had murdered her mother and forged the will to benefit from her death, she reported her strong suspicions to the local police. Upon examination of the evidence, Detective Superintendent Bernard Postles arrived at the same conclusion and an investigation was promptly initiated. In August 1998, Kathleen Grundy's body was exhumed and an autopsy revealed that she had died of a morphine overdose, most likely administered within 3 hours of her death, precisely within the timeframe of Shipman's visit to her. Shipman's home was raided yielding medical records, narcotics, an odd collection of jewelry, and an old typewriter which proved to be the instrument upon which Grundy's forged will had been created. Shipman denied the forgery claiming that the deceased had borrowed the typewriter from him on a number of occasions.

On September 7, 1998, Shipman was charged with Mrs. Grundy's murder; a highly confident Shipman denied all charges. Over the course of his interrogation, Detective Chief Inspector Mike Williams was quoted to say, "He was an arrogant type of individual to deal with. And I don't say that lightly. I've listened to the interviews, and he certainly wanted to control and dominate the interview and the officers, at times belittling them. He was treating this as some sort of game, a competition, pitting his, what he considered to be his superior intellect, to those of the officers who were interviewing him." After intense questioning of the doctor, the police became concerned that Shipman might have murdered additional patients besides Grundy. His medical records were carefully reviewed and any fatalities involving his patients following a home visit by Shipman were carefully examined. The investigation revealed that it is probable that hundreds of patients, mostly elderly women, were murdered by Shipman through the administration of morphine or heroin which in England can be prescribed by doctors. His oldest victim was 93 years old, his youngest 41. Based on the investigation, there were 218 verified victims, 171 women and 47 men. However, the Crown prosecutors decided to charge Shipman with murder in only 15 cases in which exhumation and autopsy provided iron-clad evidence for conviction. Shipman's trial started in Preston Crown Court on October 5, 1999. The prosecution asserted that Shipman had killed the 15 patients because he enjoyed exercising control over life and death and dismissed any claims that he had been acting compassionately ("mercy killing") as none of his victims were suffering a terminal illness or were in great pain.

Kathleen Grundy's daughter was the first witness for the prosecution and her testimony was very straightforward and convincing. Attempts by Shipman's defense to undermine her credibility were unsuccessful. A government pathologist described in detail the postmortem findings and the toxicological studies substantiating that morphine toxicity was the cause of death in most cases. Fingerprint analyst confirmed that Kathleen Grundy never handled the forged will and a handwriting expert dismissed the alleged signature on the will as being a crude forgery. A police computer analyst then testified how Shipman had altered his computer records within hours of the death of a patient to create symptoms or fabricate office visits or consultations that had never taken place. Like many other people, Shipman apparently had not been aware that erased electronic records can be retrieved and that changes made to computer files can be identified and dated as well. The relatives of the murdered victims testified that Shipman often demonstrated a lack of compassion when informing them of the death and he frequently disregarded the wishes of family members. He also displayed marked reluctance to attempt to revive moribund patients. In several instances, Shipman would pretend to call the emergency services in the presence of relatives, then cancel the dispatch when the patient was discovered to be dead. Police examination of the telephone records from these homes showed that no actual calls were made. Finally, evidence of implicit drug violations and abuse was introduced. Large stashes of heroin ampoules were found at his home. Falsified prescriptions for patients who did not require morphine and never received it were confiscated. Records documenting visits to the homes of recently deceased patients to collect unused drug supplies for "disposal" were uncovered; not surprisingly, there were no indications that the drugs were destroyed.

Following a meticulous summation by the judge, and a caution to the jury that no one had actually witnessed Shipman kill any of his patients, the jury unanimously found Shipman guilty on all charges: 15 counts of murder and one of forgery. Dame Janet Smith, the Superior Court Judge, sentenced Shipman to 15 life-term sentences and an additional 4-year sentence for forgery, which she commuted to a "whole life" sentence effectively removing any possibility of parole. On January 13, 2004, Shipman was discovered at 6:00 AM hanging in his prison cell, having used bed sheets tied to the window bars of his cell to form a ligature. Dr. Shipman had reportedly told his probation officer he was considering suicide so his widow could receive his generous government pension and inheritance. Indeed, following Shipman's death his widow received a pension and a lump sum from the Department of Health as well as 24,000-pound sterling in inheritance from Shipman. The doctor and his family vehemently proclaimed his innocence to the end.

Dr. Shipman's motivation for his many murders (except for the last one) is unknown, although the assumption of John Pollard, the South Manchester Coroner who knew Shipman well, seems very close to target: "The only valid possible explanation for it is that he simply enjoyed viewing the process of dying and enjoyed the feeling of control over life and death, literally over life and death." A clinical audit conducted by Professor Richard Baker of the University of Leicester at the request of England's Chief Medical Officer examined the number and pattern of patient deaths over Harold Shipman's 24 years of practice (1974–1988) and compared them with those of other practitioners. The comparison of the number of death certificates issued by Shipman vs. other general practitioners in the same locality with a similar patient mix indicated that he issued nine times as many death certificates than the average doctor. He also determined that death was due to "old age" eight times more frequently than his colleagues. Clearly, having Shipman as your doctor was a bigger risk factor for sudden death than smoking. Dr. Shipman's saving grace may have been his willingness to perform house calls. He was present at the deaths of 20% of his patients compared with a norm of 0.8%. The audit goes on to estimate that he may have been responsible for the deaths of at least 236 patients over a 24-year period. It was further speculated that Shipman might have been "addicted to killing." Harold Shipman is the uncontested Master Criminal of medical serial murders. He serves as living proof that evil doctors are not a thing of the past or limited to fiction. Though not as horrific as disembowelment, injections of morphine, (or insulin, digitalis or potassium) may be equally lethal. If we were to search for a single minimally redeeming feature of Shipman's crimes, it was that the victims were all enthralled with him as a doctor and they sank painlessly into coma and death. There is also no evidence to suggest that he billed the next-of-kin for the house call.

Shipman's motivation was not sexual/sadistic fantasy but rather, first and foremost, the feeling of power that he could choose with impunity when another person would die. It seems likely that his serial murders were either a symbolic punishment of his mother, who callously left him bereft at a very vulnerable time, or revenge against a world that permitted elderly women to live while younger women were allowed to die. Shipman was an exceptional serial killer as he was able to totally compartmentalize his murderous behavior while simultaneously living a normal life as a respected physician, husband, and a father of four children. Furthermore, he apparently committed suicide to enable his wife to receive a government pension from the Health Department which she would have lost otherwise. The record shows that this man was committed to providing money to his wife and narcotics to his patients.

Three prolific serial killers, Jack the Ripper, Dr. Thomas Neill Cream, and Dr. Harold Shipman had at least one thing in common—medical knowledge. The Ripper's crimes indicate an uncommon knowledge of anatomy. His weapon of choice may well have been a medical instrument. We will never know if he was a physician – or if he was assisted by one. Dr. Cream was obsessed with drugs and poisons from early on in his career. He put this knowledge to morbid use in his killings. Dr. Shipman used a drug that was and is readily available to presently practicing physicians. His mastery of the medical arts provided him with something that every serial killer needs—easy access to unwitting victims. Whereas the Ripper was likely a sexual sadist who gained gratification from the suffering of his victims, Shipman killed to rectify a psychological wrong that had been done to him. Shipman and Cream both enjoyed the omnipotence of choosing life or death for their victims, but the former hated women whereas the latter was a family man. Although these three killers shared some characteristics, there were more differences than similarities. It is highly unlikely that they would be able to form a partnership to run the Clinic from Hell.

Chapter 4
America's Contribution to Medical Mayhem

I think capital punishment works great. Every killer you kill never kills again.

– Bill Maher

The history of Americans (and colonists) that have been convicted of serial murder is about 350 years old, a mere trifle when compared with that of some other nations. *The Vain Prodigal Life and Tragical Penitent Death of Thomas Hellier*, a book published in London in 1680, reported the crimes of Hellier, a bonded servant in the Virginia colony, who was hanged for the murder of "his master, mistress, and a maid." He was apparently the first American "domestic killer." Until the late 1800s, murders by American physicians were practically unknown, either because the perpetrators were too good at concealing their crimes, the index of suspicion was too low, or the expectation to die under medical treatment too high. However, the 1900s and early 2000s showed a significant increase in their number. American serial killer physicians are very similar to medical deviants throughout the world and share similar motivations. Not to seem un-American, but our serial murderers aren't bigger, stronger, smarter or faster than killers from anywhere else. This is not to say our physicians have been slouches when it comes to homicide—far from it. Consider the following examples.

Dr. Holmes's House of Terror

The first, well-known American killer was Herman Webster Mudgett, not a very frightening name (how many murderers are named Herman?). He graduated from the University of Michigan's School of Medicine in 1884. While in training, he had the nasty but profitable habit of stealing corpses, mutilating them to mimic trauma caused by accidental death, and collecting insurance money on the bodies. After graduating, he traveled across the Midwest running frauds, real estate scams, and marrying an unknown number of women for their money.

In 1886, he took the name "Henry Howard Holmes" and used his medical training to get a job in a Chicago drug store owned by a Mrs. E. S. Holden. He turned the

J.A. Perper and S.J. Cina, *When Doctors Kill: Who, Why, and How*,
DOI 10.1007/978-1-4419-1369-2_4, © Springer Science+Business Media, LLC 2010

store into a success by being a deft preparer of medications and charming the lady customers with his enticing and humorous conversation all the while meticulously documenting the store's finances. Mrs. Holden seemed thrilled with the success of her business until she mysteriously vanished in 1887. Shortly thereafter, Holmes announced that Mrs. Holden had sold her store to him before leaving for the West. In truth, Holmes had murdered Mrs. Holden and had skeletonized her body.

Two years later Holmes used the income from her store, the proceeds of her life insurance policy, and the sale of her skeleton to a medical school to build himself a true castle rather than just a mansion. A crew of 800 workers under Holmes' direct supervision labored from 1888 to 1890 to build a very impressive three-story building complex with turrets, battlements, and 105 rooms. The building also featured hidden gas jets in the guest rooms, an elevator shaft with no elevator, stairs to nowhere, peepholes, secret alarm bells activated by opening apartment doors, hidden passages, soundproof asbestos-lined vaults, kilns, quicklime pits, trap doors, chemical labs, a glass-bending furnace, and a nine-room basement illegally hooked up to the city's gas mains. Holmes had repeatedly changed builders during the initial construction of the Castle to ensure that only he fully understood the design of the dungeon he had created. In addition, according to law at that time, by firing workers every 2 weeks he didn't have to pay them. When this Horror Castle was completed, Holmes started his killings in earnest. Over a period of 3 years, Holmes selected his victims from among his employees, lovers, and at least 50 paying hotel guests. Most were women but he killed a few men and children as well. Some were locked in soundproof bedrooms fitted with gas lines that permitted him to asphyxiate them at any time. Others were locked in a huge bank vault near his office; he sat and listened as they screamed, panicked and eventually suffocated. The victims' bodies went by a secret chute to the basement where many were meticulously stripped of flesh, crafted into skeleton models, and then sold to medical schools. He dissected some of the bodies, performed chemical experiments on a few, and saved pieces of several corpses in his vaults (he did not have the benefit of a freezer like Jeffrey Dahmer). He disposed of most of the evidence in his lime pits or his basement crematory. Ironically, Wade Warner, the very designer of the furnace, was reduced to ashes within it.

Holmes also had a thriving clinical practice. He picked one of the most remote rooms in the Castle to perform hundreds of illegal abortions. Many of his patients died because of his procedures and their corpses were also processed and the skeletons sold. Despite the lucrative income earned from abortion, torture and murder, the maintenance of a castle was expensive and Holmes' financial problems grew in spite of his booming business. Following the Chicago World Fair of 1893, with creditors closing in, Holmes left Chicago and apparently murdered people as he traveled around the United States and Canada. He tried to marry Minnie Williams, a wealthy Texas heiress, but her sister objected and Holmes ended up killing both of them. Holmes' murderous career came to a close after he talked a witless man by the name of Benjamin Pitezel into faking his death in order to collect on an insurance policy. When this scheme didn't pan out, Holmes killed both Pitezel and his three children and tried to claim the insurance money. Holmes was arrested when the police discovered this scam. The local authorities called the Chicago Police who then spent a month in the Murder Castle documenting the efficient methods Holmes had devised for killing his victims and disposing of the corpses. The number of Holmes' victims has been conservatively estimated between 30 and 100, though his total may have been as high as 230. The verified number of confirmed kills is 27. Police investigators stated that some of the bodies in the basement were so badly dismembered and decomposed that it was difficult to tell how many people made up his putrescent stew.

He was put on trial for homicide and eventually confessed to 27 murders (in Chicago, Indianapolis and Toronto) as well as six attempted murders. Initially he proclaimed his innocence, later he pretended he was possessed by Satan (perhaps accurately so). On May 7, 1896, Dr. Holmes was hanged in Philadelphia. Newspapers reported that the evening prior to his execution, Holmes retired at his usual hour, fell asleep easily and awoke refreshed. "I never slept better in my life," he told his cell guard. He ordered and consumed a large breakfast an hour before he was hanged. Until the moment of his death on the scaffold, Holmes remained calm and amiable, showing no signs of fear, anxiety or depression. According to the *New York Times* coverage of the execution, Holmes said to the executioner: "Take your time, old man." Unfortunately, for the doctor, his neck did not break when his body dropped as it is supposed to in a judicial execution. Instead he died slowly, twitching over 10 minutes before being pronounced dead a quarter of an hour after the trap was sprung. One of his last requests was to be buried in cement so that no one could ever dig him back up. Who would?

The Starvation "Doctor"

Linda Burfield Hazzard (1867–1938), known as the "Starvation Doctor," killed many of her patients in the 1920s by subjecting them to her patented therapy regimen designed to cure them of a variety of illnesses. Although she was technically an osteopathic nurse with little medical experience, Hazzard called herself a doctor because she had been granted a license to practice medicine due to a loophole in Washington state law. Hazzard was reported to have harshly admonished reporters that did not call her "doctor" by stating: "I have told you time and time again, it is Dr. Hazzard. Mrs. Hazzard is my mother-in-law." Sounds like a big chip on her shoulder.

In her book *"Fasting for the Cure of Disease"* Hazzard claimed that most ailments could be cured by her innovative three-prong treatment approach. First and most important was fasting – allowing the digestive system to "rest" and be "cleansed," while removing "impurities" from the body. Fasting, she maintained, could cure any disease. The real source of all disease was "impure blood" brought on by "impaired digestion." She stated emphatically "overeating is the vice of the whole human race" and convinced many readers that an empty stomach was the key to good health. Although Hazzard rightly recognized the importance of preventive medicine, a healthy diet, and the fact that people who are depressed or ill have a poor appetite, she drew the unreasonable conclusion that sick people needed minimal food and that a starvation diet could eradicate disease. In addition to fasting, her regimen included daily painful enemas that went on for hours and involved up to 12 quarts of water. The third part of her "therapy" was a violent massage that consisted of having "Dr." Hazzard slam her fists forcefully against the patients' foreheads and backs. The treatment plan was very structured. Patients were put up in Seattle hotels or in cabins on Dr. Hazzard's Olalla property for periods of weeks to months and placed on a diet consisting of small amounts of tomato and asparagus soup and an occasional teaspoon of orange juice. It is no wonder that her patients rapidly lost weight; it is amazing that more didn't die.

She appears to have killed her first patient in 1902 around the time her divorce from her first husband became final. A coroner determined death was caused by starvation and he tried to have her prosecuted for medical malpractice but failed; it is difficult to sue someone for medical neglect or malpractice if they are not really a doctor. In 1904, she married again to a rather ill-reputed gentleman who apparently "had forgotten" that he was already married resulting in a 2-year prison sentence for bigamy. In 1906, the couple moved to Olalla, a small town close to Seattle. Many locals were enticed by her medical theories and became her patients. Her sanitarium "Wilderness Heights" was nicknamed "Starvation Heights" by the locals who sometimes came across wasted escapees staggering down the road looking for food. Hazzard and her husband also had developed the profitable habit of appropriating their patients' assets through fraud, forgery, outright theft, and forcing them to sign wills naming them as beneficiaries. Apparently, her patients got what they paid for – many were "cleaned out" in more ways than one.

Hazzard's next victim was Daisey Maud Haglund who died in 1908 after a 50-day fast under Hazzard's care leaving behind a 3 year-old son. Other victims soon followed – one more in 1908, two in 1909 and one in 1910. When civil engineer Earl Edward Erdman took the cure in 1911 and died of starvation 3 weeks later, the *Seattle Daily Times* headline read "Woman 'M.D' Kills Another Patient." Nevertheless, patients kept on coming including professionals, newspaper owners and other very wealthy individuals, some of whom died after a fasting for close to 2 months. Authorities tried to step in when Lewis Ellsworth Rader, a former legislator and publisher of a magazine called *Sound Views* began wasting away. Although health inspectors tried to convince him to leave he chose to remain under Hazzard's care. She moved him to a secret location where the 5-foot 11-inch tall man died weighing less than a hundred pounds. The authorities could not intervene since Hazzard was now licensed to practice medicine and her patients were not just willing but often enthusiastic participants in their deadly therapy. Hazzard had many loyal followers and a commanding personality that deterred some of her patients from leaving once they started her program.

Although death by starvation was not uncommon in Dr. Hazzard's practice, one death under her care breaks the mold. In 1909, 26 year-old Eugene Stanley Wakelin's decomposing body was found on her property. This son of a British lord had died as a result of a gunshot wound to his head in what appeared to be a tragic suicide. Coincidentally, Linda Hazzard had power of attorney over the young man's estate. The British vice-consul in Tacoma speculated that the young man had been shot by the Hazzards who were angered to learn that, despite his nobility, he wasn't rich. It would seem that fasting cannot cure a bullet to the brain.

Pressure mounted on the Kitsap County authorities to prosecute Hazzard for her homicidal treatment of her patients. When county officials said they couldn't afford to finance a lengthy investigation, Dorothea Williamson offered to pay for the prosecution. Dorothea had strong motivation to put the starvationist out of business. Dorothea and her sister Claire were wealthy English women who had read Hazzard's book and flew to United States to try out this new health fad. Little did they know that Dr. Hazzard's cure was potentially fatal. After religiously following the treatment plan for 2 months, they had lost so much weight that they were too weak to escape. Claire died but Dorothea was rescued by her childhood nanny who had flown in from Australia when she heard of Claire's demise. When she was found, Dorothea was delirious and reduced to skin and bones. In August 1911, Linda Hazzard was arrested for the murder by starvation of Claire Williamson. The *Tacoma Daily News* headline read; "Officials Expect to Expose Starvation Atrocities: Dr. Hazzard Depicted as Fiend."

When she was tried for homicide in January 1912 the prosecutor called her "a financial starvationist" and accused her of intentionally starving her patients to death for monetary gain. Dr. Hazzard retorted that she was being persecuted because she was a successful woman and that traditional doctors, jealous of her success, conspired to oppose her natural cure. In spite of supportive testimony from her staff and some of her loyal patients, the jury convicted her of manslaughter for the killing by starvation of Claire Williamson. Dorothea's testimony was particularly damning. Not one to sit around idly, Hazzard killed two or three more patients while awaiting sentencing. She eventually served 2 years in the Washington State Penitentiary in Walla Walla prior to being pardoned by the Governor after agreeing to leave the United States and move to New Zealand. There she published another book and opened a very successful office as a "physician, dietitian, and osteopath."

By 1920, she had made enough money to come back to Olalla and build another sanitarium. Since Washington had cancelled her medical license she called it "a School of Health." The building included treatment rooms as well as a basement autopsy room. Hazzard continued to treat patients by starvation adding 12 or more victims to her death toll. The sanitarium burned down in 1935 and Dr. Hazzard died 3 years later. In the months preceding her death she hadn't been feeling well and tried her own fasting cure. It didn't help. Today, her books are still available in natural healing bookstores and some can be downloaded from the Internet. Some websites praise her as a medical visionary.

The Fugitive

In 1954, Dr. Sam Holmes Sheppard, an osteopathic physician in Bay Village, Ohio, was convicted of the murder of his pregnant wife, Marilyn, in a famous and controversial trial. Sheppard served almost a decade in the Ohio Penitentiary before his 1954 conviction was overturned and declared a miscarriage of justice. In 1966, he was acquitted in a new trial. In 2000, an attempt by his son, Sam Reese Sheppard, to have him declared innocent by finding the State of Ohio authorities guilty of "wrongful imprisonment" was rejected by a jury. The saga of Sam Sheppard was so sensational that it was the subject of a number of books, several TV reality shows and a very successful movie. The identity of the real killer is still a matter of debate – but it was likely not Sheppard.

This true-life horror story started on the eve of July 4, 1954. Dr. Sam Sheppard, a successful and reputable neurosurgeon and trauma physician, and his beloved wife and childhood sweetheart, Marilyn, were having their neighbors over for dinner. Thereafter the Sheppards watched a late movie, *Strange Holidays*, with their guests. Later, Sam fell asleep on a sofa while Marilyn went upstairs to sleep in their bedroom. Sometime after he fell asleep Sheppard awoke about 3–4 o'clock in the morning believing he had heard his wife calling his name. He ran upstairs and saw "a form with a light garment … grappling with something or someone." He heard moans or groans then suddenly he was struck from behind. When he regained his senses his wife was on the bed, face up, covered with blood with her legs apart. He checked her pulse and felt none. He ran to the next room and saw that Chip, their 7 year-old son, was still soundly asleep. He heard some noise and ran downstairs and out the door to the Lake Erie beach below his home. He then chased what he variously described as a "bushy-haired intruder," a "biped" or a "light-topped form" (no one-armed man mentioned) before he was hit and again rendered unconscious. When he woke up, he was shirtless and partly in the water. He managed to struggle home and call a neighbor for help at 6:00 AM. The neighbors arrived promptly and called the police. The Coroner arrived at the scene at about 8:00 AM, examined the deceased and told the press that the victim had 35 wounds to head. This is very impressive since modern forensic pathologists in a well-lit autopsy suite can rarely be that precise even after examining the body for many hours. Further, it was apparent to him that the killer: "…rained blow after blow on her with savage fury." He also said there appeared to be no evidence of a break-in. Neither a forensic pathologist nor a criminologist, Coroner Gerber was a general practitioner with a law degree but he fancied himself a forensic expert. Prior to his press conference, Gerber and the local chief of police had questioned Sheppard who was being treated by his brother, also a doctor, for bruises, chipped teeth, lacerations of his mouth, and neck injuries. Later, a reputable neurologist determined that Sheppard had suffered "serious damage to the spinal cord in the neck region" with a chip fracture of the cervical spine.

The police investigation of the scene revealed marked splattering of blood in the bedroom and some disarray in the house. The drawers of a cabinet were pulled out and Sheppard's medical bag was lying on the ground with some of its contents spilled out but nothing was reported missing. Sheppard later claimed that it was possible that some morphine was missing from the bag. On the beach outside the house a green bag was found containing Sheppard's watch smeared with blood. The local police felt that the case was well over their heads and asked the Cleveland police for help in the investigation. Two detectives from the Cleveland police force interrogated Dr. Sheppard at the hospital and, after the questioning, one of the detectives told Sheppard quite plainly, "I think you killed your wife." Sheppard stuck to his initial statements both publicly and during many hours of questioning by the police. However, he was unable to explain how an intruder could enter his home undetected without evidence of a break-in. And how his 7 year-old son managed to sleep through his mother's murder and his father's struggle with the "bushy-haired intruder." And why the family dog had not barked. And why the t-shirt he was wearing when his guests had left had disappeared. And how his bloodied watch ended up in a green bag on the beach. And why he survived his encounters with a vicious killer or killers with only relatively superficial wounds while his wife's head was caved in. Clearly, his defense team faced a mountain of circumstantial evidence.

Sheppard's credibility was further damaged when he lied about and later recanted allegations of affairs with a Los Angeles laboratory technician and one of his female patients and that there was no strain in his marriage or discussion of divorce. The Cleveland police recommended to the Bay Village police that they arrest Sheppard but the mayor and police chief hesitated for 25 days. Finally, under increasing pressure fanned by fiery press editorials and intense publicity, the Coroner scheduled an inquest and Sheppard was indicted for the murder of his wife. During the inquest the Coroner did not permit Sheppard's attorney to advise him and close to the end of the proceedings evicted Sheppard's lawyer from the proceedings entirely.

Sheppard's trial started on October 18, 1954. The Coroner's chief forensic pathologist, Dr. Lester Adelson, a legend in the field, testified for 2 days as to the victim's injuries. Sheppard's attorney got Adelson to admit he had made no analysis of the contents of victim's stomach, did not take microscopic samples of the wounds, and did not try to determine if she had been raped. Although the first two errors were rather trivial, the last was inexcusable. Dr. Gerber was the star witness for the prosecution. He described in detail his examination of the scene, his questioning of Sheppard and what he called a lack of cooperation by the Sheppard family. His most damning observation was his description of the bloody pillowcase from the murder bed which showed, in his expert opinion, the mark of a surgical instrument. Gerber did not say what kind of surgical instrument it could have been and didn't produce any surgical instrument which could have made the mark. The closest he came was in response to a question from the judge: "I meant that the impression could only have been made by a surgical instrument." This is the type of hyperbole currently featured on popular television crime shows. The prosecution presented the case as a simple domestic homicide carried out by an unfaithful husband who clumsily tried to disguise the murder as a robbery and faked his own injuries.

The trial took place amidst a horde of reporters, particularly the local newspapers and the *Cleveland Press*, branding the defendant as a murderer before the trial began. Most of the courtroom was occupied by the media which was seated even inside the bar separating the parties from the public. The witnesses and the defendant had to fight their way outside the courtroom through a throng of pushing and shouting journalists. The judge made no significant attempt to isolate the jury from the prejudiced publicity nor did he sequester the jury prior to their deliberation. The pictures and names of the jurors had been disclosed in the newspapers before the trial and the jurors were permitted to communicate by telephone, freely and unchecked, with anyone they chose. The circus atmosphere of the Sheppard trial made the Anna Nicole Smith media frenzy in Fort Lauderdale look like the coverage of the grand opening of a new K-Mart.

Sheppard's brother was the first witness when the defense began its case on December 2. He described his brother's injuries as being severe and took exception to the testimony of the prosecution's neurologist who tried to minimize them. He also told of seeing a floating cigarette in an upstairs toilet which apparently was never recovered or preserved. This was potentially important evidence as Sheppard was not a smoker. The defense called 18 character witnesses for Sheppard and two witnesses who said that they had seen a bushy-haired man near the Sheppard home on the day of the crime. The jury was not convinced. On December 21, 1954, after a hundred hours of deliberation, Sheppard was found guilty of second-degree murder and he was immediately sentenced to life in prison. The conviction was a combined result of the imperfect status of the available forensic analytic tools (particularly DNA); failure to disclose exculpatory evidence; mistakes and unprofessional conduct by police investigators, the local Coroner, and the forensic pathologist that performed the autopsy; and bias of the sitting judge. The media, a lead player in any high profile event, had gleefully added plenty of oil to the "lynching" fire. Soon after his conviction, Sheppard twice received devastating family news. On January 7, 1955, his mother shot herself; 11 days later, his father died of cancer. In both cases, he was permitted to attend the funerals but was required to wear handcuffs.

After more than 6 years of appeals, Sheppard's attorney died in 1961. Months later, F. Lee Bailey took over as Sheppard's chief counsel and proved his mettle as an extremely skillful defense counsel. Sheppard served 10 years of his sentence while several appeals were rejected. Finally, his petition for a writ of habeas corpus (a legal action through which a person can seek relief from unlawful detention) was granted by Judge Carl Weinman, the Chief Judge of the United States District Court of Ohio on July 15, 1964. He ordered the state of Ohio either to free Sheppard or to grant him a new trial. Judge Weinman's decision discussed in great detail the improprieties of the law enforcement authorities and the lower court judge in the investigation and trial of Sam Sheppard. Without addressing the question of guilt or innocence, he carefully documented the inflammatory, pervasive and biased nature of the local newspapers and *Cleveland Press* that likely affected the outcome of the investigation and ultimately the jury's decision at trial. Judge Weinman supported his conclusions with extensive quotations from newspaper articles and cited in detail the following discussion between Dorothy Kilgalen, a well-known journalist, and Judge Blythin who presided over the trial:

> She stated that on, what was to the best of her recollection, the first day of trial, someone told her that Judge Blythin would like to see her in Chambers. The following is Miss Kilgallen's statement regarding her conversation with the judge: He was very affable. He shook hands with me and said, 'I am very glad to see you, Miss Kilgallen. I watch you on television very frequently and enjoy the program.' And he said, 'But what brings you to Cleveland?' And I said, 'Well, your Honor, this trial.' And he said, 'But why come all the way from New York to Cleveland to cover this trial?' And I said, 'Well, it has all the ingredients of what in newspaper business we call a good murder. It has a very attractive victim, who was pregnant, and the accused is a very important member of the community, a respectable, very attractive man.' And I said, 'Then added to that, you have the fact that it is a mystery as to who did it.' And Judge Blythin said, 'Mystery? It's an open and shut case.' And I said, 'Well, what do you mean, Judge Blythin?' I was a little taken aback because usually, I have talked to many judges in their chambers, but usually they don't give me an opinion on a case before it's over. And so I said, 'What do you mean Judge Blythin?' And he said, 'Well, he is guilty as hell. There is no question about it.'

Judge Weinman concluded that the Sheppard trial had been "a mockery of justice" because of numerous legal flaws. There was no way Sheppard could have had a fair trial since the jury had been prejudiced by the media and the judge presiding over the trial had convicted him prior to the opening arguments.

On June 6, 1966 the U.S. Supreme Court held that Sheppard's conviction was the result of a clearly unfair trial in which the defendant was denied due process, that a "carnival atmosphere" had permeated the trial, and that the trial judge had refused to sequester the jury or order them to ignore and disregard media reports of the case. The Justices' opinion accepted Dorothy Kilgallen's claim that the judge had told her on the very first day of trial that Sheppard was "guilty as hell" and the defense's contention that Coroner Gerber had said on the morning of the crime, "Well, men, it is evident the doctor did this, so let's go get the confession out of him." The Supreme Court instructed "that Sheppard be released from custody unless the state puts him to its charges again within a reasonable time." Therefore, the State of Ohio put Dr. Sam Sheppard on trial again on November 1, 1966. The prosecutor's brief opening statement was notable for what he did not mention – no faked injuries, no "surgical instrument," and no talk of affairs or impending divorce. It was during this trial that Paul Kirk, a well-known criminologist, presented blood spatter evidence he collected in Sheppard's home in 1955 which proved crucial to his eventual acquittal. He further contended that Marilyn had broken two teeth when she bit the assailant and that Sheppard did not have any bite marks. He also documented that some of the blood on the stairs could not have been from Marilyn but had to be from the fleeing assailant (a claim later verified by DNA fingerprinting). Following new federal guidelines, the jury was sequestered for the duration of the trial, their phone calls were monitored, and their newspapers were censored. No television cameras were allowed in the courtroom and seating for news reporters was markedly restricted. The trial concluded in a matter of days with a unanimous verdict of "not guilty."

Sam Sheppard was again a free man but obviously not the successful doctor who had gone to jail 12 years before. A 2 year attempt to return to medical practice failed after he was sued by two patients for malpractice. Later, Sheppard briefly worked as a professional wrestler, going by the ring name "The Killer". Just 6 months before his death, Sheppard married his wrestling partner's 20-year-old daughter. He died on April 6, 1970 of liver failure due to chronic alcoholism 4 years after his release from prison. Sam Sheppard never was a free man after all.

Years later, aided by a Supreme Court ruling that required prosecutors to disclose exculpatory evidence, police records that were suppressed in the 1954 and 1966 trials were made available to Sam R. Sheppard, the doctor's son. Among the evidence collected by the police in 1954 was a plaster impression of a freshly made pry mark found on the basement door of the Sheppard house with a copy of a detective's report describing evidence of forced entry with a wedge-like tool. Given that the prosecution's case against Sam Sheppard was based, to a great extent, on the lack of evidence of forcible entry into the home, this disclosure would have been critical during the initial trial. More significantly, a wood chip from the Sheppards' stairway with blood on it was made available for examination. It was recovered from a trail of blood leading from the bedroom to the main floor and down the basement steps. Prosecutors assumed it was Marilyn's blood that had dripped from the murder weapon. However in 1997, DNA testing determined that the blood on the stairway was not Marilyn's. Rather, it was consistent with Richard Eberling's DNA, a window-washer for the Sheppards. When questioned, Eberling told authorities he had dripped blood on the Sheppards' steps 2 days before the murder when he had accidentally cut himself. However, a former employee of Eberling's, Vern Lund, had since testified that he washed thes' windows on July 2, not Eberling. Another former employee, Ed Wilbert, told of the hostile feelings Eberling had for Marilyn because she had caught him stealing and threatened to spread the word. He was arrested by authorities in 1959, 5 years after the murder, with Marilyn's ring in his possession. Eberling's history suggests periods of psychotic anger in association with a string of suspicious deaths, culminating with his arrest and conviction for the murder of an elderly woman in 1989. His fellow inmates have recounted Eberling's admission that he killed Marilyn Sheppard, wearing a bushy wig to cover his premature baldness and to avoid recognition. He said that when Dr. Sheppard came to her aid, he knocked him out twice. He may have been telling the truth – or he may have been trying to increase his stature in the prison hierarchy.

Some experts still vehemently deny Sheppard's innocence but their arguments are not watertight. Although there are still many unanswered questions, given the recently released exculpatory evidence and the newly available DNA analysis, it would be a stretch to conclude that Dr. Sheppard was "guilty beyond a reasonable doubt." Armed with this new evidence, Sam R. Sheppard sued the state of Ohio for wrongful imprisonment. He not only wanted his father to be considered not guilty, he sought a proclamation of innocence. To his dismay, the jury denied his claim.

Dr. Poison

Between 1984 and 1997, Dr. Michael Swango (nicknamed "Dr. Poison") of Tacoma, Washington, became one of America's most prolific serial killers. Over that time span, he likely killed between 30 and 60 patients both in the United States and Africa by poisoning them with arsenic. Swango graduated from the Southern Illinois University Medical School in April 1983 and was admitted into the internship program at the Ohio State University Hospital that July. While working as an intern he murdered Cynthia McGee by injecting her with a lethal dose of potassium in January 1984. One month later, Swango assaulted another patient by injecting her with poison but she survived the attack. After suspecting him of the latter crime, the hospital removed him from the residency program and the Ohio authorities began a covert murder investigation. No charges were filed and Swango left the state, leaving his past behind him. In 1985, Dr. Swango started working at the Adams County, Illinois, Ambulance Service as an emergency medical technician. While there he poisoned several of his co-workers with arsenic. He was arrested for aggravated battery and subsequently sentenced to 5 years in prison.

In 1992, after he falsified facts about his prior criminal conviction, he was hired by the University of South Dakota and assigned to work as a resident at the Veterans Affairs Medical Center in Sioux Falls. However he was promptly discharged from the program after hospital administrators became aware of his criminal record. A year later, Swango applied for and obtained a position at the State University of Stony Brook Medical School which ran a residency program at the Northport VA Medical Center. During the application process, he explained that his criminal conviction in Illinois stemmed from a barroom brawl. Once on the job, Swango murdered three patients by injecting them with toxic substances. Swango also injected poison into another hospital patient who fortunately survived the incident. In October 1993, Dr. Swango was discharged from his position and applied for a job as a physician at the Zimbabwe Association of Church Hospitals before charges were filed. He flew to Africa and started working at Mnene Hospital in Zimbabwe. There he continued his murderous ways by administering injections of a variety of poisons into two of his patients who luckily survived the attacks. Swango was suspended from practice at Mnene Hospital in July 1995 but could not be prosecuted in the United States for his crimes for technical reasons. In 1997, after once again lying about his past. Swango obtained employment as a physician through KAMA Enterprises, Inc., an employment agency in Portland, Oregon. He was assigned to work as a physician at the Royal Hospital in Dharan, Saudi Arabia and in June 1997 booked a flight from Africa to Chicago en route to Saudi Arabia.

Upon arrival to the United States he was arrested and indicted on six counts of making false statements to the government and violating controlled substance statutes. In March 1998, he plead guilty to one of the six charges and was sentenced to a 3½-year prison term which was scheduled to expire on July 15, 2000. While still incarcerated, Swango was indicted for the murder of three of his victims as well as attempted murder. In announcing the indictment, United States Attorney

Loretta E. Lynch stated, "Through a web of lies and deception, Michael Swango inveigled his way into the confidence of hospital administrators across the country and the world. Once in their trust and employ, he utilized his skills to search for victims and take their lives." Swango was tried and convicted of only one murder and sentenced to life without parole. Dr. Swango's final death tally is unclear. What is certain is that several murders could have been avoided if his employers had followed proper procedures and looked into his past. Dr. Michael Swango should be considered the poster boy for criminal background checks.

Chapter 5
International Men of Mystery: Other Medical Murderers

When a doctor does go wrong he is the first of criminals.
He has nerve and he has knowledge.

– Sir Arthur Conan Doyle

While the vast majority of physicians attempt to optimally perform their duty to care for the sick, a very small minority of physicians are involved in nefarious activities including homicide. In most of Western society, a police investigation culminates in an arrest followed by a trial by jury. In dictatorial countries, the situation is quite different. First of all, medical murders may be more difficult to commit because of the tight social controls and governmental intervention in the practice of medicine. Those physicians who succeed in carrying them out, however, may benefit from such regimes' tendencies to cover up any social or public ills or perceived flaws in the system and to protect members of the ruling, elite class from disgrace. Alternatively, the murderer may be summarily executed and placed on public display as a deterrent to future crimes. No locale is free of physician killers except perhaps the Arctics and very sparsely populated areas with too few physicians and too few potential victims.

East Versus West

In previous chapters we described some of the criminal deeds of the famous (or in famous) doctor serial killers, most of them from United States and England. The USA, with around 6% of the world's population, has given rise to more than three quarters of all recognized serial killers and trends indicate that their prevalence is increasing. Between 1900 and 1959, there were about 1.7 new serial murder cases per year in the United States. Through the 1960s the figure grew to five a year and by 1980 it had tripled. By 1990, there were 36 cases per year representing a rise of 940% in the space of just three decades. Europe was second with 17 new serial murders per year. Men accounted for 90% of the perpetrators and women were 65% of the victims.

Serial killers can be found all over the world although at a lower frequency. It may be argued that in developing countries the lower reported rates of serial

J.A. Perper and S.J. Cina, *When Doctors Kill: Who, Why, and How*,
DOI 10.1007/978-1-4419-1369-2_5, © Springer Science+Business Media, LLC 2010

killers in general and of serial killer physicians in particular are the result of less effective police monitoring and investigation. Though this is likely true, it also seems likely that the disproportionately high rate of serial killers in developed countries may be related to the celebrity status they are afforded by the media. If you kill one person, you may make the local news. If you kill five, you will probably end up on national television for a week (maybe longer if nothing else is going on in the world). If you are a physician-murderer, you will probably get a juicy book contract and have your life immortalized in a made-for-TV movie.

Eastern Europe has had a number of murderous physicians, men of mysterious motives rather than compassionate healers. Dr. Maxim Petrov, a Russian physician and a serial killer, is a case in point. Petrov, born in 1962, worked as an emergency room physician in St. Petersburg, Russia. His modus operandi was to visit elderly patients at their homes, unannounced or on short notice, when he was off duty and when all relatives were likely to be at work. He would usually measure their blood pressure and tell the patients that they needed an injection. He then drugged them and while they were unconscious stole their possessions, taking even the rings and earrings from the victims' bodies. In all, he anesthetized and robbed about 50 elderly women pensioners. The first few victims did not die – they awoke several hours after his visit to find themselves several rubles poorer. One of the victims, Anastasia Plotnikova, was quoted by newspapers as recalling, "I remember a call at my flat at about 2 p.m. The young man presented himself as a doctor from the local clinic. The doctor took my blood pressure, which appeared to be high, and offered an injection. He spent a lot of time trying to find the vein, and I thought, "how can a doctor have problems with such a thing?" When I woke, there was fire around me. I cried for help on the balcony. The fire service came but the flat was badly burned." Plotnikova later discovered that her gold earrings, wedding rings and two packets of tea had been stolen. Another survivor, Valentina Pleshikova, told the local media that she was only saved because her husband returned home early from work. She claimed she also was injected with a substance by Dr. Petrov and fell asleep. When she was awakened, she discovered the gas oven had been turned on and all the windows shut. They later discovered that a set of silver forks and 200 rubles (less than $20) were missing – plus some coffee. The trend toward stealing caffeinated beverages is rather curious. Perhaps the perpetrator was tired after a long shift in the ER. Alternatively, there were no Starbucks stores in St. Petersburg at the time.

On February 2, 1999 during his thirtieth robbery, Dr. Petrov graduated to murder after being surprised by the daughter of an anesthetized patient who returned home unexpectedly and interrupted his robbery. He stabbed her with a screwdriver and then strangled the patient with a stocking. After this incident, he began to inject his victims with lethal mixtures of a variety of different drugs including propanolol (a high blood pressure medication). This drug is not detected on routine toxicology screens; specialized test are required to find it in the blood and you have to be looking for it. He then set fire to their homes to destroy any evidence. The police did not release a drawing of the suspect's face thinking that he would soon be caught.

The police investigation resulted in the discovery of a common denominator in these crimes. All of the victims were elderly patients with lung disease who had received chest x-rays at a local health clinic. The police identified 72 possible future victims who had been seen at the clinic and developed "Operation Medbrat" ("Medical Brother"), a sting involving 700 police officers. They finally arrested Petrov when he visited one of those patients on January 17, 2000. Initially, Petrov confessed to the murders but a few months later he recanted his confession and fiercely denied the accusations. He claimed that he had been coerced into falsely admitting the charges by the intense psychological pressure he had endured while in custody. He even wrote a protest letter to the television channel NTV (no, not MTV) from his jail cell complaining that a series of documentaries about him portraying him as a killer were "libelous." The media claimed that Dr. Petrov loved his fame (or infamy) and dubbed him Dr. Killer or Dr. Death (the Russians aren't very creative). In 2002, he was convicted of 12 murders and sentenced to life in prison.

Jean Claude Romand, a Frenchman who impersonated a doctor, killed his entire family in 1993 out of fear that his elaborate charade would be revealed. He was born in 1954 in Lons-le-Saunier, once an old Roman salt city, about a 4 hour drive from Paris. Located in the heart of the Jura vineyards, it is a picturesque and historic city with a population of about 18,000. Romand's father was a forest ranger and his mother a very fragile woman who had to be gingerly treated in order not to become upset and ill. Romand was an only child, calm with no apparent problems, and a very good student. In many ways, he was a model child – except that he was an introvert who only confided in his dog. He did well in high school and earned his baccalaureate degree. His final thesis was, ironically, an exploration of the concept "What is Truth?"

In 1971, he enlisted in Agronomic University preparatory classes in Lyon, but dropped out after one semester. He told his parents that he had to stop taking the classes for health reasons. Afterwards he enrolled as a medical student and passed the exams at the end of the first year but did not take the exams required to finish the second year. Between 1975 and 1986, Romand re-enlisted himself no less than 12 times in the second year of medical school, later on stating that he himself "was surprised that this was possible." This practice ended when a new chief of medicine discovered his scam and asked for an explanation from the "ghost student." After this inquisition he no longer haunted the campus. Having failed to finish medical school Romand brazenly pretended that he had graduated as a doctor, and succeeded in fooling everyone he knew for years. His family and friends genuinely believed that he was a successful medical professional and researcher in the World Health Organization. In search of sympathy and as an additional cover, Romand also pretended that he suffered from lymphoma (a type of cancer) and complained periodically of severe pain. To make his lies more credible, Romand spent his time visiting the local World Health Organization offices as a visitor and gathering all the free information documents he could find to prove that that he worked there. Romand occasionally told his family that he had to leave his (imaginary) local office for classified work trips but only traveled to Geneva's Cointrin International Airport where he spent a couple of days in a hotel room.

He spent these mini-vacations studying medical journals and travel guides pertaining to the country he had supposedly visited. Upon return from these fictitious trips, Romand showered his wife with expensive gifts. Romand derived his income from a number of sources including money he and his wife had made by selling an apartment, his wife's salary, his parents' bank accounts, and money given to him by various relatives who believed he was investing in hedge funds and foreign ventures on their behalf. He succeeded in bilking them out of more than 2.5 million francs. His luck seemed to have run out, however, when his father-in-law asked for a partial return of his invested funds. To Romand's good fortune, however, his father-in-law experienced a fatal fall on the steps of his home and the request was forgotten. It could never be proven whether Romand played a role in this death.

By January 1993 Romand greatly feared that his family was about to discover the truth of his deception from a debt collector. One afternoon, "Dr." Romand went to his villa a few miles from Geneva and suggested to his wife and kids that they watch a taped movie entitled "The Three Little Pigs." While they were viewing the movie, Romand shot all three dead and killed his dog as well. That evening he went to have dinner with his parents. After the meal, Romand told his father that there was an apparent leak in an upper room and when the father bent down to check the pipes, Romand shot him with a .22 caliber long rifle in the back. He then called his mother upstairs and shot her too. Before being shot the mother had the time to ask "Jean Claude what happened to you?" Soon after Romand also made an attempt to kill an ex-lover by spraying tear gas in her face and shocking her with a Taser™ (a disabling electrical control device discharging 50,000 V) in the stomach. When she screamed and struggled, he released her and drove her home, apologizing for trying to harm her. He then returned to his home and set it on fire after taking an overdose of barbiturates, likely intending to incinerate himself with his family. Local fire fighters, who were alerted by road cleaners at 4 o'clock in the morning, rescued him. Romand's trial began in June 1996 and he was sentenced to life imprisonment several weeks later. A subdued and contrite defendant, the 42-year-old Romand asked for forgiveness for his crimes both from the victims and the paltry remainder of his living family. He also apologized for living a lie.

Germany contributed Dr. Gard Wenzinger to our Wall of Ignominy. In June 1997 this 53-year-old German doctor was arrested in Brazil for torturing and killing 13 women in Germany and four others in Brazil. Wenzinger unsuccessfully attempted to kill himself after learning that German police had found a videotape showing him cutting a woman into small pieces. When Brazil's Supreme Court approved his extradition to Germany, Wenzinger hanged himself. Considering the size of Germany, it is surprising that more murderers have not made it on to these pages so far. They will make up for it later.

Witch Doctors

In some regions of the African continent witch doctors are treated as both healers and spiritual guides. Though not doctors in the traditional sense, these revered figures still have the power over life and death in some cultures. It is likely that their powers of healing are due to a combination of placebo effect and actual medicinal properties of certain herbal remedies. As in any other part of the world, this power to heal is invariable associated with the power to kill.

Many people in Southern Africa, particularly in South Africa's villages, firmly believe in the existence of a Zulu water spirit by the name of Tokoloshe. *Time* magazine reported that in the backcountry natives' bicycles are built with a small extra seat in the back should Tokoloshe want a ride. Tokoloshe is usually invisible but can materialize at any time, mostly to witch doctors and especially to children with whom he likes to play but occasionally hurts. He is alternatively described as a small teddy bear-like beast with very sharp teeth or a small furry dwarf. When he manifests himself as a human, he enjoys milk and sexual intercourse with women. This little rascal is said to have a penis so long that it has to be slung over its shoulder! Both men and women are afraid that he may hide under their bed and rape them at night (sounds like a legitimate fear given the anatomy described above) so they place their beds on stacks of bricks to thwart his attacks. Sometimes the spirit can be summoned by a witch doctor and requested to possess men to murder the witch doctor's foes. While the South African government tries to respect traditional beliefs under the aegis of cultural diversity it is somewhat stumped when faced with homicides in which the murderers sincerely claim that they were compelled by Tokoloshe to commit the crime. In sporadic cases the South African Courts have recognized the beliefs of the accused and sentenced them to only a few years of prison, instead of a life sentence or execution.

The courts were much sterner in a case where a serial killer posed as a healer. A burly Zulu named Elifasi Msomi came to be known as South Africa's Axe Killer. He was a young witch doctor who was not doing very well at his trade so he went to another witch doctor for advice. While there he found Tokoloshe masquerading as the man's son. "You will go with this son of mine," said the elder doctor "and get me the blood of 15 people … First I want the blood of a girl." For the next 18 months, Tokoloshe and Msomi wandered throughout South Africa's Natal province looking for a suitable victim. At last they found a girl whose blood was to Tokoloshe's liking. Msomi killed her and collected some of her blood in a bottle as instructed. Msomi was captured and put in jail but soon afterward, thanks to Tokoloshe it was believed, he escaped and his bloody hunt went unabated sowing terror in Zulu villages. During the following months, 14 more people were killed by Msomi's knives, clubs and axes until one day Tokoloshe announced: "You have rendered good service; now we will wash in the river and part." Later arrested for petty theft, Msomi was identified as the killer wanted for 15 of South Africa's most horrific murders. He readily admitted his crimes and even helped the police to find the skull of one of his victims. The first night in jail, he slept soundly stirring only to make room on his bed of rags for some unseen being. "It's a friend," he smiled to his jailers, "just a friend."

At his trial Msomi claimed that Tokoloshe jumped on his shoulder and ordered the killings to fulfill the wishes of the elderly witch doctor. However, two leading psychologists testified that Msomi was very intelligent and derived sexual pleasure from inflicting pain on others (a classic sexual sadist). In January 1956, Msomi was found guilty of first-degree murder and was sentenced to death by hanging in

Pretoria. Nine local Zulu chieftains, who were afraid that Tokoloshe might save Msomi, asked and were granted permission to stand by and watch when Msomi was hanged. After the execution, Zulu Chief Manzo Iwandla breathed relaxedly and reportedly said, "I am satisfied. Tokoloshe did not save him." The dead body of "Dr." Msomi was put on display in a small village to reassure the restless natives that he would never escape again.

Witchcraft murders continue to happen on the African continent. In November 2007, a "witch doctor", Sipho Kumalo, killed a baby claiming that it was Tokoloshe. He force-fed the infant wax mixed with herbs prior to beating it to death. In 2008, the President of Tanzania publicly condemned the alarming increase in the number of murdered African albinos. It turns out that witch doctors believe their organs have magical powers. Sounds like bad medicine.

Chapter 6
To Catch a Killer: Investigating Serial Murders

The darkest souls are not those which choose to live within the hell of the abyss, but those who choose to break free from the abyss and move silently among us.

– Dr. Samuel Loomis at the beginning
of the movie "Halloween"

Just because you kill 10, 50, or 1,000 people doesn't make you a serial killer. There is a big difference on several levels between serial killers and individuals who kill a lot of people. Murderers of multiple people are classified in three major groups:

1. Spree killers or rampage killers are individuals who kill multiple victims over a short period of time (hours or days) in an outburst of rage, either at random or targeting specific groups or individuals. The US Bureau of Justice Statistics defines spree killings as "killings at two or more locations with almost no time break between murders." There are no reported cases of spree killings by physicians. Most spree killers are apprehended or killed by the police within a short time and others commit suicide. For example, Charles Joseph Whitman, a student at the University of Texas at Austin, killed 14 people and wounded 31 others as part of a shooting rampage from the observation deck of the University's 32-story administrative building on August 1, 1966. He did this shortly after murdering his wife and mother. He was eventually shot and killed by Austin police. An autopsy revealed a malignant brain tumor which might have precipitated the murderous rampage. Another tragic killing spree occurred on Tuesday, April 20, 1999 at Columbine High School in Colorado. Twelve students and a teacher lost their lives in a nationally publicized bloodbath. Two alienated Columbine students, Eric Harris and Dylan Klebold, were the perpetrators. As is often the case, Harris and Klebold committed suicide after committing their crimes in what was likely a suicide pact. The Columbine event was unusual in that most killing sprees involve a single murderer. The more recent mass killing of 32 people at Virginia Tech University in 2007 also ended in the suicide of the assailant, Seung-Hui Cho. Doctors don't tend to go on killing sprees.
2. Serial killers are different from spree killers in many ways, including the characteristic "cooling periods" between attacks when they act in an apparently

normal fashion (the so called "mask of sanity"). Their crimes may be horrible but they are done in privacy rendering detection difficult. Serial killers may hone their sadistic fantasies for decades and their crimes may span continents. Most of the high-profile physician killers fall into this category.

3. Mass murderers kill large numbers of people typically at the same time or over a relatively short period of time. Mass murders may be committed by individuals acting on their own or on the behalf of a government faction, sect, or other group. Many mass murders are associated with the genocide of people of a different race, philosophy, religion or ethnic origin. The terrorists of September 11, 2001, would be included in this category. Unfortunately, a number of physicians have assisted, either willingly or under duress, in mass murders. The role physicians played in Nazi concentration camps is a case in point.

The most dangerous serial murderers are obviously the ones who never get caught and are still out there today. Their patterns are so subtle that it may be virtually impossible to link a diverse group of victims over a large geographic area to a single assailant. The detection of physicians committing clinicide (intentional murder in the setting of providing care) is also very difficult but it can occasionally be discovered following unexplained increases in morbidity (patient illness) or mortality among a physician's patients. Clinicide can also be detected by the substantiation of injurious, unnecessary, and potentially lethal medical procedures or treatment. Autopsies, considered the "Gold Standard" for discovering homicidal injury, cannot identify every type of poison or chemical in every case and testing may be equivocal or inaccurate in some settings, such as following embalming or in the setting of advanced decomposition. Crafty medical serial murderers are likely those who use poisons or medications with lethal consequences on patients who are expected to die and whose deaths will not arouse suspicion. These killers likely will never come to trial.

Early identification of physician murderers, particularly serial killers, is difficult since many of them have the ability to completely conceal their true persona. The best serial killers have a very pleasant personality and a flawless image of a "nice guy" especially towards their families, patients, and fellow physicians. This explains the adulation of some patients for some murderous doctors and their refusal to believe the charges against them despite insurmountable evidence to the contrary. When the practice patterns of these killers are viewed in the retrospectoscope, many of these perfect doctors display episodic, violent "explosions" that most often surface when they are frustrated. Of course, most physicians exhibit this behavior on occasion (consider the heart surgeon who is told that his OR is not ready for him) and the vast majority of these are not serial killers to the best of our knowledge. It is absolutely imperative to identify physicians who have gone bad. Once they have killed a single patient, the genie is out of the bottle and they may murder again and again.

In recent decades, criminologists have become very interested in serial killers and their social and psychological characteristics. One of the most prevalent classifications has been devised by Holmes. His typology classifies serial killers as being "disorganized", "organized" or mixed-type offenders and as either "asocial" or "nonsocial". The labels "disorganized" and "organized" refer to the degree of personality dysfunction which correlates with the degree of chaos at the crime scene. "Asocial" and "nonsocial" refer to whether the person is a loner because of inborn psychopathology or by choice. The characteristics of "disorganized" serial killers would be atypical for most physicians and other highly educated or intelligent murderers.

Disorganized killers usually have a low or borderline IQ of 80–95, are socially inadequate (admittedly, this does not exclude some physicians), live alone, had no strong father figure, may have been subjected to familial emotional abuse, live or work near the crime scene, have minimal interest in the media, often drop out from school, exhibit poor hygiene and housekeeping skills, keep a secret place at home, tend to be nocturnal, drive low-quality cars or trucks, and have no interest in police work. Disorganized serial killers attack in a blitz-like pattern, usually kill at one site, leave the body fairly intact at the scene, and leave a messy crime scene that usually contains significant evidence. As to post-crime behavior, disorganized murderers often have a need to return to the crime scene to relive memories, may contact the victim's family to play "games", and respond best to counseling interviews when captured. Ed Gein was a disorganized serial killer who skinned his victims and made articles of clothing and furniture from them. His crimes influenced the development of fictional characters such as Leatherface of *The Texas Chainsaw Massacre*, Norman Bates, and Buffalo Bill from *Silence of the Lambs*.

On the other hand, "organized" serial killers are almost the inverse image of the disorganized killers and are much more consistent with the profile of doctors involved in such crimes. They have an above average IQ of 105–120 or more, are socially adequate, frequently live with a partner, had a stable father figure, have a history of harsh physical family abuse, are geographically and occupationally mobile, follow the news media, often have a college degree or higher education, have good hygiene and housekeeping skills, do not usually keep a hiding place, have diurnal habits, drive flashy cars, and are interested in police activities (sometimes becoming police groupies or "wannabes"). John Wayne Gacy, Thomas Neill Cream, and Ted Bundy fit this profile. In regards to the methodology of crime, organized serial killers usually attack using seduction followed by restraint. They routinely kill at one site and dispose of bodies at another. Occasionally they will dismember the body and they generally leave a controlled crime scene that contains little physical evidence. As to post-crime behavior, organized murderers need to return to the crime scene to see what the police have done, usually contact the police to play games, and respond best to direct interviews.

Although many physicians perpetrating serial murders display general traits common amongst organized serial killers, others showed mixed-type features. These killers may have done poorly in school at times, had trouble holding down jobs, come from markedly unstable families, may have been neglected or abandoned by their fathers and raised by domineering mothers, or have been abused psychologically, physically or sexually. These killers may harbor deep feelings of hatred towards their parents and often have a history of psychiatric problems requiring treatment or hospitalization, an interest in sadomasochistic pornography, fascination with fire, and a propensity to enjoy hurting or killing small animals. These latter characteristics are shared by some of the more widely known, non-physician serial killers. These disturbed individuals commonly evolve into sexual sadists and commit the most horrific of crimes.

The motivation of serial killers may be classified as being either "Act Focused" (quick kills) or "Process Focused" (prolonged kills). The Act Focused murderer includes two subcategories:

1. The Visionary often hallucinates and hears voices or sees visions that order them to kill (classic psychotic features). The voices, usually coming from God or the devil, legitimize the violence and
2. The Missionary who has been placed on earth to eradicate a group of people (prostitutes, gays, minorities, etc.) because the perpetrator sees them as social pollution or enemies

In contrast, the Process Focused serial killer includes four subcategories:

1. The comfort-oriented hedonist that takes pleasure from killing, but also gets some profit or personal gain from it. This variety of killer is more common among females
2. The lust-oriented hedonist who associates sexual pleasure with murder. Sex while killing and necrophilia are viewed as eroticized experiences
3. The thrill-oriented hedonist who gets a "rush" or "high" from killing and feels euphoric at the victim's anguish and suffering, and
4. The power/control freaks that take pleasure from manipulation and domination of another human being (a true sociopath) and experiences a "rush" or "high" from the victim's misery

The motivation of the perpetrators of medical homicide is often complex and multifactorial. Some are Act Focused "missionaries" whereas others are "control freaks" best fitting the Process Focused model. Physician killers tend to be self-centered sociopaths disdaining or indifferent to other people's suffering. They are often narcissistic, arrogant and patronizing to both their victims and the police. In his book "*The Psychopathology of Serial Murder: A Theory of Violence*" Stephen Giannangelo discusses the characteristics of serial murderers that kill simply for the joy of killing. Their hallmark is "the ultimate control of another human being and the accompanying catharsis" and a narcissistic personality is at the core of their psyche. Freud's designation of narcissism is based on a pathological self-love as exemplified by the legend of Narcissus. According to myth, Narcissus, a young Greek, was so unusually handsome that everyone he met fell in love with him. Echo, a beautiful nymph fell under his charms but was cruelly ignored by him, breaking her heart. As a punishment the God of Revenge, Nemesis, put a curse on him that caused Narcissus to fall in love with his own reflection in a pool of water. He stayed mesmerized by his own reflection until he died and was then turned into a flower by the gods. It logically follows that characteristics of narcissistic personality disorder include a grandiose sense of self-importance; preoccupation with fantasies of unlimited success, power, brilliance, beauty or ideal love; a firm belief that she or he is "special" and unique and can only be understood by other special or high-status people; a need for excessive admiration; a sense of entitlement; a decided lack of empathy; intense envy of others while believing that others are envious of him or her; and consistent arrogant, haughty behavior. Some of these traits are common among physicians who don't kill their patients as well as those who do.

Lawrence Miller, a police psychologist, contends that predatory killing is linked to the typical hunting behavior of males, pathological only in terms of degree. Serial murderers feel intoxicated by their power over helpless victims and crave this "high" just as males in battle or in athletics pursue the adrenaline rush that has been called "the thrill of victory." They eventually become addicted to the psychologically rewarding homicide, a powerful addiction similar to that of gambling, BASE jumping, and other potentially harmful, obsessive behaviors. Furthermore, their initial capability to avoid apprehension by the authorities is also a thrill which prompts them to take progressively more and more risks to maintain their "buzz." This escalating athrill-seeking behavior ultimately gets some serial killers arrested. In the end, it almost seems that they wanted to be caught.

Nature or Nurture?

As with any severely aberrant behavior there is a deeper question behind the stereotypical motivations and behavior of serial killers – are serial murderers born or made? Are they the product of an inborn genetic defect or of some deep-seated emotional trauma inflicted during an impressionable period? Some experts such as Helen Morrison, an American forensic psychiatrist, believe in a very strong genetic influence; others disagree and emphasize early adverse environmental factors. To date, no familial cases of serial murderers have been reported and no "killer" gene has been discovered, but absence of evidence is not evidence of absence. The psychiatric environmentalists point to the very troubled childhood and adolescence experiences of several serial murderers. However, traumatic personal events, some very severe, are common in the lives of many individuals and very, very few turn into serial killers. The truth is that nobody knows what triggers the killing behavior in some individuals but not in others. No one knows what experiential catastrophic event or events amalgamate with an inborn susceptibility to reach a critical mass that releases powerful demons locked in the unconscious mind. Once the emotional avalanche begins, however, the most basic feelings of compassion and respect for human life are eradicated and a monster is born.

It seems likely that the creation of a serial murderer is akin to the development of cancer. In both cases, there is an underlying genetic problem that either encourages abnormal development or fails to inhibit abnormal growth (this may be applied to cells or personality traits). An external factor in the environment, such as cigarettes (or a physically abusive father), can then mutate the cells making up the lining of the to create a benign tumor stomach (or foster an interest in sadistic pornography by a 10-year-old). A third environmental insult, such as nitrates in hot dogs (or an overly domineering mother) results in the transformation of the benign tumor into cancer (or leads to a teenager setting fire to puppies). Any additional biochemical insult to the cancer cell (or emotional trauma to the incipient serial murderer) can result in an aggressive malignancy capable of killing.

The majority of serial killers does not fulfill the legal definition of insanity as they fully appreciate the criminality of their acts and plan their actions very carefully. This is particularly true of the organized killers. However, to the average person the behavior of serial killers is light-years away from any resemblance of sanity. The repulsive nature of the gruesome attacks, especially those accompanied by mutilation or disemboweling of the victims, protracted torture, and the consumption of body parts is way outside of society's norms.

How Do You Catch Them?

The type of victim selected by a medical murderer serves as a marker of how their crimes and their psychological profile are likely to resemble or differ from other serial killers. Physician serial killers that murder strangers fit the profile of non-medical, organized serial killers and the crimes can be investigated in an identical manner. However, doctors that murder their own patients may show significant deviations from the common pattern of serial killers in general. The investigation of their crimes and their eventual conviction is much more complex and challenging compared to the investigation of other murderers.

In the majority of serial killings done by non-physicians the major forensic questions that must be addressed involve the specific identification of the deceased, the circumstances of death, the scene characteristics, the survival time of the victim, the time of injury and death, the pattern and significance of injuries, and the commonalities of the dead person with other similar crime victims. The major and central goal is to identify the unknown assailant by integrating the facts of the investigation with physical evidence present on the victim's body or at the scene (such as fingerprints, hair, DNA, etc.). A great deal of effort is directed at generating a "profile" of the murderer so he can be promptly identified and arrested prior to killing again. While this approach works well when it is obvious that people have been murdered, when doctors kill a series of patients it can be quite difficult to identify the victims because they blend in with the general patient population. Since sick people often die unexpectedly the murders may continue for years or decades before any crime is suspected. Discovery of the homicides may be triggered by a serendipitous observation of an abnormally high mortality rate in a certain physician's practice (possible in small towns, very unlikely in larger cities), increasingly bold behavior on the part of the egotistical killer, or choosing the wrong victim at the wrong time. Once homicide is suspected, there is really no need for profiling since the suspect can usually be apprehended at his office or in the hospital or on the golf course without a struggle.

In non-medical serial murders, except in the case of some exotic modalities of death, an autopsy readily identifies the cause of death (e.g. blunt trauma, stabbing, gunshot wounds, etc.). Determination of the manner of death in these cases, homicide, also does not require Sherlock Holmes or Kay Scarpetta. In serial murders by non-physicians, once the murders are uncovered the case becomes a "Whodunnit" rather than a "How Did They Do It?" In contrast, since most murders of patients by physicians are done by poisons, excessive medications, or unwitnessed, inappropriate medical procedures (such as the injection of air into the bloodstream or disconnecting medical devices) substantiating both the cause and manner of death can be very difficult. In these cases, if an autopsy is performed it may show significant natural disease, no evidence of trauma, and no indication of homicide. Only thorough toxicological analysis can detect the presence of toxins, poisons or excessive amounts of medications in the victim's blood. In many jurisdictions, this exhaustive testing is not routinely performed on apparent natural deaths. In fact, most "natural" deaths never even come to the Medical Examiner's Office for examination. For these reasons exhumation of potential victims may be required when a murderous physician is apprehended.

Some homicides can be missed even if the body is autopsied and appropriate toxicological tests are performed. Certain toxins are not detected in the blood unless highly sophisticated tests are ordered. Heavy metals (such as lead, mercury or thallium), a variety of poisons including arsenic, certain narcotics (such as "China White"), and overdoses of naturally occurring substances (like insulin) will only be detected if someone tells the toxicologist to specifically look for them. Even if homicide has been confirmed and the lethal substance is known postmortem artifacts including decomposition and embalming may affect the accuracy of the test or render any results inconclusive. In the absence of a confession, even if there is no doubt a murder was committed, there may be little or no physical evidence to link a doctor to his murdered patient. In democratic societies the conviction of serial killer physicians is fraught with difficulty and it may take years to develop an "air tight" case.

Since murderous physicians tend to kill their own patients the best way to detect these killers is to monitor physician performance to detect any "red flags." In our computerized era such monitoring is possible. Any given physician can be tracked by the number of death certificates they generate and the number of patients they send to the Medical Examiner or Coroner. The more difficult problem is the determination of the expected mortality rate for the patients of that physician taking into account the age of the patients, their medical conditions, the particular procedures performed by the doctor, and the medical specialty of the practitioner. It would be unfair to compare an oncologist's patient death rate with that of a pediatrician (or at least one would hope so). Elaborate software could probably be developed to take into account all of these variables and develop a "most wanted doctor" list but this has not yet happened (at least we, as doctors, don't know about it). Perhaps such a program will be a part of sweeping healthcare reform; there is no doubt that universal electronic medical records would make this approach easier. Until then patients may derive a degree of consolation in that murders by physicians, and in particular serial murders, are extremely rare and few are sadistic murders.

The ancient Greeks, aware of the spectrum of evil, believed that the Gods punished crimes in accordance with the degree of depravity involved. Some criminals were relegated to the regular abode of the dead (Hades) but others were sent to a much deeper and more terrifying place, Tartarus. The Greek poet Hesiod asserted that a bronze anvil dropped from heaven would fall 9 days before it reached the Earth. The anvil would take nine more days to fall from Earth to Tartarus, making it approximately 25,920 miles deep (under normal gravitational conditions with a free-fall velocity of 120 mph, of course). In the Iliad, Zeus says that Tartarus is "as far beneath Hades as heaven is high above the earth." An icy cold place, far away from the sun and buried deep in the earth, Tartarus was said to be surrounded by an impenetrable bronze wall and isolated by three layers of night. It was a dark and horrendous endless pit engulfed by gloom and terror. For some criminals, including doctors who betray the trust of their patients and rob them of their lives, an eternal medical convention in Tartarus would not be too harsh a punishment.

Chapter 7
The Nazi Murders

Humanitarianism is the expression of stupidity and cowardice.

– Adolf Hitler

Most of the world is aware of the awful crimes committed by the Nazis during the Second World War. In addition to the horror of the Holocaust resulting in the death of six million Jews and the murder of countless Russians, Poles, and other Europeans, many disabled, "undesirable," or otherwise flawed Germans were also categorically eliminated. The active participation of German physicians in the serial murder of thousands of innocent men, women, and children has not been adequately exposed.

German professionals made up the highest percentage of enrollment in the ranks of the Nazi Socialist-National Party and its paramilitary terror troops, the SA Storm Troops and the SS. The SS, short for Schutzstafel (defense squadron), was initially Hitler's personal guard unit. After 1929, under Heinrich Himmler, it became a strongly committed, elite Nazi corps modeled after the Jesuits with absolute sworn obedience to Hitler. The SS had a number of sections, mostly operative in extermination camps and in occupied territories. Forty-five percent of German physicians became members of the Nazi party and, as officers in the SS, were active participants in the killing of the "unfit" and "undesirable racial pollutants." Though the killings started gradually in 1939, they progressed geometrically from late 1942 until the end of the War in 1945. Thousands of people were packed like sardines into locked cattle trains and shipped for days or weeks to the death camps in Poland. Each train wagon had only one open toilet for all the occupants and some of the oldest and youngest passengers died of exhaustion, thirst and hunger before reaching the destination. They received no medical care during this ordeal. Initially the doctors were supposed to cover up the serial murders by justifying their necessity on medical grounds and by issuing false death certificates. Later on, with hundreds of thousands moving quickly through the meat grinder of the death camps, the issuance of fraudulent death certificates was abandoned and the victims were cremated without any further identification or documentation of their death. People simply ceased to exist.

A major role of the physicians in the concentration camps was in the so-called "selection" process. Upon arrival, the inmates were chased out of the

J.A. Perper and S.J. Cina, *When Doctors Kill: Who, Why, and How,*
DOI 10.1007/978-1-4419-1369-2_7, © Springer Science+Business Media, LLC 2010

wagons, greeted with cries of "Raus, Raus" ("Out, Out"), and harshly prodded and battered into "receiving lines" for medical review. Doctors in elegant SS uniforms selected which prisoners should be immediately gassed and those who were to survive as slave laborers. As we have seen before, some doctors have the need to "play God" – these Nazi physicians were no exception. Older men, ill people and pregnant women were immediately killed, as were small children unless they were needed for "the advancement of science." Some prisoners were selected for involuntary medical experimentation often culminating in death. The reviewing physician sorted the throng by flipping his hand; to the right meant "death", and to the left "temporary survival". The selection was done casually with the screening doctors often smiling, joking or laughing. The more vicious doctors did not hesitate to brutalize some of the slower moving inmates. Some reports suggest that crying children were thrown alive into cremation fires during this screening procedure.

In the early stages of the War, physicians were responsible for turning on the gassing apparatus. These physicians were also supposed to witness the exterminations to assess the efficacy of the process. Once the bodies were removed from the chamber, German dentists extracted gold teeth from victims. Some of the victims' bodies were stripped of their flesh with the skeletons submitted for anthropological studies to German universities. Many of these specimens were found in the university museums at the end of the War, before the local staff had a chance to dispose of them. In addition to the role they played in the concentration camps, Nazi physicians also participated in other progressively injurious or murderous programs including coercive sterilization, the killing of "impaired" children in hospitals, and the eradication of "defective" adults mostly from mental hospitals or institutions in special centers.

Coercive sterilization was done under the direction of the German Hereditary Health Courts. Men were forcibly vasectomized whereas women were initially sterilized by removal of their ovaries—sometimes with the uterus. Experiments on forced sterilization by radiation were performed on hundreds of women detained in concentration camps. By the end of the Nazi regime, over 200 Hereditary Health Courts (Erbgesundheitsgerichten) in which two of the three members were physicians were operating. Under their rulings, over 400,000 Germans had been sterilized including 200,000 deemed mentally deficient; 100,000 with mental illness; 60,000 epileptics; 10,000 alcoholics; 20,000 with body deformities; and others afflicted with Huntington's chorea, hereditary blindness or deafness. The Nazis also considered Blacks inferior and despised their culture, including Black music and jazz. They decided to take action against people of color in the Rhineland. In 1937 some 400 children of mixed parentage were arrested and sterilized.

In the beginning of the so called "euthanasia" program, the Nazis were very careful to present to the German public only the most egregious cases of disability and deformity. This government response was marketed as a compassionate response to frantic pleas from parents wishing to put a suffering child out of his/her misery. In many of these cases, the pleas were either fabricated by the government or were made after coercion. The actual child euthanasia program started with a family petition for the "mercy killing" ("Gnadentod") of an infant by the name of Knauer. He had been born blind, mentally retarded, and with one or both legs and part of one arm missing. Hitler himself ordered the killing only after Karl Brandt, his personal physician, verified the accuracy of the facts and consulted with the treating physicians who approved euthanasia. Hitler granted the physicians assisting the government in this project immunity from prosecution.

By late 1938, only months before the preparations for war accelerated, the Nazi regime authorized mercy killings of babies born deformed or with brain damage. A Reich Committee for the Scientific Registration of Serious Hereditary and Congenital Diseases (Reichsausschuss zur wissenschaftlichen Erfassung von erb- und anlagebedingten schweren Leiden), was made responsible for monitoring the registration of all children under 3 years of age with any suspected "serious hereditary diseases" including a variety of mental and physical challenges. Midwives were required to make these reports at the time of birth and doctors were to report all such children up to the age of three on questionnaires of the Reich Health Ministry. The physicians staffing the euthanasia commission made their determination of "lebensunwertes leben" (life unworthy of life) solely on the basis of the questionnaire without examining the children or reviewing their medical records. A red cross marked on the form indicated that that the child had to be killed, a blue one that it will be allowed to live. If the commission could not unanimously decide the fate of a child based on the questionnaire, the child was shipped to one of six psychiatric "euthanasia" sites including the Hadamar Psychiatric Clinic. While in the care of the Clinic, children were killed by either gradual starvation or by the administration of increasing doses of Luminal (phenobarbital – a type of sleeping pill). In the end, 70,000 German children thought to be abnormal were forcefully taken from their homes, institutionalized, and eventually killed. The parents were told by the doctors that their offspring died of natural conditions or of unavoidable complications of necessary surgical or medical therapy. The bodies were burned en mass and comingled ashes were sent to the families.

The Nazi serial murders soon snowballed and the "euthanasia" program was expanded to include inmates of psychiatric facilities, adult patients with severe neurological disorders and other "undesirables." In October 1939, Hitler issued a decree increasing "the authority of certain physicians to …(identify) persons who, according to human judgment, are incurable … (and can) be accorded a mercy death." Anyone who suffered from schizophrenia, manic-depressive disorder, epilepsy, senility, paralysis, syphilis, retardation, encephalitis, Huntington's chorea, and other neurological conditions had to be reported to the Nazi Health Authorities. The criminally insane and patients who had been institutionalized for 5 or more years were also on the hit list. Patients who did not have German citizenship or were not of German descent, including Jews, blacks, and Gypsies, were to be reported as well. Obviously, if you were not German, something had to be wrong with you. This seems curious since Hitler was Austrian.

By 1941, public outcry regarding the government's euthanasia program ("Aktion T4") had reached a fever pitch and Hitler suspended the program. Over 100,000 men, women and children had been killed. The Nazis were no longer able to kill institutionalized patients with mass gassings. Drugs and starvation were used instead – it was much more discreet. Hitler still tried to influence the public view of euthanasia through a clever, emotionally charged movie entitled *Ich Klage* (I Accuse), which was shown in theatres all over Germany. It depicted the tribulations of a good and charitable physician and a loving husband whose wife suffered from disabling multiple sclerosis. The wife begged her husband to end her misery and help her to commit suicide and the husband reluctantly agreed. The husband was then charged with murder and he in turn accused the State of failing to help the disabled to die and thereby relieve their suffering. Obviously, the Nazis could not turn a blind eye to this poor fellow's plight.

Why Did They Do It?

It is difficult to understand how normal human beings could have, would have, and did willingly take part in this orgy of medical mayhem and murder, particularly physicians who have taken an oath to do no harm. The Nazi doctors were not isolated psychopathic or sociopathic physicians but rather throngs of hundreds if not thousands of practicing doctors assimilated into the Nazi movement. In her 1963 work *"Eichman in Jerusalem,"* Hannah Arrendt argued that the explanation is what she termed "the banality of evil." Her theory suggests that great evils in history in general, and the Holocaust in particular, were not largely executed by fanatics or by sociopaths, but by ordinary people. Each small, human, cogwheel accepted the commands of the State as a matter of routine and complied with their instructions without much critical thinking. While such an attitude clearly facilitated some of the Nazi atrocities, it is not the sole explanation. The metamorphosis of Germans doctors from healers to killers was a much more complex, multifaceted and gradual process, and an intrinsic outcome of very clever indoctrination of the German people by Hitler and his National-Socialist Nazi Party. Many German physicians were also strongly influenced by Hitler's charisma.

In 1929, Hitler had appealed directly to German physicians to assist him in his campaign of "racial hygiene" and in response, a group of 40 German doctors formed the Nationalist Socialist Physician League to support the Nazi racial policy designed to "purify" the medical establishment. Almost 2,790 physicians, 6% of the entire medical profession, joined the League well before Hitler came to power. Hitler's appeals also prompted many physicians to join the Nazi Party. Between 1924 and 1944, the physicians' membership in Hitler's National Socialist Party was threefold that of the general German population, with most of the supporters being young physicians below 40. Like moths attracted to a burning light, many German physicians blindly followed the Nazi myths and practices. Those that did not march to the tune of the State could well become a future "patient" of the regime.

Duty

The enthusiasm with which the Nazis carried out their onerous tasks in the extermination camps varied from bland indifference to undisguised pride. Although it was not uncommon for newly assigned doctors to be upset by the skeletonized appearance of starving inmates and mounds of murdered victims ready for cremation, in time most were capable of efficiently carrying out their duties (although some resorted to heavy drinking). The small number who complained that they were unable to carry out their assignment were re-educated about their duty as "medical soldiers" and the need to unquestioningly follow the instructions of their beloved Fuehrer. Many other doctors fulfilled their duty with maximal devotion looking forward to every new arrival of victims. Some displayed unusual cruelty towards the inmates, especially doctors with innate narcissistic or sadistic personality traits. Such was the case of Dr. Joseph Mengele, a Bavarian physician who became the "Angel of Death."

In 1945 Mengele was stationed at the Auschwitz–Birkenau concentration camps where numerous Poles, homosexuals, Soviets, Jews, and Romanians met horrible and untimely deaths. Mengele would inspect incoming camp prisoners and assign them to work, experimentation, or the gas chambers. He believed fanatically in the Social Darwinism of Nazi racism and generally carried out his odious duties in a very obsessive fashion, usually with marked indifference to the suffering around him. He made a special point of greeting every load of incoming prisoners, as he wanted to be sure that he was not going to miss sets of twin prisoners up on which he was always burning to experiment. Mengele apparently enjoyed the dramatic contrast between his elegant officer's clothing and the dirty rags worn by most prisoners. Psychiatrists who have studied Mengele have asserted that this infatuation was a marker of a narcissistic personality with sexual gratification overtones. Even Mengele, however, displayed short-lived flashes of humane behavior, a phenomenon known as doubling. For example, Mengele had a protégé among the Gypsy camp inmates, a young boy, who he provided with better food and clothing. Despite this apparent kindness, on the night when he was ordered to exterminate all the Gypsies in the camp, Mengele himself relentlessly hunted for the boy throughout the camp and personally saw to it that he was gassed with the rest of the prisoners.

After the war Mengele fled to South America (Paraguay and Brazil) where he eventually died by drowning decades after the War. Despite the insinuations made in "The Boys from Brazil" movie, there is no firm evidence to suggest that after Mengele relocated to South America he attempted to clone Hitler. However, it should be noted that in a 2009 book entitled *"Mengele: an Angel of Death in South America"* an Argentine historian argued that Mengele's activities after the War were the explanation for the high proportion of twins in the tiny Brazilian town of Candido Godoi. Further, although the natives resembled their neighboring South Americans, most of the twins were blond-haired and blue-eyed. The residents of the town apparently reported that Mengele made repeated visits there in the early 1960s. He first claimed to be a veterinarian but then offered free medical treatment to women, providing them with unidentified elixirs and pills and taking blood samples.

Shortly after the end of the war, a small group of Nazi physicians were brought before an Allied tribunal at Nurenburg and tried for war crimes including human medical experimentation. Some were sentenced to death by hanging, some to long prison terms, and a few were acquitted. In truth, a very small number of culpable German physicians were brought to justice and most escaped punishment. Many esteemed physicians from reputable German universities had collaborated shamelessly with the Nazi authorities and had received organs, tissue and skeletons of the murdered camp victims which they used in their research. Despite the advances made in the name of science, they could not justify the atrocities committed and an indelible mark of Cain was emblazoned on the body of German Medicine.

Preservation of the Race

Many Germans physicians of the 1930s were strong supporters of eugenics. This branch of science has as its goal the improvement of the human race through manipulation of genetic hereditary traits. It discourages the propagation of negative hereditary traits (negative eugenics) and encourages propagation of positive traits (positive eugenics). The term was coined in 1865 by Sir Francis Galton in a social application of his cousin Charles Darwin's *On the Origin of Species*. On the face of it, eugenics seems to be a well-intentioned and beneficial philosophy to humankind. In modern times, it has played a formative role in pre-natal testing and screening, genetic counseling and molecular correction of genetic diseases. Unfortunately, the Nazis used eugenics as a model for coercive state-sponsored discrimination, forced sterilization of persons with disabilities and/or genetic defects (real or conveniently assumed), the killing of disabled or institutionalized people and, in some cases, outright genocide of populations perceived as inferior or undesirable. Malignant eugenics and pseudo-eugenics practices were at the very heart of Nazism.

In an 1895 book entitled *"Das Recht auf den Tod"* (the Right to Death) Adolf Jost argued that the State should have the ultimate authority to decide who should live and who should die since it has the responsibility of efficiently handling the society's resources "in order to keep the social organism alive and healthy." He argued that the State already exercised such rights in war, when throngs of individuals are sent to die for the good of the State. Jost advocated that for the collective good, the State's right to decide death should be extended to peacetime and that the euthanasia of the disabled is not an act of cruelty but of mercy. Though morally repugnant, similar arguments are currently being made by some extremists who are trying to figure out how to deal with millions of aging "baby-boomers."

In 1920 Karl Binding, a law professor from the University of Leipzig, and Alfred Hoche, a professor of psychiatry at the University of Freiburg, authored *"Die Freigabe der Vernichtung lebensunwerten Lebens"* (The Permission to

Destroy Life Unworthy of Life). The authors included in the category "unworthy life" not only the incurably sick but large segments of the mentally ill, the feebleminded, and retarded or deformed children. They claimed that the termination of life unworthy of life is "purely a healing treatment" and a "healing work." Many German physicians accepted such argumentation as being rational and ethically justified. As early as 1922, the popular writer Ernst Mann (a pseudonym of Gerhardt Hoffman) defended direct medical killing commenting that illness is "a disgrace to be managed by health control" and that "misery can only be removed from the world by painless extermination of the miserable!" Mann wrote that, "all the weaklings and the sick must be exterminated" and suggested to the Reichstag that anybody who was a burden on society and unable to contribute to it should die. After all, if they weren't exterminated, they would be miserable anyway. He argued that a combined plan of eugenics and euthanasia would bring about a triple benefit for Germany:

1. It would be seen as an act of mercy by society in general;
2. It would improve the stock of the Aryan race and;
3. It would be financially sound for the State.

His euthanasia extremism was also evident in his book "*Moral der Kraft*" (The Morality of Strength) in which he advocated that war veterans should commit suicide in order to reduce public welfare costs. In 1936, Gerhardt Wagner, the head of the Nazi Health System and of the Reich's Physicians Chamber to which all physicians were mandated to belong, held informal discussions about killing "idiotic children" and "mentally ill" people. The group also advocated producing propaganda films for the German audiences emphasizing the humanity of such an approach. He also identified as the task of his Public Health Office "the promotion and perfection of the health of the German people ... to ensure that the people realize the full potential of their racial and genetic endowment." An influential manual by Dr. Rudolf Ramm of the University of Berlin proposed that each doctor was to no longer be merely a caretaker of the sick but to become a "cultivator of the genes," a "physician to the Volk," and a "biological soldier."

Ramm criticized the widespread belief that a doctor should under no circumstances take a patient's life, arguing that "euthanasia" was the most "merciful treatment" and "a central obligation to the Volk." Ramm's manual (which was mandatory reading for medical students) also specified that a doctor was to be a biological militant, "an alert biological soldier" living under "the great idea of the National Socialist biological state structure." Further, "National Socialism, unlike any other political philosophy or Party program, is in accord with the natural history and biology of man" and "biology and genetics are the roots from which the national-Socialist world view has grown." Many doctors joined the Party immediately after hearing Deputy Party Leader Rudolf Hess convincingly claim at a meeting in 1934 "National Socialism is nothing but applied biology." Many physicians saw themselves as professional flag bearers of the biological (racist) doctrine of Nazism.

The Nazis also implemented a number of "positive eugenics" policies such as rewarding Aryan women who had large numbers of children and fostering practices in which "racially pure" single women could deliver illegitimate children. Nazi eugenists kidnapped thousands of Polish and Czech children that they considered "racially valuable" or "racially pure" because they had the required blonde hair and blue eyes and brought them to Lebensborn centers were they were forced to forget their parents and adopt the Nazi beliefs. Those who refused were beaten or killed; SS families adopted the ones who accepted the "re-education". It is estimated that up to 250,000 such children were brought to Germany but after the war, only 25,000 were returned to their families.

Dr. Fritz Lenz, a notable Nazi physician, advocated sterilizing people with minimal signs of mental disease. He soon recognized that a radical application of this principle would result in the sterilization of 20% of the total German population – some 20 million people. Although one could argue that Hitler showed some subtle signs of mental imbalance, it seems very unlikely that Dr. Lenz would want to force his boss to get a vasectomy.

Anti-Semitism

Hatred and organized persecution of Jews started in Germany with the German Crusade of 1696. This was part of the First Crusade in which zealous peasants from France and Germany attacked many Jewish communities despite Pope Urban II condemning any such violence. Although anti-Semitism had existed in Europe for hundreds of years, this was the first recorded organized mass extermination program. This vat of anti-Semitism continued to simmer over the following centuries, heightening during harsh economic and social times and ebbing when societal conditions improved. In his biography and blueprint of Nazism "*Mein Kampf*" Hitler relentlessly emphasized the pernicious nature of Jews as a Public Enemy of the Reich and "poisoners" of the German-Aryanic racial purity. For the good of Germany they had to be liquidated. Many German doctors accepted and agreed (or at least went along) with this virulent anti-Semitism and the persecution of Jews that followed. In many instances, this incidentally improved their own economic status by eliminating competition by Jewish physicians.

Hitler was successful in tapping the overt and covert feelings of racial hatred and professional jealousy prevalent in the German medical community and German physicians rewarded him by joining the Nazi Party in droves. By supporting the Nazi approach to the "Jewish problem," German doctors were following a long tradition of intellectual anti-Semitism. Prior to Hitler's rise to power, Jewish doctors represented 13% of all German physicians, and in some large cities, they reached almost 50%. By 1941, the number of practicing Jewish physicians had essentially dropped to zero. Jewish physicians were referred to as "healers" rather than "doctors" and they could treat only Jewish patients under penalty of law.

Could This Nightmare Happen Again?

Genocide was not invented by the Nazis. There were despicable genocides before and after they soiled the world stage including the Armenian slaughter by the Turks, the Chinese genocide by the Japanese before the Second World War, the Sarajevo killings of Moslems by Serbs, and the murder of thousands of Africans in Sudan by local Arabs. The Nazis distinguish themselves by the methodical nature of their killings and the integration of physicians into the extermination of millions of human beings. When doctors are willing to stand by and watch or, worse, participate in the elimination of the very people they have sworn an oath to help, will the rest of society behave any better?

Section 3
In the Name of Science

Chapter 8
Hitler's "Scientists"

Among the experiments that may be tried on man, those that can only harm are forbidden, those that are innocent are permissible, and those that may do good are obligatory. It is immoral then, to make an experiment on man when it is dangerous to him, even though the result may be useful to others.

– Claude Bernard, French physiologist, 1865

Medical experimentation on humans began many centuries ago. The first "volunteers" were slaves, considered at that time to be property rather than human beings. One of the first experimenters was the famous Greek physician Herophilos (335–280 BC), co-founder of the great medical school of Alexandria and widely regarded as the "father of anatomy" (though Vesalius may argue this point). He was the first researcher to base his anatomic studies on dissection of the human body. Though this was scientifically valid and led to a greater understanding of the human body, he carried out the procedures on living slaves which raises questions about his ethics. Tertullian, a prolific Christian writer (AD 197–220) claimed that Herophilos had performed vivisections on more than 600 slaves.

The Egyptians also participated in scientific inquiry. In the first century BC, Queen Cleopatra devised a series of experiments to test the accuracy of the theory that it takes 40 days to fully fashion a male fetus and 80 days to create a female fetus. Whenever one of her handmaids were sentenced to death, Cleopatra had them impregnated and subjected them to subsequent operations to open their wombs at specific times of gestation. The results of these experiments have never been published. Eighteen hundred years later King George I offered free pardons to any inmate of Newgate Prison who agreed to be experimentally inoculated with infectious small pox. This might have turned out to be a fair trade given the condition of prisons of that era. John Hunter, the brilliant Scottish physician and scientist made many advances in surgery, anatomy and physiology. He also stole the skeleton of Charles Byrne, a 7′ 7″ Irish giant against his deathbed wishes. For £500 Hunter successfully bribed a member of the funeral party for the bones which he studied, wrote about, and subsequently published. The unfortunate giant never received the burial at sea he had hoped for;

J.A. Perper and S.J. Cina, *When Doctors Kill: Who, Why, and How*, DOI 10.1007/978-1-4419-1369-2_8, © Springer Science+Business Media, LLC 2010 his skeleton still resides in the Hunterian Museum at the Royal College of Surgeons in London. Though these select historical examples range from the callous to the abhorrent, they were at least designed to advance science. The Nazis, however, conducted a myriad of horrific experiments to answer a different calling – curiosity-based sadism.

The Nazi Experiments

Children are afraid of terrifying monsters hiding in the dark, under the bed, or in the closet. At any moment, these living nightmares may pounce and bury long claws and sharp teeth into their shivering flesh. Caring adults switch on a light, tenderly hug the panicky tots and assure them that their fears are groundless. As they fall back to sleep, they are reassured that there are no monsters or that they have departed never to return. This usually works and life goes on. However, one could not have extended such comfort to the victimized children in Nazi Germany. Infants, toddlers and older children died on cold surgical tables after experiencing unimaginable pain as "scientific experiments" were performed without the distraction of anesthesia. Thousands of children died in the name of science during the Third Reich. Monsters do exist.

SS doctors carried out Nazi "medical" experimentation primarily in concentration camps often with the direct assistance and cooperation of civilian academicians from reputable medical schools and universities. These criminal experiments had three avowed goals:

1. To produce in healthy camp inmates bodily injuries or illnesses to which Nazi soldiers may be exposed and to try to reverse them
2. To expose inmates, adults and children, to different poisons in order to observe what are the lethal doses and survival times, and
3. To try to scientifically substantiate the genetic inferiority of so called inferiority races

With few exceptions, the scientific value of the experiments was virtually nil for a number of reasons. These included doubts about the integrity of the data provided by scientists/physicians who either felt pressure to provide the desired results or who wanted to substantiate the truth of their own racial beliefs; inconsistency of some of the results and the fact that they were never published in reputable journals; and the lack of reproducibility of these tortuous experiments that can never be replicated in any civilized society.

Between 1939 and 1945, more than 70 types of research projects involving dangerous experimentation on human subjects were conducted in Nazi Germany. More than 7,000 Jews, Poles, Roma (Gypsies), political prisoners, Soviet prisoners of war, homosexuals, and Catholic priests were among the victims. It would be difficult to list all of the forms of experimentation performed on these unwilling volunteers in a single chapter so we will attempt to highlight some of the more heinous acts committed by Nazi doctors in the name of science.

Freezing Experiments

Nazi doctors conducted the freezing/immersion hypothermia experiments for the German High Command and at the request of Air Force Field Marshall Erhard Milch. The experiments were conducted on young healthy prisoners of various religions and nationalities under conditions simulating the biting and disabling, freezing weather faced by the invading German Army in Russia and by pilots shot down over the North Sea. It was estimated during postwar testimony that 360–400 hypothermia experiments were conducted on 280–300 victims. The experiments were conducted at the Birkenau, Dachau (near Munich) and Auschwitz extermination camps by a number of SS physicians under the supervision and direction of Dr. Sigmund Rascher, an Air Force physician who reported directly to Himmler.

The freezing experiments were designed to establish how long it would take for a subject to die after exposure to cold and, secondly, to learn how to resuscitate frozen victims. The "experimental" subjects were exposed to sub-zero temperature by immersing them naked or fully dressed into long narrow tanks filled with ice water or by exposing them strapped naked to a stretcher in freezing weather. An insulated probe, which measured the drop in the internal body temperature, was inserted in their rectum and anchored to the intestinal wall. Most victims lost consciousness and died in exquisite pain when the body temperature dropped to 25°C (77°F). Though most victims were lucky enough to die at this point, some of the volunteers were rapidly enrolled in the resuscitation or warming experiments. Several techniques were applied including forceful irrigation of the stomach, intestines, or bladder with very hot, almost boiling, water and rapid immersion of the entire body in hot water resulting in death by shock of the near-frozen victims. In a few cases, gradual exposure to heat in a warm bath resulted in some survivals. The surviving subjects were then eligible to participate in additional studies.

Heinrich Himmler, who was a close friend of Dr. Rascher's wife suggested that he try to use sexual activity to warm up the frozen men. Rascher agreed to test this theory by placing semi-frozen males between two naked women and prompting them to engage in sex. These rewarming exercises failed miserably, perhaps due to impotence issues associated with exposure of the male sexual organs to cold. In 1942, Rascher presented the results of his freezing experiments at a medical conference entitled "Medical Problems Arising from Sea and Winter" claiming that the hypothermia experiments were not designed to produce fatalities and "only" a total of 13 deaths occurred. This is in conflict with the post-war testimony of two of his assistants who estimated that "at least 80 to 90 victims died during the experiments, and only two were known to have survived the war, both of whom became 'mental cases.'" Like Dr. Rascher.

Genetic Experiments

Dr. Joseph Mengele, "The Angel of Death", pioneered the Nazi genetics program. His list of "experimental" murders is truly stunning. He dissected live infants; injected chemicals into the eyes of children in an attempt to change their eye color; sterilized and castrated inmates without anesthetics; burned prisoners with incendiary bombs to examine their injuries; inflicted high-voltage electric shocks upon subjects of varying ages; froze inmates to study the effects of hypothermia; injected malaria-contaminated blood into test subjects; and exposed inmates to mustard gas and other poisons. After he had gassed any survivors of the experiments, he defleshed and skeletonized the victims for measurements of the bones to satisfy his interest in human anthropology.

Mengele had a particular interest in twins and always hunted for them upon the arrival of new batches of Auschwitz inmates. Initially the twins were extensively photographed for several days with special attention paid to their hair patterns. They were forced to stand, bend, and kneel for hours in many uncomfortable positions to document their appearance and characteristics from all angles. They were then showered and shaved from head to toe and returned nude for a thorough physical examination. If any of the camp physicians performing the examinations missed any details they were likely to be harshly punished. Each twin then had full body x-rays resulting in exposure to carcinogenic levels of radiation. The next stage of the examination consisted of removing all of the twins' remaining hair in a very cruel and painful manner. The twins were placed repeatedly in vats with very hot water to soften the skin then strapped to a table in order to have each hair plucked out including the roots. The next "medical" procedure consisted of forcing a gas though the nose and upper airways of the torture victims until they coughed and expectorated deep sputum which was collected for analysis. The twins then received a series of enemas each consisting of several liters of water which caused them much pain and discomfort. Once they had been cleansed, prison doctors forcefully distended the anus to facilitate a lower intestinal examination. This procedure was so painful that the victims had to be gagged to muffle their screams. The male subjects received a thorough urological examination with no anesthesia and tissue samples were taken from the testicles, prostate, and kidneys. After 3 weeks of "medical experimentation" and collection of all available data, the twins were taken to an execution room and killed simultaneously by an injection of chloroform in the heart administered by SS physicians. The murdered twins were then autopsied and their organs were sent for further examination to the Institute of Biological, Racial, and Evolutionary Research in Berlin.

High-Altitude Experiments

In 1942, experiments were conducted for the German Luftwaffe to investigate the effect of flying at high-altitude. The "volunteers" were prisoners at the Dachau concentration camp who were subjected to conditions designed to simulate those faced by German pilots forced to eject at high altitude. The experimenters placed camp inmates into low-pressure chambers that simulated altitudes as high as 68,000 ft and monitored their physiological response as they suffered, succumbed and died. Under conditions approximating parachuting from an altitude of 8 miles without an oxygen supply, spasms began almost immediately and the victims rapidly lost consciousness. At 9 miles (15 km) they had additional breathing problems and there were instances when they stopped breathing altogether. Nevertheless, the experiments went on to an altitude of 13 miles. Dr. Sigmund Rascher, the main experimenter, dissected the victims' brains after their skulls were broken open while they were still alive and conscious to demonstrate the formation of tiny air bubbles (air emboli) in the blood vessels of the brain. Of 200 people subjected to these experiments, 80 died outright and the remainder were murdered and autopsied.

Antibiotic Experiments

Between July and September 1943 experiments were conducted at the behest of the German Army whose frontline soldiers often sustained infections of their wounds with resultant gas gangrene. Nazi physicians at the Ravensbruck concentration camp under the direction of Dr. Herta Oberheuser performed studies testing the efficacy of sulfanilamide and other drugs in curbing these highly lethal infections. They intentionally injured many prisoners causing battlefield-like wounds which were inoculated with bacteria including *Clostridium perfringens*, the microorganism responsible for gas gangrene. The doctors aggravated the resulting infections by rubbing ground glass and wood shavings into the wounds. In most of these cases, the response to this antibiotic was insufficient to avoid loss of limbs, sepsis, and death.

Experimental Poisoning

Nazi researchers studied a variety of methods of execution by injecting Russian prisoners with phenol and cyanide, placing different poisons in their food, and shooting them with poisoned bullets. Victims who did not die during the experiments were killed and autopsied with their remains analyzed for the presence of poison and evidence of tissue injury.

Phosgene Experiments

In an attempt to find an antidote to phosgene, a toxic gas used as a weapon by the Germans during World War I, Nazi doctors exposed 52 concentration camp prisoners to the gas at Fort Ney near Strasbourg, France. Phosgene gas causes extreme irritation to the lungs and severe shortness of breath, chest pain and disability. Many of the prisoners, who according to German records were already weak and malnourished, suffered pulmonary edema after exposure and four of them died from the experiments. In essence, they drowned in their own body fluids. The survivors had severe lung damage for the rest of their lives. There is no record that any antidotes were given to the prisoners though that was the stated goal of the experiment.

Bone, Muscle and Joint Transplantation

Between September 1942 and December 1943, physicians conducted a series of surgical experiments in order find out whether a limb or joint from a person could be successfully attached to an amputee. Nazi doctors at Ravensbruck concentration camp amputated legs and shoulders from Polish inmates in futile attempts to transplant them onto other victims who been intentionally maimed. They also removed sections of bones, muscles, and nerves from prisoners to study regeneration of these body parts. Victims suffered excruciating pain, mutilation, and permanent disabilities.

Sterilization Techniques

The Nazis attempted to find out which sterilization method was the easiest, most rapid, and most effective to use on the millions of people deemed "enemy" populations. Experiments were conducted on both men and women prisoners at Auschwitz and Ravensbrueck under the direction of the Nazi doctors Carl Clauberg and Horst Schumann. The sterilization was done by drugs, surgery, and x-rays to the genitals at different intensities resulting in severe burns and infected sores. Some women had caustic substances forced into the cervix or uterus, and experienced severe abdominal pain and bleeding. The degrading, forced sterilization also resulted in severe depression for many of the victims. After the war, Dr. Schumann fled to Africa where, in a remarkable change of heart, he worked tirelessly in remote areas saving victims of sleeping sickness. He later described himself as "having found the serenity and the calm necessary for the moral balance of a human being." He was repatriated to Germany in 1966 where he was imprisoned for several years for his crimes decades earlier. He was eventually released without standing trial because of a very poor state of health. In custody, he alternated between statements such as "It was terrible what we did" and others defending or denying his actions. He died in 1983.

Artificial Insemination Experiments

After hearing that Dr. Carl Clauberg had successfully treated a high-level SS officer's infertile wife, Heinrich Himmler ordered Clauberg to conduct artificial insemination experiments. Some 300 women at Auschwitz subsequently underwent artificial insemination at the hands of Clauberg. In addition to the physical humiliation of the procedure, he reportedly taunted his victims by informing them that he had just inseminated them with animal sperm and that monsters were now growing in their wombs. Clauberg was ultimately arrested and imprisoned in the Soviet Union, then repatriated to Germany where he returned to medical practice. Due to an outcry by survivor groups, he was arrested in 1955 and died mysteriously in his cell in a West German prison in 1957.

Seawater Experimentation

In 1944, Dr. Hans Eppinger and others Nazi doctors at the Dachau concentration camp conducted experiments on how to make seawater drinkable. The doctors forced roughly 90 Gypsies to drink only seawater while also depriving them of food. The Gypsies became so dehydrated that they reportedly licked floors after they had been mopped just to get a drop of fresh water. The cruel experiments caused extreme pain and suffering and resulted in serious bodily injury and death. Dr. Eppinger killed himself by poison on September 25, 1946, exactly 1 month before he was scheduled to testify in the Nuremberg trial.

Incendiary Bomb Experiments

Experiments were conducted at Buchenwald extermination camp in order to test pharmaceutical treatments for phosphorus burns on prisoners. Phosphorus from bombs was applied to the skin of camp prisoners and then ignited. The skin was allowed to burn for more than a minute before the flames were extinguished.

Human Petri Dishes

German soldiers contracted many typhus cases after invading the Soviet Union. Experiments were designed to test the efficacy of vaccines against typhus, smallpox, cholera, and other diseases on camp prisoners who had been purposely injected with the respective infectious agents. More than 90% of the inmates involved in these studies died. Other experiments involved infecting the subjects with malaria and tuberculosis. Many of these experiments involved Catholic priests. More people died of the treatments than of the diseases themselves.

Polygal Experiments

When Himmler was told that the cause of death of most soldiers on the battlefield was uncontrollable bleeding, he ordered the dependable Dr. Rascher to develop a blood clotting agent to be administered to German troops before a battle. Rascher conducted experiments to test the effectiveness of polygal, a blood coagulant, which he developed for the treatment of bleeding wounds. After infusing his subjects with this medication, he quantified it effectiveness by measuring the rate of blood drops oozing from freshly cut amputation stumps of living and conscious prisoners at the Dachau crematorium.

German Academicians

Professors in the highest institutions of medical learning in Germany supported the Nazi theories of racial eugenics and racial selection and participated to various degrees in the murder of innocent men, women and children. It is likely that some of the support radiated from a fear of the regime taking away their positions, livelihood, family, and life if they did not cooperate with the government. It is also likely that some academic physicians truly believed in the Nazi cause and did everything they could to help. Dr. Carl Schneider (1891–1946), Professor and Chairman of the Department of Psychiatry of the University of Heidelberg, psychologically assessed children he knew would be killed under the Nazi eugenics programs and had their brains collected and dissected after they were murdered. Schneider committed suicide after the war. Dr. Hermann Stieve, a leading anatomist and professor at the University of Berlin and the Berlin Charité Hospital, investigated the impact of fear and stress on the menstrual patterns of women who had been informed that the Gestapo would kill them on a particular date. Upon the women's execution, their pelvis was opened and the uterus excised for microscopic examination of the endometrium (the lining of the womb that eventually sheds at the end of the menstrual cycle). Shamelessly, Stieve published reports of his findings and even lectured about them to medical students in East Berlin after the war. Dr. Eduard Pernkopf, the Chair of The Institute of Anatomy of the University of Vienna and Dean of the associated medical school, possessed all the anatomic illustrations portraying the murder victims of the Nazi terror regime. In 1998, an investigation reluctantly conducted by the University after the repeated requests of Jewish organizations and the Israeli government reported that the Institute of Anatomy had received almost 1,400 cadavers from the Gestapo execution chamber in the Vienna Regional Court

(Landesgerichte). While the Institute's collection was destroyed by a bomb near the end of the War, the investigation did identify approximately 200 specimens from the Nazi era that were still in other University's collections.

Are the Results of Nazi Criminal Experimentation Reliable?

As we pointed out before there are many that question the accuracy and reliability of most of the Nazi medical research done in the death camps or elsewhere on unwilling victims. Brigadier General Telford Taylor, Chief Counsel for the prosecution at Nuremberg, stated unequivocally that the Nazi experiments were unscientific, "a ghostly failure as well as a hideous crime . . . Those experiments revealed nothing which civilized medicine can use." Arnold Relman, editor of the *New England Journal of Medicine*, similarly stated that the Nazi experiments were such a "gross violation of human standards that they are not to be trusted at all" and for this reason, the Journal would not publish material related to the criminal research.

Doctor Leonard Hoenig, Assistant Professor of Medicine at the University of South Florida College of Medicine, categorized the Nazi experiments as "pseudo-science" since the Nazis blurred the distinction between science and sadism. The Nazi data was not derived from scientific hypothesis and research, but rather inspired and filtered through a racial ideology of genocide. Doctor Hoenig maintained that nothing scientific could have resulted from sadism.

Nevertheless, the ethical question remains as to whether one should reject all of the results, even if some of the research could be determined to be scientifically valid and potentially helpful. There are two opposite points of view on this issue. The first is that the Nazi experiments are clearly so abhorrent in their disregard of the prisoners' pain, suffering, health and life, that by using their results a scientist would brand himself or herself an accomplice to their crimes. Whatever the benefit to the public might be, one should relegate such results to oblivion and not use them. Dr. Henry Beecher, the late Harvard Medical School Professor, analogized the use of the Nazi data to the legal inadmissibility of tainted evidence. Dr. Beecher said that even though suppression of the data would constitute a loss to science in a few specific areas, "this loss, it seems, would be less important than the far reaching moral loss to medicine if the data were to be published." An alternative point of view is that one should not forget the terrible crimes of the Nazis, but that at least the victims who died or were injured did not die in vain and their suffering might in some measure help humanity.

Perhaps an unbiased, reputable panel of scientists could critically evaluate the results of Nazi medical research and, if reliable results are found, they should be disclosed. The original experimenters should not be given personal credit for these atrocities. If there is any credit to be claimed for any useful scientific data it should go to the unwilling subjects and the names of the criminal researchers should be blotted out of memory forever. The obvious disadvantage of this philosophical approach is that any evaluation process implicitly confers some scientific validity to these monstrous acts of cruelty that have deeply debased the art and practice of medicine.

Modern Day Human Experimentation

The purpose of medicine is to relieve human suffering, heal the sick and injured, promote health, improve the quality of life, and delay the inevitable death that awaits us all. In trying to achieve those lofty goals, even physicians harboring the best intentions may cause temporary or permanent distress, pain, disease, injury and occasionally death. We call such untoward effects of healing efforts iatrogenic diseases (from the Greek words "iatros" meaning doctor and "genesis" meaning formation). Obviously ethical physicians try their best to avoid iatrogenic complications of treatment but they may be compelled to attempt dangerous surgery or infuse a potentially toxic medication if the risk-to-benefit ratio is substantially in favor of the patient.

Any experimental or investigational treatment is more likely to cause iatrogenic injuries than standard therapy because it treads into unknown territory. In contrast to risky, heroic measures designed to save a given patient's live, experimental treatment regimens are not necessarily designed to benefit the test subject. If they were, why would have of the patients be given a placebo and the remainder be given the potential cure? Rather, the experiment is conducted to determine the efficacy of treatment for many potential future patients – a good response in the patient receiving the drug is a welcome bonus. Rather than enrolling volunteers into programs most accurately deemed "human experiments" researchers have euphemistically christened medical experimentation on humans as "clinical trials." Many modern, voluntary clinical trials, though described as "your only chance" or "the right thing to do," are inherently dangerous and are, ultimately, human experimentation. This does not mean that we disapprove of these studies – they are the cornerstone of medical progress. Criteria for ethical and scientifically valid human experimentation have been established to minimize the risks to participants. Studies must be approved by a hospital's IRB (Institutional Review Board) prior to enrolling any patients. International policy also dictates that medical experimentation on humans must be truly voluntary and adhere to strict guidelines. Informed consent is the key to compliance with these rules.

Nazi doctors committed the most egregious violations of the basic principles of ethical medical experimentation during the Second World War. Their research crossed the line between science and sadism again and again. On a smaller scale, more surreptitious but equally lethal experiments are still going on today throughout the world. Moreover, you may own stock in some of the perpetrating companies.

Chapter 9
Made in Japan: Unethical Experiments

Heresies are experiments in man's unsatisfied search for truth.

– H.G. Wells

Before and during the Second World War, from 1935 to 1945, Japanese physicians engaged in criminal medical experimentation on thousands of human beings. These doctors dedicated themselves to the development of biological weapons at the direction of and with the full support of the Japanese Government. Their activities were little different from the medical atrocities committed by the Nazi physicians. The involuntary subjects of experiments were mainly Chinese soldiers and civilians but also included members of other nationalities including Koreans, Burmese, Russians, Mongolians, and Americans.

The Japanese WMD Program

The Japanese Government became interested in the possibilities of biological warfare at the conclusion of World War I in 1918, when the medical bureau of the Japanese army assigned Major Terunobu Hasebe to head a research team to explore the potential of microbial weapons. Dr. Ito, who directed a team of 40 scientists, soon succeeded Hasebe. However, the real beginning of Japan's biological warfare came only when Ishii Shiro entered the scene.

Dr. Shiro Ishii (1892–1959), a medical graduate of Kyoto Imperial University, was the central figure in the planning and execution of criminal biological experimentation on prisoners and in directing the use of biological weapons of mass destruction in attacks against China. He had a reputation of being brilliant but arrogant, rude towards his peers and obsequious towards his superiors. Upon graduation from medical school, he promptly joined the Japanese Imperial Army and after 3 years of postgraduate studies, he earned a PhD degree with expertise in the fields of bacteriology, immunology and preventive medicine. Beginning in 1928, Ishii took a 2-year tour of the West as a military attaché. In his travels, he did extensive research on the effects of biological and chemical warfare from World War I. It was a highly successful mission and it helped win him the patronage of Sadao Araki,

J.A. Perper and S.J. Cina, *When Doctors Kill: Who, Why, and How*,
DOI 10.1007/978-1-4419-1369-2_9, © Springer Science+Business Media, LLC 2010

Minister of the Army. Upon his return, he was appointed professor of immunology at the Tokyo Army Medical School and was given the rank of major. While there, Ishii quickly made a name for himself by inventing an effective water purification filter that he demonstrated before the Emperor. On a less noble front, Ishii urged the military to develop biological weapons to be used against the Chinese.

By the end of August 1932, Ishii led a group of ten scientists from the Army's Medical College on a tour of the Chinese territory of Manchuria, which had been invaded by the Japanese a year earlier. The Japanese Army gave him control of three biological research centers, including one in the city of Harbin in Manchuria. The preliminary experiments in biological warfare began as a secret project for the Japanese military with Ishii placed in command of the Army Epidemic Prevention Research Laboratory, at the Zhong Ma Prison Camp in Beiyinhe, a village south of Harbin. Ishii organized a covert research group, "Togo Unit," to conduct chemical and biological weapons research. In 1935, a jailbreak and an explosion (believed to be an attack) forced Ishii to shut down this facility. He moved to Pingfang, approximately 24 km south of Harbin, to set up a new and much larger facility. A year later, Ishii built a huge compound for "Unit 731" that included more than 150 buildings over 6 km². The research was top-secret; the official story was that the unit was engaged in water-purification work. A special project code, "Maruta," was used for experiments performed on human beings. Test subjects were gathered from the surrounding population and were sometimes referred to euphemistically as "logs" (maruta). This term originated as a 'joke' on the part of the staff because the official cover story for the facility provided to the local authorities was that it was a lumber mill. The tests were done in large underground rooms beneath a huge isolated building with subjects including male and female adults, infants, children, the elderly, and pregnant women.

Many experiments and vivisections (autopsies on living people) were performed without the use of anesthetics because it was believed that it might affect the results of the experimentation. The Commander of the Kuantung Army in Manchuria, Major General Hideki Tojo, supplied unit 731 with plenty of live experimental victims. He was a staunch supporter of Ishii and of biological warfare and he later became Japan's Prime Minister. The unfortunate victims were infected with different contagious diseases and were killed at different time intervals following infection in order to study the various stages of plague, cholera, tuberculosis, and other serious illnesses.

Although the Geneva Convention of 1925 had banned both chemical and biological warfare, Japan had refused to sign the treaty and had deployed poison gas bombs at the beginning of the Second Sino-Japanese war in August 1937. Shiro Ishii was instrumental in the planning, manufacturing and testing of these weapons on humans. In 1940, Ishii was appointed Chief of the Biological Warfare Section of the Kwangtung Army, holding the post simultaneously with that of the Bacteriological Department of the Army Medical Academy. From 1940 to the end of the Second World War in 1946, Ishii directed his specialized units to engage in biological warfare by attacking the Chinese Ningpo, Chinhua, and Chechiang provinces.

In October 1941, Prime Minister Tojo personally presented an award to Ishii for his contributions to developing biological weapons and had his picture taken with him which appeared in major newspapers. Early in November 1941, Unit 731 dispatched an airplane to spread bubonic plague at Changte, Hunan, an event verified by Dr. E. J. Bannon of the American Presbyterian Church hospital at Changte. Chinese authorities had long known that Japan had used biological warfare against them and had repeatedly appealed to the international community for help to no avail. In 1942, Ishii began field tests of germ warfare agents and used various methods of dispersion (i.e. firearms, bombs etc.) first on Chinese prisoners of war and then operationally on battlefields and against civilians in Chinese cities.

Some historians estimate that tens of thousands died as a result of exposure to these bioweapons which included bubonic plague, cholera, anthrax and other biological agents. His unit also conducted physiological experiments on human subjects, including vivisections, forced abortions, and simulated strokes and heart attacks. Decades later, in 1986, surviving American P.O.W.s testified before a U.S. House of Representatives' subcommittee that captured Americans, along with several hundred British and Australian soldiers, were met in Mukden on November 11, 1942 by a team of Japanese medical personnel wearing masks. They sprayed liquid into the prisoners' faces and gave them injections. One prisoner reported that after release from confinement he experienced episodes of unexplained high fever until a blood culture confirmed a diagnosis of the typhoid. Other cruel experiments included inserting glass rods to their rectum.

At Unit 731 alone, the central experimentation center, at least 3,000 people were tortured and murdered during such experiments. Similar experiments were carried out at the four regional branches of Unit 731, at the Manchuria Medical School and in military hospitals. All of these sites were under the direction of the highly decorated Lt. General Shiro Ishii. Shamelessly, Ishii produced scientific papers describing the results of his criminal experiments on prisoners. Circulated throughout the Japanese medical and scientific community, the experimental "logs" were referred to as "monkeys" in the publications. Despite this concealing strategy, it was well known that humans were the real experimental subjects. In all, Ishii personally patented over 200 discoveries, benefiting financially from his "medical" research. From 1942 to 1945, Ishii was Chief of the Medical Section of the Japanese First Army. In 1945, in the final days of the Pacific War and in the face of imminent defeat, Japanese troops blew up the headquarters of Unit 731 in order to destroy evidence of the research done there. As part of the cover-up, Ishii ordered 150 remaining subjects killed. In all, between 3,000 and 10,000 "maruta" were murdered.

Before making their escape immediately prior to the Japanese surrender, Unit 731 set free many thousands of infected rats that caused widespread plague in 22 counties of the Heilungchiang and Kirin provinces that took more than 20,000 Chinese lives. Ishii faked his own death in late 1945 and went into hiding. When American occupation forces learned that Ishii was still alive, they ordered the Japanese to hand him over, which they did. Investigators from Camp Detrick, the center for the study of biological weapons in the United States, questioned Ishii thoroughly. At first, Ishii denied performing any human testing but, aware that he may be handled over to the Soviets who were also very interested in "talking" to him, he relented. Ishii agreed to reveal all the details of his bio-warfare weapons program in exchange for immunity from war crimes prosecution. Anxious to learn the results of experiments that they themselves had been unable to perform, the American military accepted Ishii's offer. Ishii and his team were granted immunity from prosecution before the Tokyo Tribunal of War Crimes by General McArthur in 1946. This agreement was kept secret from the American people until 1993, when U.S. Defense Secretary William Perry, under pressure, promised to declassify the records of the WWII experiments.

The Japanese officers and scientists who worked in the Manchurian labs during World War II re-entered civilian life unscathed. The military officers retired on respectable pensions and the civilian scientists continued their work with large chemical and medical companies in Japan. Some of them became presidents and professors at leading universities, others became prominent industrial leaders. Ishii was never prosecuted for any war crimes and the Army allowed him to keep his lieutenant general pension. Although publicly shunned because of his infamous bio-warfare reputation he continued to be visited at his home by many of his military and scientists friends. He died of throat cancer at the age of 67 in Tokyo.

It is interesting to note that in 1985 a former U.S. Army officer, Dr. Murray Sanders, claimed he persuaded General MacArthur to approve the immunity deal with members of Unit 731. Sanders was a microbiologist who served as an advisor on biowarfare at Fort Detrick and had taught at the College of Physicians and Surgeons of Columbia University before joining the Army. 'I feel terrible about it," the 75-year-old Sanders told reporters shortly before his death. He said he did not know at the time that the Japanese had experimented on humans. "If we had known they used human guinea pigs, I doubt we would have given immunity," he said. The released medical documentation from that period, however, seems to clearly indicate that the American authorities were aware of the extent of medical experimentation on humans.

The State War Navy Coordinating Committee (SWNCC), responsible for coordinating and overseeing the war crimes trials in Japan, supported the intelligence community's stance in this matter and stated, "Data already obtained from Ishii and his colleagues has proven to be of great value in confirming, supplementing and complementing several phases of U.S. research in BW, and may suggest new fields for future research. This Japanese information is the only known source of data from scientifically controlled experiments showing direct effect of BW [bacteriological warfare] agents on man. In the past, it has been necessary to evaluate effects of BW agents on man from data through animal experimentation. Such evaluation is inconclusive and far less complete than results obtained from certain types of human experimentation...It is felt that the use of this information as a basis for war crimes evidence would be a grave detriment to Japanese cooperation with the United States occupation forces in Japan. For all practical purposes, an agreement with Ishii and his associates that information given by them on the Japanese BW program will be retained in intelligence channels is equivalent to an agreement that this Government will not prosecute any of those involved in BW activities in which war crimes were committed. Such an understanding would be of great value to the security of the American people because of the information which Ishii and his associates have already furnished and will continue to furnish." The rather icy conclusion stated "The value to the U.S. of

Japanese BW data is of such importance to national security as to far outweigh the value accruing from `war crimes' prosecution. In the interests of national security, it would not be advisable to make this information available to other nations, as would be the case in the event of a `war crimes' trial of Japanese BW experts. The BW information obtained from Japanese sources should be retained in intelligence channels and should not be employed as `war crimes' evidence." One must wonder how many of these people eventually worked for the CIA.

Basic Japanese Medical Experiments

Mahasira Morioka, a Japanese ethicist and professor of philosophy, categorized the criminal experiments performed by Japanese doctors into four major groups:

1. Training inexperienced military surgeons on Chinese prisoners
2. Studies of chemical and biological weapons such as plague, typhoid and cholera, on Chinese villages and towns
3. Studies of new treatments on deliberately injured subjects, and
4. Studies on the tolerance of the human body to extremely adverse environmental conditions

Japanese Army doctors in training performed surgery without anesthesia on living and conscious prisoners. These procedures were justified by the need to mimic more accurately battle conditions where it may not be possible to anesthetize patients prior to emergency surgery. Insensitive to the pain and cries of their victims, the trainees performed various medical procedures including tracheostomies, internal organ surgery, amputations of healthy arms and legs, re-attachments of amputated limbs to the opposite sides of the body (it is not clear how this would be a wartime advantage), and repair of deliberately inflicted gunshot wounds. At the end of the procedures, the experimental subjects were all killed.

Nicholas D. Kristoff, a *New York Times* newspaperman who penned an article entitled "Unmasking horror – A special report: Japan confronting gruesome war atrocity" soberly described his interview with a Japanese medical professional that had assisted in the horrific medical experimentation. The interviewee is described as "a cheerful old farmer who jokes as he serves rice cakes made by his wife, and then he switches easily to explaining what it is like to cut open a 30-year-old man who is tied naked to a bed and dissect him alive, without anesthetic." The article continued: "The fellow knew that it was over for him, and so he didn't struggle when they led him into the room and tied him down," recalled the 72-year-old farmer, then a medical assistant in a Japanese Army unit in China in World War II. "But when I picked up the scalpel, that's when he began screaming. I cut him open from the chest to the stomach, he screamed terribly, and his face was all twisted in agony. He made this unimaginable sound, he was screaming so horribly. Then finally, he stopped. This was all in a day's work for the surgeons, but it really left an impression on me because it was my first time." At the end of the story, the old man, who insisted on anonymity, explained the reason for the vivisection. The Chinese prisoner had been deliberately infected with the plague as part of a research project and the researchers decided to cut him open to see what the disease does to a man's inside. No anesthetic was used, he said, out of concern that it might have an effect on the results. The activities of Dr. Ishii and Unit 731 have been described in detail. Other prisoners were exposed to chemical warfare agents such as mustard gas, hydrogen cyanide, acetone cyanide and potassium cyanide. Hydrogen cyanide was given extensive study because of its potential for ease of delivery into water supply. In some instances, live and conscious experimental victims were surgically opened to observe the changes caused by the chemicals.

Many prisoners were killed during clinical trials of experimental treatments including poorly developed vaccines. Other cruel experiments seemed more designed to satisfy curiosity than to advance science. One of the arguably more practical experiments involved transfusion of horse blood to prisoners to determine its suitability for administration to wounded Japanese soldiers when human blood was in short supply. Although it may have seemed a good idea at the time, we now know that the immune response to this foreign blood would result in rapid, painful death. The ubiquitous Unit 731 performed air decompression experiments similar to those used by the Nazi concentration camp doctors. In these studies, experimental subjects were killed by lowering the air pressure in the sealed chambers causing their blood to boil. Some Japanese doctors studied the effects of injecting large syringes full of air into their patient's bloodstream in order to induce air emboli, a condition encountered during rapid decompression. Dr. Hisato Yoshimura studied the effects of intense cold and attempted to treat intentionally inflicted severe frostbite of the arms and legs by warming them with hot water. Observations of the physiological changes occurring in prisoners exposed to freezing outdoor temperatures were also documented. Additional unethical experiments involved choking people who had been suspended upside down, injecting horse urine into the kidneys, starvation and water deprivation, electrocuting subjects to determine the maximal strength of an electrical current that humans can stand, bleeding prisoners to determine the amount of blood loss likely to kill, placing prisoners in centrifuges and spinning them to death, placing glass rods in their rectums, exposing subjects to lethal doses of radiation, and injecting sea water into the blood. It wasn't always good science – it was always lethal.

Human Target Practice and Other Atrocities

While physicians and scientists conducted many experiments independently, others were undertaken by the military with assistance from doctors. In some studies, restrained prisoners were used to test the range and destructive power of grenades positioned at various distances from their bodies. In other cases, flame throwers were discharged at living humans to document the extent of injury and survival time. Other volunteers were tied to stakes and used as targets for chemical and biological weapons as well as explosives. Autopsies were performed on prisoners who had been used as target practice to determine the extent of injuries imparted by a variety of weapons and ammunition at various ranges of fire.

Why Did They Do It?

Why did Japanese doctors become murderers during World War II? Was it possible to stop the experimental massacre, limit it or avoid participation? It would seem that in wartime, funding and equipment for research at the major universities was limited. Cooperation with the likes of Dr. Ishii could ensure an institution of a stream of experimental data and the supplies they would need to conduct their own research. In return for the assistance of the military, the professors promised to send Ishii their best disciples to staff his death factories. In addition to this mutually advantageous professional relationship, several other factors likely encouraged the participation of Japanese physicians in unethical experimentation:

1. There was a widely held belief that in wartime everything was justified for the purpose of winning the war. Japanese people believed anything was excusable if it was done for the sake of the country and "Tenno Heika" (the emperor)
2. A deep and widespread prejudice was harbored by the Japanese against the Chinese, and foreigners in general
3. The Japanese had a utilitarian approach of not wanting "to waste" suspected spies or other enemies who would be executed anyway. They would make ideal "guinea pigs"
4. The philosophy of the leadership and sense of mission inculcated in the participants led to a collective loss of compassion and humanity toward the victims
5. Traditional Confucianism includes a high respect for authority including boundless submission to the Emperor. If the government said this behavior was acceptable, an obedient citizen was bound to follow suit
6. The belief that honor in serving the Emperor was much more important than a person's life and their personal morality, and
7. Human subjects could be treated worse than animals with no penalties. The participation of these unwilling volunteers allowed for studies which could rapidly advance the practice of Japanese medicine. For the aggressive, creative thinker, human experimentation could facilitate a fast track within academia.

There were other factors in play during World War II in Japan. Japanese citizens were taught that cooperation with the military should not be questioned. Conscientious objectors or critics of the government or its policies were labeled as "Hikokumin" (traitors). Therefore, virtually all the physicians recruited during the War accepted their fate without resistance, even when they knew they would be assigned to do unethical acts or outright atrocities. The hierarchical structure of Japanese medical schools also played a role in assuring the Japanese military of a steady stream of talented, young scientists. Traditionally, in Japanese medical schools the head professors exercised supreme power over their staff. Usually, there was only one professor in each "Ikyoku" (department). Even after earning a doctoral degree, lower-level researchers devoted themselves totally to the Ikyoku and to its head professor hoping to be nominated as a successor in the future. Rejection of a professor's order, including an assignment to a remote medical facility, would unfailingly result in excommunication from the Ikyoku, in effect compelling the "Hikokumin" to abandon his academic career. Another draw to Ishii's factories was the luxury of his well-funded facilities. For example, the annual budget of Unit 731 was 10 million yen (about 9 billion yen in modern currency). Half of this budget was for research, and the other half was for labor costs for about 3,000 employees. The salaries were quite high compared to the academic institutions in this war-torn country and the living conditions were very good for the scientists and physicians performing the experiments.

After the War, the Japanese medical and scientific community shied away from human experimentation of any type for several years. Over the past several decades, international ethical standards applying to human experimentation have been strictly followed (probably more closely than in the United States). Professor Thakashi Tsuchiya from the Faculty of Literature and Human Sciences at Osaka City University stated that in mainstream Japan "Jintai-Jikken" (human experimentation) is often regarded as a very deviant practice performed only by evil doctors. Consequently, "Jintai Jikken" has become a taboo utterance in the Japanese medical establishment since the end of the War. Experimentation on humans should be taboo in all languages.

Chapter 10
Good Old Fashioned American Ingenuity—and Evil

*Never perform an experiment which might be harmful
to the patient even though is highly advantageous
to science or the health of others.*

– French physiologist Claude Bernard

Both before and after the Second World War a significant number of American physicians have conducted unethical experiments on vulnerable humans resulting in serious injuries and deaths. Both the American public and the government in later years unequivocally condemned these experiments. While these studies never reached the level or magnitude of depravity manifested by the Nazis and Japanese during World War II, they nevertheless deeply marred the image of American medicine. Unethical medical experiments continued in civilian and military research establishments unabated for 35 years after World War II and more sporadically into the early 2000s. This was in spite of the 1945 Nuremberg Code and American legislation that forbid unethical and involuntary medical experimentation. The subjects of the unethical experimentations were mostly minorities, the poor and the disadvantaged as well as veterans and "captive populations" including members of the military, prison inmates and institutionalized patients, both adults and children.

In 1995, Justice Edward Greenfield of the New York State Supreme Court ruled that parents do not have the right to volunteer their mentally incapacitated children for non-therapeutic medical research studies and that no mentally incapacitated person whatsoever can be used in a medical experiment without informed consent. In *Higgins and Grimes v. Kennedy Krieger Institute* The Maryland Court of Appeals made a landmark decision regarding the use of children as test subjects, prohibiting non-therapeutic experimentation on children on the basis of "best interest of the individual child." In 1998 Professor Adil E. Shamoo of the University of Maryland and the organization Citizens for Responsible Care and Research testified to the U.S. Senate's Committee on Governmental Affairs and to the U.S. House of Representatives' House Committee on Veterans' Affairs that: "This type of research is ongoing nationwide in medical centers and VA hospitals supported by tens of millions of dollars of tax payers money. These experiments are high risk and are abusive, causing not only physical and psychic harm to the most vulnerable groups but also degrading our society's system of basic human values. Probably tens of

J.A. Perper and S.J. Cina, *When Doctors Kill: Who, Why, and How*,
DOI 10.1007/978-1-4419-1369-2_10, © Springer Science+Business Media, LLC 2010

thousands of patients are being subjected to such experiments." Clearly, if these incidents occurred as recently as a decade ago, this is a persistent problem.

The number and type of unethical medical experimentation carried out by American physicians over the past 150 years, is rather stunning. The following examples of unethical medical research, although not totally inclusive, are representative of the various studies performed by our own physicians and scientists.

Experiments in the Old South

Between 1845 and 1849 Dr. James Marion Sims, a South Carolinian from Lancaster County, was one of the first American physicians documented to have performed numerous unethical and virtually criminal medical experiments. He was not condemned or prosecuted at the time because his victims were black slaves, which were considered property rather than humans with rights. His imposing bronze bust statue stands today in a peaceful shady corner on the statehouse grounds in Columbia, South Carolina bearing three highly praising epitaphs. One is a quote from Hippocrates, "Where the love of man is, there is also the love of art." On the panel to the right, the inscription notes "He founded the science of gynecology, was honored in all lands and died with the benediction of mankind." Etched on a left panel, an inscription proclaims "The first surgeon of the ages in ministry to women, treating alike empress and slave." Well not exactly. When he treated Princess Eugenie of France during a trip to Europe, she received a higher level of care than did the slaves.

Dr. Sims, an 1835 graduate of Jefferson Medical College in Philadelphia, was interested in the possible surgical treatment of women with vesicovaginal fistula, an abnormal communication between the urinary bladder and the vagina that results in continuous involuntary discharge of urine into the vagina. Black slave women often contracted it after traumatic, unattended labor, which reduced considerably their selling value as producers of further slaves. In Montgomery, Alabama Sims initially "treated" three Alabama slave women (Anarcha, Betsy, and Lucy) with over 30 operations each. The surgery was performed without the use of ether anesthesia that had recently become available, because Sims believed that unlike sensitive white females, black ones could easily handle a little pain. After additional experiments resulted in the death of several more slaves as a result of post-surgical infections, Sims finally perfected his technique and operated on white women with fistulas (using anesthesia, of course).

Another of Dr. Sims's experiments was prompted by his belief that the movement of the skull bones during protracted births caused "lockjaw" in infants, an inability to open the mouth fully due to spasm of the jaw muscles. Today this is known as being an early symptom of neonatal tetanus, an infection occurring in newborns following septic deliveries. Slaves were particularly at risk for infections associated with childbirth because their deliveries often took place under suboptimal conditions, in some instances close to manure contaminated with tetanus bacteria. Sims tried to correct this condition surgically (obviously with poor results) by using a shoemaker's awl to reposition the skull bones of babies born to enslaved mothers.

It is true that Sims discovered a number of useful gynecological procedure and tools including the first speculum for examination of the vagina, but all those were achieved on the backs of suffering black slaves. It is worthy to note that after moving to New York, Sims apparently cognizant of the repugnant nature of his medical experiments never admitted publicly that he experimented on involuntary black patients. He is the only American physician having the dubious distinction of having practiced vivisection and experimental surgical procedures on involuntary patients. His ends did not justify the means.

Experiments on Filipino Prisoners

After the successful conquest of the Philippines in 1902, the American forces found that their soldiers were exposed to a very unsanitary environment. The country was rampant with a variety of severe infections and there were very poor nutritional conditions. The medical corps found its hands full treating both our soldiers and the Filipinos. In an effort to better understand the risks facing our troops, a series of experiments were devised that led to the death of many Filipinos.

U.S. Army doctors working in the Philippines withheld proper nutrition from 29 prisoners in order to induce Beriberi, a nutritional disease due to lack of vitamin B1; four test subjects died. Later that year, Army physicians working in the Philippines infected five prisoners with plague and in 1906 Dr. Richard P. Strong, a professor of tropical medicine at Harvard, experimented with cholera on other prisoners. The most infamous of these studies was Strong's inoculation of 24 inmates with a new live cholera vaccine that had somehow become contaminated with plague organisms. Strong had conducted the inoculations "in the convalescent ward [where] he ordered all the prisoners there to form a line ... without telling them what he was going to do, nor consulting their wishes in the matter." All the men became sick and 13 died. These experiments were all the more unusual in that neither cholera nor plague was prevalent in the area at the time. An investigating committee suggested that Strong had forgotten "the respect due every human being in not having asked the consent of persons inoculated." It enjoined the Governor General to order that no one would be subjected to "experiment without prior determination of the character of that experiment by authorities ... nor without having first gained the expressed consent of the person subject to it." Nonetheless, at the conclusion of the investigation, Strong was exonerated of any wrongdoing. During the Nuremberg Trials, Nazi doctors cited this study to justify their own medical experiments.

Experiments on the Disadvantaged

Our government continued its work for the betterment of humanity in other countries as well. In 1900, the famous Dr. Walter Reed injected 22 Spanish immigrant workers in Cuba with the agent for Yellow Fever, paying them $100 dollars in gold if they did not contract the disease and $200 if they contracted it. Between 1932 and 1972, the U.S. Public Health Service in Tuskegee, Alabama carried out a clinical study entitled "The Tuskegee Study of Untreated Syphilis in the Negro Male" later known as the Tuskegee Syphilis study. The study had selected 399 infected subjects (plus 201 patients without syphilis to serve as a control group) who were poor and mostly illiterate, black sharecroppers after screening more than 4,000 of them for the disease. In exchange for being in the study, the participants were provided free medical treatment, rides to the clinic, meals, and burial insurance in case of death. Initially, the intention of the study was to study the prevalence of the disease, its natural history, and the effectiveness of available treatments. When the study started, the fatal outcome of syphilitic infections was well known but standard treatments for the disease (including Salvarsan, mercury ointment and bismuth) were toxic, dangerous, and of questionable effectiveness. Part of the original goal of the study was to determine if patients were better off if not treated with these toxic remedies. Some of the infected men would be treated for the disease and others would serve as a control group. If one of the treatments was proven to be effective, it would become the standard of care for this killer disease.

Unfortunately for the men in Tuskegee, the 1929 Stock Market Crash resulted in loss of funding for the treatment component of the study which then changed into an observation of the effects of untreated syphilis. This study became infamous because the uneducated sharecroppers enrolled in the program had never given informed consent. Further, they were not informed of their diagnosis or told they had a sexually transmitted disease. Instead, the United States Public Health Service informed the men that vitamins, tonics, and aspirins would help cure their "bad blood" and that these treatments would be provided free in the study. Over the first years of the project, a few men received sporadic treatment with arsenicals and bismuth but they were never told when treatment was discontinued. In some instances, they were openly lied to and informed that they had been treated when in fact they had received placebo tablets. Occasionally, uncomfortable diagnostic procedures were misrepresented to them as actual treatments. For example, midway through the study, 400 subjects were sent a letter entitled "Last chance for a free treatment" which told them that a spinal tap could help cure their symptoms.

By 1947 penicillin had become the standard treatment for syphilis but rather than starting to treat all of the study subjects with this drug the Tuskegee scientists withheld the drug and continued to study how the disease spread and killed. The subjects were also prevented from receiving syphilis treatments that were available to other people in the area by notifying hospitals and the military not to provide participants with penicillin. During World War II, 250 of the men registered for the draft and were consequently diagnosed and ordered to obtain treatment for syphilis; however, the Public Health Service blocked this directive and stated: "So far, we are keeping the known positive patients from getting treatment." The study continued until 1972, when leaks to the *Washington Star* and *New York Times* resulted in public turmoil, congressional hearings and the appointment of an ad hoc advisory panel which determined the study was medically unjustified and ordered its termination. The Public Health Service remained unrepentant claiming the men had been "volunteers" and "were always happy to see the doctors." An Alabama State Health officer dismissed the criticisms as insignificant stating that "somebody is trying to make a mountain out of a molehill." Dr. John R. Heller who had led the study program in later years, including the period coincident with the routine successful treatment of syphilis with penicillin, stated "The men's status did not warrant ethical debate. They were subjects, not patients; clinical material, not sick people." By the end of the study, only 74 of the test subjects were still alive. Twenty-eight of the men had died directly of syphilis, 100 were dead of related complications, 40 of their wives had been infected, and 19 of their children had been born with congenital syphilis. The victims' families were never told that they could have been treated. As part of a settlement of a class action lawsuit subsequently filed by the NAACP, the surviving participants and family members who had been infected as a consequence of the study were awarded 9 million dollars in damages as well as free medical treatment.

The Tuskegee Syphilis Study led to the establishment of the National Human Investigation Board, and the establishment of Institutional Review Boards in 1979. On May 16, 1997, President William J. Clinton called the Tuskegee survivors and descendants to the White House for a formal apology for the United States' role in the study. Ernest Hendon, who was to become the last survivor, was watching from his home in Tuskegee, as President Clinton said: "The United States government did something that was wrong – deeply, profoundly, morally wrong. It was an outrage to our commitment to integrity and equality for all our citizens … and I am sorry" He added unequivocally: "What was done cannot be undone, but we can end the silence … We can stop turning our heads away. We can look at you in the eye, and finally say, on behalf of the American people, what the United States government did was shameful and I am sorry."

Paying a Debt to Society

When a person is sent to prison for rehabilitation, the intent is not to give them a disease to rehabilitate from. Nonetheless, over the past century American physicians have found prison inmates to be handy subjects for a variety of experiments. In 1915, Dr. Joseph Goldberger, induced pellagra, a niacin deficiency that damages the skin and the central nervous system, in 12 Mississippi inmates in an attempt to find a cure for the disease. One test subject later said that he had been through "a thousand hells." In 1935, the director of the U.S Public Health Office admitted that officials had known for some time that pellagra was caused by niacin deficiency but did nothing about it apparently because most victims were poor African-Americans. During the Nuremberg Trials, Nazi doctors used this study along with Dr. Strong's trials in the Phillipines to try validate their experiments on concentration camp inmates. While the Nazis do have a point, the subjects in the Mississippi study were truly volunteers who were eventually treated in an attempt to restore their health. In the Nazi experiments, there was usually no health left to restore.

Between 1919 and 1922 researchers performed testicular transplant experiments on 500 inmates at San Quentin State Prison in California, inserting the testicles of recently executed inmates and goats into the abdomens and scrotums of living prisoners. This of course begs the question "why?" In 1942, U.S. Army and Navy doctors infected 400 prison inmates in Chicago with malaria to study the disease and hopefully develop a treatment for it. The prisoners were told that they were helping the war effort not that they are going to be intentionally infected with a potentially fatal disease. Three years later another 800 prisoners were inoculated with the same pathogen. In 1942, Harvard biochemist Edward Cohn injected 64 Massachusetts prisoners with cow blood in a Navy-sponsored experiment. The rejection of this foreign material by the victims was catastrophic. In 1944, Dr. Captain A. W. Frisch, a well-known microbiologist, performed experiments on four volunteer inmates from the state prison at Dearborn, Michigan inoculating them with hepatitis-infected specimens obtained in Northern Africa. One prisoner died; two others developed hepatitis but lived, and the fourth developed severe symptoms but did not actually contract the disease. In a follow-up study in the 1950s Dr. Joseph Strokes of the University of Pennsylvania infected 200 female prisoners with viral hepatitis to study the disease. The list goes on and on.

In 1952, at the famous Sloan-Kettering Institute, Dr. Chester M. Southam injected live cancer cells into prisoners at the Ohio State Prison to study the progression of the disease. Half of the prisoners in this National Institutes of Health-sponsored (NIH) study were black, igniting racial suspicions stemming from the Tuskegee incident which was also an NIH-sponsored study.

In 1956, Dr. Albert Sabin tested an experimental polio vaccine on 133 prisoners in Ohio. This was prior to his receiving the Nobel Prize for his efforts. In 1963, researchers at the University of Washington directly irradiated the testes of 232 prison inmates in order to determine radiation's effects on testicular function. When these inmates later left prison and had children, at least four fathered babies with birth defects. The exact number is unknown because researchers did little follow-up on the men to see the long-term effects of their experiment. In 1967, researchers injected 64 prison inmates in California with a neuromuscular compound called succinylcholine, a chemical which paralyzes the diaphragm leaving a person suffocating. When five prisoners refused to participate in the experiment, the prison's special treatment board gave researchers permission to inject them with the drug against their will.

Between 1964 and 1968, the U.S. Army paid $386,486 to University of Pennsylvania Professors Albert Kligman and Herbert W. Copelan to run medical experiments on 320 inmates of Holmesburg Prison to determine the effects of seven mind-altering drugs. The researchers' objective was to determine the minimum effective dose of each drug needed to disable 50% of any given population. Though Drs. Kligman and Copelan claimed that they were unaware of any long-term effects the mind-altering agents might have on prisoners, documents released later proved otherwise. The same Dr. Albert Kligman conducted skin product experiments on hundreds of inmates at the same prison. "All I saw before me," he said about his first visit to the prison, "were acres of skin." Between 1964 and 1967, the Dow

Chemical Company paid Dr. Kligman $10,000 to learn how dioxin – a highly toxic, carcinogenic component of Agent Orange – and other herbicides affected human skin. Workers at the Dow chemical plants were developing an acne-like condition called chloracne and the company wanted to know whether the chemicals they were handling were to blame. As part of the study, Kligman applied dioxin to the skin of 60 prisoners but was disappointed when the prisoners showed no skin lesions. A follow-up study involved 70 volunteers at the same prison. Without the company's knowledge or consent, Kligman increased the dosage of dioxin he applied to ten prisoners' skin to 7,500 mg, 468 times the dosage Dow official Gerald K. Rowe had authorized him to administer. As a result, the prisoners developed acne-like lesions that progressed into purulent boils. These skin lesions were not treated and remained for up to 7 months. None of the subjects were informed that they would later be studied for the development of cancer at these sites. Based on his vast experience, the U.S. Army paid Dr. Kligman to apply skin-blistering chemicals to the faces and backs of the inmates to "learn how the skin protects itself against chronic assault from toxic chemicals, the so-called hardening process." The bottom line is that death row at Holmesburg Prison may have been safer than Kligman's clinic in the 1960s.

Taking Advantage of the Weak and Innocent

America has not gone as far as the Nazis by recommending the extermination of the weak and infirm. Instead, they became unwitting subjects for a series of experiments that sound worse than euthanasia. In 1943 in order to "study the effect of frigid temperature on mental disorders," researchers at University of Cincinnati Hospital kept 16 mentally disabled patients in refrigerated cabinets for 120 hours at 30°F. It should be intuitive that hypothermia affects both geniuses and the alternatively gifted. Between 1956 and 1972, Dr. Saul Krugman of New York University, conducted a study funded by The Armed Forces Epidemiological Board which attempted to induce hepatitis into mentally disabled children at Willowbrook School on Staten Island by injecting serum into their veins or by feeding them an extract distilled from the feces of infected patients. Krugman had the parents sign an informed consent document which fraudulently suggested the children would be receiving a vaccine to prevent hepatitis without disclosing that they would need to be infected intentionally beforehand. In 1972, Krugman became President of the American Pediatric Society.

In 1963 Dr. Chester M. Southam, who had injected Ohio State Prison inmates with live cancer cells in 1952, performed the same procedure on 22 senile, African-American women at the Brooklyn Jewish Chronic Disease Hospital in order to watch their immunological response. Southam told the patients that they are receiving "some cells" but left out the fact that they were the seeds of cancer. He claimed he did not obtain informed consent from the patients because he did not want to frighten them by telling them what he was doing. Despite his good intentions he temporarily lost his medical license because of these experiments.

Yet he still became the President of the American Cancer Society. Clearly, innovative experimentation looks good on a resume.

In 1950, Dr. D. Ewen Cameron published an article in the *British Journal of Physical Medicine* in which he described experiments that entailed forcing schizophrenic patients at Manitoba's Brandon Mental Hospital to lie naked under 200-W red lamps for up to 8 hours per day. His other experiments included placing mental patients in an electric cage that heated their internal body temperatures to 103°F. His interest in physiological responses went beyond a study of hyperthermia. He also induced comas by giving patients large injections of insulin.

In our society, children hold a sacred place. They are dependent upon the care of adults and look to them for safety and security. Many parents have had to console a child when faced with a visit to a doctor. In some instances, their fear is justified. In 1941, Dr. William C. Black infected a 12 month-old baby with herpes as part of a medical experiment. At the time, the editor of the *Journal of Experimental Medicine*, Francis Payton Rous, called it "an abuse of power, an infringement of the rights of an individual and not excusable because the illness which followed had implications for science." In 1962, researchers at the Laurel Children's Center in Maryland tested experimental acne antibiotics on children and continued their tests even after half of the young test subjects develop severe liver damage because of the experimental medication. More recently, in 2002, 2 year-old Michael Daddio of Delaware died of congestive heart failure. After his death, his parents learned that doctors had performed experimental surgery on him when he was 5 months old rather than using the established surgical method for repairing his congenital heart defect. The established procedure had a 90–95% success rate. The inventor of the procedure performed on baby Daddio was fired from the hospital in 2004. In the BBC documentary "Guinea Pig Kids" and the article of the same name, reporter Jamie Doran reported that children in the New York City foster care system had been unwitting human subjects in experimental AIDS drug trials starting in 1988. In response to the BBC documentary and article, the New York City Administration of Children's Services admitted in a press release that foster care children had been used in experimental drug trials, but claimed that the last trial took place in 2001 and thus the trials were not continuing. No wonder kids are scared of people in white coats with needles.

It Takes a Village

Occasionally, larger populations are needed to obtain scientific validity of experiments. When a prison or hospital contains too few subjects, the government has turned to our cities for its subjects. Most people don't know that Federal law authorizes the conduct of such experiments by the government:

> "The use of human subjects will be allowed for the testing of chemical and biological agents by the U.S. Department of Defense, accounting to Congressional committees with respect to the experiments and studies," and "The Secretary of Defense [may] conduct tests and experiments involving the use of chemical and biological [warfare] agents on civilian populations [within the United States]." (Public Law 95-79, Title VIII, Sec. 808, July 30,

1977, 91 Stat. 334. In U.S. Statutes-at-Large, Vol. 91, page 334; Public Law 95-79. Public Law 97-375, title II, Sec. 203(a)(1), Dec. 21, 1982, 96 Stat. 1882. In U.S. Statutes-at-Large, Vol. 96, page 1882).

Here are a few examples of the application of this law.

In order to determine how susceptible an American city could be to biological attack, the U.S. Navy sprayed a cloud of *Bacillus globigii* bacteria from ships over the San Francisco shoreline. According to monitoring devices situated throughout the city to test the extent of infection, 8,000 residents of San Francisco inhaled 5,000 or more bacterial particles and many contracted a pneumonia-like illness. In 1950 the Army staged another mock attack on San Francisco this time covertly spraying the city with the microbe *Serratia marscenses* and other agents thought to be harmless. At least one patient died after a flu like illness caused by this germ. The experiment, which involved blasting a bacterial fog over the entire 49-square-mile city from a Navy vessel offshore, was documented with clinical nonchalance: "It was noted that a successful BW [biological warfare] attack on this area can be launched from the sea, and that effective dosages can be produced over relatively large areas," the Army wrote in its 1951 classified report on the experiment. These experiments were made public in Senate subcommittee hearings in 1977. Obviously, earthquakes are not the only concern around the Golden Gate Bridge.

The rest of the country has not gotten off the hook. Between 1956 and 1957, U.S. Army doctors and scientists released mosquitoes infected with Yellow Fever and Dengue Fever over Savannah, Georgia and Avon Park, Florida to test the insects' ability to carry disease. After each test, Army agents posed as public health officials to track the effects of the trial. These experiments resulted in a high incidence of fevers, respiratory distress, stillbirths, encephalitis and typhoid among the residents of both cities as well as several deaths. As part of a test codenamed "Big Tom" the Department of Defense sprayed Oahu, Hawaii's most heavily populated island, with *Bacillus globigii* in order to simulate an attack. *Bacillus globigii* causes infections in people with weakened immune systems but this was not known to scientists at the time. Or they simply didn't care. In 1966, U.S. Army scientists dropped light bulbs filled with *Bacillus subtilis* through ventilation gates into the New York City subway system exposing more than one million commuters to the bacteria. The Army's justification for the experiment was the fact that there are many subways in the (former) Soviet Union, Europe, and South America and we need to consider all possibilities in the event of war. There is no record of any fatalities associated with this military science project but the details of the experiment are still classified. At least there is no way this kind of thing could happen today. Yeah, right.

Willing to Die for Your Country?

The government essentially owns the bodies of its military personnel. As such, they are vulnerable to experimentation if it will best serve the interests of our country. Ironically, some of the worst tests performed on our own soldiers were designed to test the effects of poisons on our soldiers before our enemies had the chance to do so.

In response to the Germans' use of chemical weapons during World War I President Woodrow Wilson created the Chemical Warfare Service (CWS) as a branch of the U.S. Army. Twenty-four years later the CWS was still performing mustard gas and lewisite experiments on over 4,000 members of the armed forces. "The Manhattan Project" gave birth to the atomic bomb and led to an interest in the effects that radioactive materials had on people. The Project's medical team led by Dr. Safford Warren injected 4.7 mg of plutonium into soldiers and several civilians at the Oak Ridge facility, 20 miles west of Knoxville. In 1977, the government issued an official apology to the families of the test subjects and paid $400,000 to Jeanne Connell, the sole survivor from these clinical trials.

Between 1954 and 1975 U.S. Air Force medical officers assigned to Fort Detrick's Chemical Corps Biological Laboratory were involved in "Operation Whitecoat" – a study exposing human test subjects to a variety of dangerous biological agents including plague. The volunteers were 2,300 Seventh Day Adventist military members who chose to become human guinea pigs rather than potentially kill others in combat. Over the 20-year period, the Army used them to test vaccines against the various biological agents to which they were exposed. Long-term follow up of about a quarter of all "White Coat" volunteers found an increased incidence of asthma and headaches but no well-documented deaths.

Some ripples of military experimentation still permeate our society and occasionally make headlines. In 1996, the Department of Defense admitted that American soldiers were exposed to chemical agents during Operation Desert Storm in 1990. More than 400,000 of these soldiers were ordered to take an experimental nerve agent antidote called pyridostigmine which some now believe to be the cause of Gulf War Syndrome. The afflicted war veterans developed a variety of symptoms including skin disorders, neurological problems, incontinence, uncontrollable drooling and vision problems. This disease is real and is not a figment of some shell-shocked veteran's imagination.

A Piece of Your Mind

No doubt you have been wondering when the CIA was going to emerge in this chapter. Wait no longer. Between 1955 and 1960, the CIA conducted a mind control and brainwashing program with the code name "MKULTRA" using psychoactive drugs such as LSD and mescaline at 80 institutions on hundreds of subjects. MKULTRA was started on the order of CIA director Allen Dulles on April 13, 1953, largely in response to alleged Soviet, Chinese, and North Korean use of mind-control techniques on U.S. prisoners of war in Korea. The CIA wanted to use similar methods on their own captives and possibly to manipulate foreign leaders with such techniques.

The project was run by the Office of Scientific Intelligence under the direction of Dr. Sydney Gottlieb, a psychiatrist and chemist. Prior to MKULTRA a number of secret U.S. governmental studies had been conducted to study mind-control, interrogation, behavior modification and related topics including Project CHATTER in 1947, and Project BLUEBIRD and Project ARTICHOKE in 1951. Because most MKULTRA records were deliberately destroyed in 1973 by order of then CIA Director Richard Helms, it is difficult if not impossible to have a complete understanding of the more than 150 individually funded research sub-projects sponsored by MKULTRA and related CIA programs. The Agency invested millions of dollars into studies probing dozens of methods of influencing and controlling the mind by chemical, biological and radiological means. Experiments included administering LSD to CIA employees, military personnel, doctors, other government agents, prostitutes, mentally ill patients, and members of the general public in order to study their reactions. LSD and other drugs were usually administered without the subject's knowledge and informed consent, a violation of the Nuremberg Code that the U.S. had agreed to follow after WWII.

In 1965, the CIA and the Department of Defense began Project MKSEARCH, a program to refine the ability to manipulate human behavior through the use of mind-altering drugs. Some of these agents were later used in government-sponsored interrogations. As this would be considered a form of torture by inducing mental and psychological hardship, this could not be used by the CIA today. But demos of the technique can be seen on "24".

On November 28, 1953, Army scientist and experimental subject Frank Olson died after falling 13 stories from the Pennsylvania Hotel in Manhattan. The CIA's internal investigation claimed that Olson had prior knowledge of the details of the experiment, although, in fact, neither Olson nor the other men taking part in the experiment were told of the exact nature of the drug until some 20 minutes after they ingested it. The investigative report suggested that the experimenter was somewhat at fault for the death and deserved a reprimand for failing to take into account suicidal tendencies Olson was known to have had. LSD and other mind-altering substances can aggravate suicidal ideation. While the government claimed Olson committed suicide, a forensic scientist determined in 1994 following an exhumation and autopsy that Olson had suffered head trauma from a blunt source prior to his death. Frank Olson's family received $750,000 by a special act of Congress and both President Ford and CIA director William Colby met with Olson's family to apologize.

In Operation "Midnight Climax" (very catchy and aptly named) the CIA set up several brothels to obtain subjects for an experiment on mind-altering drugs. The men were dosed surreptitiously with LSD and their sexual behavior under the influence of this hallucinogenic drug was filmed for later viewing and study via two-way mirrors. These films were also used to keep the participants from talking about the experiment if they found out about it. A good fiction writer could not think this stuff up.

Between 1957 and 1964, MKULTRA experiments were exported to Canada where the CIA had recruited Scottish physician Dr. Donald Ewen Cameron, creator of the "psychic driving" concept, which the CIA found particularly interesting. Psychic driving was a theory of treating insanity by erasing existing memories and rebuilding the psyche completely. It was like deleting your hard drive and reinstalling the software. After being recruited by the CIA, Cameron was paid $69,000 to conduct his work at the Allan Memorial Institute of McGill University.

The experiments were carried out primarily on thousands of unsuspecting Canadian patients and on some US citizens. Often the patients entered the Institute for minor problems such as anxiety disorders and post-partum depression and were unwittingly subjected to Cameron's experiments.

The "psychic driving" experiments consisted of putting subjects into sensory deprivation rooms or drug-induced comas for weeks (up to 3 months in one case) and electroshocking them several times a day at higher voltages than usual. This resulted in incontinence, total amnesia, loss of speech, and an erasure of memory that left the patients thinking the doctors were their parents. The "blank slate" deprogramming was followed by reprogramming in which the patients were subjected to hearing repetitive messages (both negative and positive) to direct their behavior and "reform" their minds. The CIA was obviously very interested in these "brain washing" experiments. It was during this era that Cameron became known worldwide as the first chairperson of the World Psychiatric Association as well as President of the American and Canadian Psychiatric Associations. Interestingly, Cameron had also been a member of the Nuremberg medical tribunal where he hypocritically villified Nazi medical experimentation merely a decade prior to his own unethical research. Cameron retired suddenly in 1964 and his successor organized a team to evaluate Cameron's "psychic driving" theory of treatment. The team found it worthless. Cameron died in 1967 in a tragic mountain climbing accident. The *American Journal of Psychiatry* published a long and glowing obituary with a full-page picture.

The MKULTRA projects resulted in a number of deaths but the exact number will never be known. The details of many of the experiments fall into the "I could tell you but I would have to kill you" category. Of all the hundreds of human test subjects used during MKULTRA, only 14 were ever notified of their involvement and only one receives a paltry compensation of $15,000.

Doing Your Civic Duty

Between 1962 and 1973 the U.S. Department of Defense conducted a variety of experiments with a variety of code names such as Whistle Down, Elk Hunt, Devil Hole, Sun Down, Swamp Oak, Red Cloud, Watch Dog, Dew Point, Rapid Tan, DTC Test 69-75, Tail Timber, Pine Ridge, Green Mist, and DTC Test 68-53. These catchy nicknames involved exposing civilians to some "simulated" agents as part of a control group examining the effects of live chemical and biological agents. The land-based tests were conducted in Alaska, Florida, Hawaii, Maryland, Utah, Canada, and the United Kingdom. Sea-based tests that were part of Project SHAD (Shipboard Hazard and Defense) were also conducted. The tests used both live chemical or biological agents and "simulants" (ostensibly non-harmful materials that behaved in a manner similar to real agents). Some of the substances included in this study were very toxic such as Sarin, VX, Soman, Tabun, ester of benzilic acid, and bacterial organism such as *Francisella tularensis* and *Puccinia graminis var. tritici*. The government began investigating the records of these experiments in September 2000 at the request of the Department of Veterans Affairs and acknowledged that unwitting civilians were used in the study on October 9, 2002. In a public statement William Winkenwerder, the Assistant Secretary of Defense, stated: "The purpose of these operational tests was to test equipment, procedures, military tactics, et cetera, and to learn more about biological and chemical agents. The tests were not conducted to evaluate the effects of dangerous agents on people." He added, "Things were learned at that time that would have been useful" for the offensive use of chemical or biological agents against our enemies. Further, he was "highly confident that civilians were not exposed to live chemical or pathogenic biologic agents." Nevertheless, civilians in Hawaii, Alaska, Florida, and Puerto Rico, might have been exposed to biological and chemical stimulants that were considered harmless at the time of the tests, but were later found to pose a potential health risk to people with weak immune systems. In addition to the civilian "volunteers" approximately 5,000 service members were involved in the sea-based tests and another 500 in land-based studies.

Before we become nostalgic for the good old days of government experimentation, let us understand that studies are still going on in this decade. In 2001, the U.S. Air Force and rocket maker Lockheed Martin sponsored a Loma Linda University study that paid 100 Californians $1,000 each to eat a dose of perchlorate. This is a toxic component of rocket fuel that causes cancer, damages the thyroid gland, and hinders normal development in children and fetuses. To test the effect of cumulative dosage, these Westcoasters snacked on this noxious chemical every day for 6 months. The dose eaten by the test subjects was 83 times the safe dose of perchlorate set by the State of California which has trace amounts of perchlorate in some of its drinking water. This Loma Linda study was the first large-scale study to use human subjects to test the harmful effects of a water pollutant. Though the environmentalist goals were laudable, these experiments border on unethical. Even on Californians.

Why Did American Doctors Perform Unethical Medical Experimentation?

As Mr. Spock said in *Star Trek 2: The Wrath of Khan*, "The good of the many outweighs the good of the few – or the one." This excuse has been used by many doctors accused of unethical medical experimentation or fudging on the Informed Consent paperwork. The crux of this argument centers on the fact that although a few people may be damaged or killed during a risky clinical trial or while undergoing an experimental surgical procedure, many will be saved if it works. This mentality has been a driving force behind a great deal of American and international human experimentation. This rationale is quite logical, of course, unless you are one of the "few" or the very unlucky "one".

It may well be that the way to Hell is paved with good intentions, but in the annals of American medical experimentation the good intentions were very rarely directed towards the experimental subjects. In many cases, the only potential beneficiary of the results of these tests was the U.S. military. Although some physicians truly believed that a little human suffering now could avert global tragedy later, most American doctors performing illegal or unethical experiments on people most often did so for one of the following three reasons:

1. An excessive curiosity to better understand the causes, mechanisms, and development of diseases and injuries in order to determine how they can be effectively treated. In the case of military-oriented programs the study of injury patterns and the effects of drugs can lead to more effective warfare and espionage. While it is questionable whether curiosity ever killed a cat it is certainly very true that scientific curiosity may kill any sense of humanity and make researchers see human beings as life support systems for organs, "acres of skin" or "objects" of research
2. A motivation to advance professionally and, occasionally, to get rich. We have seen examples of several prominent physicians who were involved in questionable research but rose to the pinnacle of their respective specialties, or
3. Moral blindness and a complete lack of sensitivity to the suffering of the human subjects. These physicians conveniently forgot that once these patients enrolled in an experiment under a doctor's control they were automatically covered under the umbrella of the Hippocratic Oath

How American society could produce such insensitive physicians is not easy to answer. One possibility is that American medical schools, like many other institutions throughout the world, have historically concentrated obsessively on teaching the cold, hard facts with little focus on the ethical aspects of medical care. Many schools have argued that the requisite memorization of a mountain of medical information does not leave students time for the exploration of the seemingly less important hills of the moral vista. This is a grave mistake which should be promptly corrected since a physician without a caring soul cannot be a humane provider of medical care. Only recently have allopathic ("M.D.") medical schools added medical ethics to the curriculum and given adequate consideration to the feelings and emotional needs of vulnerable human beings. In many ways, schools of osteopathic medicine ("D.O.") have been ahead of the game on this front by taking a more holistic approach to patient care.

Experimentation and the Law

Although Americans were instrumental in the drafting of the Nuremberg Code establishing the guidelines for the performance of ethical medical experimentation, the actual implementation of its provisions through federal legislation and enforcement of the law proceeded at a snail's pace. Unethical human experimentation is and has been officially and publicly condemned by our government and its leaders; however, the main offenders in this arena appear to be governmental agencies and the U.S. military. Thirty-five years after Nurenberg, Secretary of Defense Charles Wilson issue the "Wilson Memo", a top-secret document establishing the Nuremberg Code as the official Department of Defense policy on human experimentation. The Wilson memo required voluntary, written consent from a human medical research subject after he or she had been informed of "the nature, duration, and purpose of the experiment; the method and means by which it is to be conducted; all inconveniences and hazards reasonably to be expected; and effects upon his health or person which may possibly come from his participation in the experiment." If this has been the government's position for over two decades, one must ask why unethical experiments are still going today.

There have been some signs that the situation is improving. Medical experiments performed at academic institutions have to be approved by institutional review boards (IRBs). An IRB is an independent ethics committee (also known as an ethical review board) that is formally charged with approving, monitoring, and reviewing medical and behavioral research involving humans in order to protect the rights and welfare of the subjects. The composition of these Boards is specifically regulated to ensure their objectivity and fairness. Many reputable journals will not publish the results of a study without documentation that an IRB has reviewed the experiment prior to its inception. Of course, many experimenters, such as those employed by the CIA, may not care if their research is published and may see little need for IRB approval.

There have also been significant actions at all levels of government in the past few decades. In 1969, President Nixon officially ended the United States' offensive biowarfare program including the human experimentation studies at Fort Detrick. Nixon wouldn't lie about this. In 1971, the biowarfare lab was converted to the Frederick Cancer Research and Development Center, now known as the National Cancer Institute (NCI). In addition to cancer research, scientists at the NCI now study virology, immunology and retrovirology (including the HIV). The site also has become home to the U.S. Army Medical Research Institute which studies drugs, vaccines and countermeasures for biological warfare. It would seem that the old Fort Detrick could not completely free itself from its biowarfare past.

There have been other significant steps toward limiting the abuse of humans through unethical medical experimentation. In 1977, the Senate Kennedy Hearings led to a Presidential Executive Order prohibiting intelligence agencies from experimenting on humans without informed consent. The enforcement of this Order is still questionable. In 1977, the National Urban League held its National Conference on Human Experimentation. They succintly stated the shared sentiments of many scientists and physicians: "We don't want to kill science but we don't want science to kill, mangle and abuse us." In 1979, the National Commission for the Protection of Human Subjects of Biomedical and Behavioral Research released the Belmont Report. This publication mandates that researchers follow three basic principles:

1. Respect the subjects as autonomous persons and protect those with limited ability for independence (such as children)
2. Do no harm, and

3. Choose test subjects equitably and justly – being sure not to target certain groups because they are easily accessible or easily manipulated, rather than for reasons directly related to the tests

For any physician remotely familiar with the Hippocratic Oath these truths should be self-evident.

In 1980, the FDA finally prohibited the use of prison inmates in pharmaceutical drug trials leading to the advent of the experimental drug testing centers industry. Many college students have earned invaluable "beer money" by participating in these studies. However, in 2006 the New York Times reported that "An influential federal panel of medical advisers has recommended that the government loosen regulations that severely limit the testing of pharmaceuticals on prison inmates, a practice that was all but stopped three decades ago after revelations of abuse." Ethicists are firmly against such relaxation of these rules pointing out that an imprisoned population lacks the ability to give free and unfettered consent. College students would also be very upset.

In 1995, President Clinton formed the National Bioethics Advisory Committee. The role of this body is to advise the President on ethical issues that may emerge as a consequence of advances in medical science and technology. In connection with its advisory role, the mission of the Council includes the following functions:

1. To inquire into the human and moral significance of developments in medical and behavioral science and technology
2. To explore specific ethical and policy questions related to these developments
3. To provide a forum for a national discussion of bioethical issues (such as ethical issues related to fetal research, cloning, growing of organs from isolated tissues)
4. To facilitate a greater understanding of bioethical issues, and
5. To explore possibilities for useful international collaboration on bioethical issues

It is then up to the President to do something with this information. Presumably, this type of bioethical advisory input was sought by President Obama when he gave the O.K. for stem cell research.

In 1997, California prefaced the *Protection of Human Subjects in Medical Experimentation Act* by stating, "The Legislature hereby finds and declares that medical experimentation on human subjects is vital for the benefit of mankind, however such experimentation shall be undertaken with due respect to the preciousness of human life and the right of individuals to determine what is done to their own bodies." This should be simple common sense and reaffirms our inalienable rights stated so eloquently in the Constitution. This being the case, why do our own scientists and doctors violate them again and again? It may be shocking to read the chapters in this book describing Nazi and Japanese scientific atrocities in the 1940s. Perhaps the hypocrisy of American morality is even more disturbing.

Chapter 11
Physician Kill Thyself: The Story of Dr. Gwinn E. Puig

Suicide may also be regarded as an experiment – a question which man puts to Nature, trying to force her to answer.

– Arthur Schopenhauer

Humans are self-experimenters from birth. In fact, we cannot prevent ourselves from being so. Our entire life is a string of self-experiments, whether pleasurable or painful, beneficial or disastrous. As children we are fearless and simply don't appreciate danger. It is the duty of our parents to train us to recognize and avoid the hazardous situations that we invariably seek out. As adults, if we have learned our lessons, we avoid treacherous experiments that may cost us life or limb based on the experience (often tragic) of others and our own reasonable but not infallible judgment. "Not infallible" would be the key words in that sentence.

Self-Experimenting Physicians

When physicians attempt to discover the causes of disease and mechanisms of injury or devise treatments through self-experimentation, it is obvious that they are engaged in medical research (rather than masochism). There is virtually unanimous agreement that physician self-experimentation has been of great benefit to the development of medicine. Many experiments that physicians have performed on themselves were potentially fatal. A successful experiment meant a great leap forward for medicine; a failure led to a pine box. Prior to the eighteenth century medical research was based on studies of just a few people with a given condition, sometimes only one, resulting in conclusions of dubious scientific merit. In modern times, this somewhat subjective "research" has been replaced by clinical trials and retrospective analysis of large groups of people with the same disease giving rise to statistically sound data. Accordingly, self-experimentation (on a sample size of one) is generally frowned upon these days and its scientific validity may be harshly questioned.

Nevertheless, medical self-experimentation continues to occur. Some modern self-experimenters have clearly contributed to medical progress and have enjoyed universal fame. Others have paid for their achievements with their lives and many more have failed miserably despite their sacrifice and died in obscurity. There is one consistent truism regarding self-experimentation; it always seems to involve significant discomfort, risk, and/or pain to Dr. Guinea Pig, the victim of his own experiment.

Boldly Going Where No Man Has Gone Before

British physicians have a penchant for self-destructive chivalry in the name of Science. In 1767, Dr. John Hunter, a surgeon to King George III, injected venereal pus from a prostitute with gonorrhea into his penis. He then successfully treated himself with mercury and eradicated the infection. Unfortunately for him, the woman also had syphilis and Hunter died subsequently of late complication of this disease. Had he explained the experiment to his wife he likely would have died much sooner.

In 1769, Dr. William Stark, a London physician, studied the benefits of a simple vs. complex diet. He began the experiment by placing himself on a very strict diet of bread, water and meat. He was adding different food groups to the regimen in order to study the impact of the nutrients afforded by various consumables. Much to his consternation, just before adding fruits and vegetables to his diet he died of scurvy, a disease caused by lack of vitamin C, a critical vitamin found in citrus fruits and in vegetables.

In the nineteenth century, the medical establishment still believed that a woman's pain during labor was a biological necessity, a conviction perhaps also influenced by the biblical injunction punishing Eve for eating the forbidden fruit from the tree of knowledge. A young Scottish obstetrician, Dr. James Simpson, did not believe that this agony was an immutable punishment and applied himself to the idea of facilitating a painless delivery. In one of the seemingly more enjoyable self-experiments in this chapter, he sniffed a large number of substances in search of one that would dull or eliminate pain. To test the analgesic effect of each agent he pricked himself with a sharp instrument or asked a colleague to kick him in the shin. Eventually he found chloroform most suitable and in 1848 he tried it on 30 women in labor; all experienced a painless delivery. Simpson's colleagues were scandalized by his unorthodox treatment, which they believed was a danger to both mother and fetus. The criticism quickly died down after Queen Victoria allowed Simpson to use chloroform on her to deliver her eighth child, Prince Leopold (as if she needed it by then). She subsequently knighted Dr. Simpson.

In 1885, Daniel Carrion, a 26-year-old Peruvian medical student, proved that two Central American diseases believed to be distinct, were actually caused by the same bacterium. The diseases were Verruca Peruana, characterized by the development of warts, fever and joint pains and Oroya Fever, manifested by a high fever, chills, and abdominal pain that progressed to severe anemia and heart disease. In spite of strong disapproval by his professors and friends, Carrion had blood taken from a patient's wart injected into his arm. He eventually developed and died of Oroya Fever, now named Carrion's Disease in his honor.

In 1900, Dr. Jesse Lazear, an American surgeon who had extensively researched Yellow Fever, attempted unsuccessfully to infect himself with the disease through multiple stings by mosquitoes exposed to patients with Yellow Fever. Despite carefully controlled conditions, he could not contract the disease. Ironically, he died of Yellow Fever from the sting of a wild mosquito shortly thereafter.

Dr. August Bier, a German surgeon, was the pioneer of spinal anesthesia. He volunteered to be the guinea pig of an experiment in which his assistant, Dr. Hildebrandt, was supposed to inject him with cocaine into his spinal canal. Initially the assistant performed the procedure properly but he could not continue because the needle he was using was the wrong size. The roles were then inverted with Dr. Hildebrandt turning into the experimental subject. The procedure was very successful with Dr. Hildebrandt reportedly feeling nothing below the level of the injection. Dr. Bier wanted to be sure that the anesthesia was effective, so he stabbed Hidebrandt in the legs with pins, squeezed his skin with a hooked forceps, hammered his shin bone, burned his legs with a cigar, pulled his pubic hair and, for good measure, forcefully squeezed his testes. Apparently, the two had a close working relationship. After the cocaine effects wore off, in spite of lingering pain, the experimenters celebrated their achievement with plenty of booze and dinner – and perhaps some mood music.

In 1961, Dr. Victor Herbert almost died after he attempted to prove that megaloblastic anemia (an anemia associated with abnormally large red blood cells and neurological damage) was caused by a folic acid dietary deficiency. This B vitamin is found in fresh vegetables and is easily destroyed by boiling or cooking. He lived on a monotonous and tasteless diet of thrice-boiled vegetables for 5 weeks prior to developing irritability, forgetfulness, and, ultimately, megaloblastic anemia as intended. Unbeknownst to him, his diet was also deficient in potassium. He developed paralysis and cardiac abnormalities that probably would have killed him if he had not been treated by a meat-eating colleague.

Few self-experimenters have earned worldwide recognition and fame for their achievements. The stories of Dr. Werner Forssmann, the innovator of cardiac catheterization, and Dr. Barry Marshall, who discovered the infectious nature of stomach ulcers, are exceptions. For their individual efforts, they were each awarded Nobel Prize in Medicine.

In 1929 in a small town of Northeast Germany, just 30 miles away from Berlin, Dr. Werner Forssmann became intrigued by drawings he saw in a French physiology book that depicted a man standing beside a horse and inserting a catheter into its jugular vein to reach the heart. Forssman believed that a similar procedure could be performed on humans in order to inject life saving drugs during resuscitation efforts. He relayed his theory to his supervisor, Dr. Richard Schneider, and asked permission to test it on either terminal patients or on himself. Dr. Schneider categorically rejected Forssman's requests, as it was believed at the time that any entry into the heart would be fatal. Forssman decided to test his theory anyway to either refute or confirm this medical myth. As he needed access to a suitable catheter to reach his heart, he convinced a nurse, Gerda Ditzen, to assist him in his efforts.

The nurse consented on the condition that she would be his first experimental subject. Forssman agreed, but at the last moment distracted her, anesthetized his own elbow, and inserted a urinary catheter into a vein in his arm and pushed until he felt that that the catheter reached his heart. Though Gerda was initially furious she eventually relented and took Forssman to the hospital's basement where an X-ray proved that it had entered the heart's upper right chamber with no adverse effects. When Forssmann self-experimentation became known he was immediately fired for insubordination.

Despite the significance of his discovery he was forced to switch from cardiology to urology. The popular press highly praised his achievement and considered him a hero, but the medical establishment saw his work as unreliable trickery and for more than a decade refused to acknowledge its value. However in the mid 1940s two cardiologists, Drs. Andre Cournard and Dickinson Richards, re-discovered his work and applied it successfully first to volunteers and then to real cardiac patients. In 1956, all three of them were jointly awarded the Nobel Prize. Hundreds of thousands of patients worldwide have reaped the benefits of Forssman's self-experimentation.

In July 1984 Dr. Barry Marshall, a medical resident at Freemantle Hospital in Perth, Western Australia, attempted to decisively prove that many stomach ulcers are related to a bacterial infection. In contradistinction to the mainstream belief that bacteria could not survive in the stomach because of the high acidity of the gastric juices and that ulcers were only a result of stress and diet, he theorized that infection with *Helicobacter pylori* could wreak havoc with the gastric lining. He was unwilling to experiment on human volunteers as he stated later that he "was the only one informed enough to give consent." Having obtained the appropriate consent from himself, he drank a cocktail containing millions of *Helicobacter* microorganisms from a lab beaker. For 3 days, Marshall experienced "rumbling" of his stomach, bloating, and fullness after evening meals. This was later followed by vomiting and halitosis (putrid breath). To solidify his theory, 10 days later he developed gastritis (an inflammation of stomach's lining) and a stomach ulcer. He subsequently treated himself successfully with Tinidazole, an antibiotic which kills *Helicobacter*. Marshall documented the results of his experiments very carefully by repeated gastroscopies, x-rays, bacteriological cultures, and evaluation of gastric biopsies (small samples of the stomach lining that are pinched off and examined microscopically) obtained both before and after his experiment.

Initially the medical community rejected Dr. Marshall's findings until they were repeatedly verified. Ultimately, Dr. Barry Marshall and his colleague, pathologist Dr. Robert Warren, were awarded the Nobel Prize and congratulated by the Nobel Committee of Sweden's Karolinska Institute for their "tenacity and a prepared mind to challenge prevailing dogmas." Despite the fact that their research has led to the treatment of millions of people with gastritis, ulcers, and gastric lymphomas, ethical condemnation by some peers did not fade away. The critics chided that self-experimenters had a moral duty not to put their life and limb at almost suicidal risk in order to advance medicine. Sounds like a bit of sour grapes to us. It also reminds us of those whiners who don't want to drill for oil somewhere because it may endanger the indigenous Rhodesian striped wombat.

The latest self-experimentation worthy of note was that of Indian virologist Pradeep Seth, a leading researcher at the All India Institute of Medical Sciences (AIIMS), in New Delhi. Having already successfully tested a vaccine directed at the Human Immunodeficiency Virus (HIV) in mice and on monkeys, Dr. Seth was very eager to know the human body's reaction to his formulation. Unfortunately, human trials were not due to start until 2005. When he injected himself with the vaccine in 2003, India's medical community considered the experiment unethical because the vaccine had yet to be cleared for human trials. Despite the fact that Dr. Seth showed no ill-effects from the vaccine, it has not yet been used in India although millions are infected with the virus.

Some self-experiments have been based on incorrect hypotheses or misconceptions. For example, in 1882 a German physician by the name of Max von Pettenkofer stubbornly believed that cholera, a potentially fatal intestinal disease, was not caused by an infection with *Vibrio cholera*. He chose to ignore the experiments of the famous German bacteriologist Robert Koch who grew the organisms from polluted water in India two decades before. Dr. Pettenkoffer believed, as did many others at that time, that cholera was the result of a "miasma," an airborne invisible emanation possibly coming from dirty soil or from decomposition of the feces of cholera patients. So certain was Pettenkofer of his theory that he publicly drank a test tube with a bouillon containing myriads of the bacteria. He promptly became sick with profuse diarrhea, the hallmark of cholera, but recovered rapidly (probably because he was immune to the disease having had prior exposure to a mild form of the illness). Despite this apparent cause-and-effect experience, he and his supporters did not abandon their mistaken belief in the "miasma" theory.

Similarly, Stubbing Firth (1784–1820), an American medical student from the University of Pennsylvania believed that Yellow Fever was caused by heat and stress rather than a virus since it was more common in summer than in winter. To prove it, he smeared black vomit from patients with yellow fever on cuts in his arms and on his eyes, inhaled vapors from boiled vomit, and even swallowed black vomit, sweat, urine and other waste products of patients with Yellow Fever. As he did not acquire the disease, he concluded that his hypothesis was correct and even published papers and books on the topic. Despite his good luck (and probably bad breath) his grotesque self-experimentation was in vain as Yellow Fever was ultimately proven to be an infectious disease transmitted by mosquitoes. Firth's fundamental error was that he had collected samples from patients who were already in the recovery process and were no longer contagious. Yet he did make a valuable contribution to medicine – he set the standard for what we can expect medical students to go through over the course of their training.

What Were They Thinking?

An aggregate of factors may be at play in motivating these self-experimenters. The doctors seem to share a sense of altruism, adventurism of spirit, an almost fanatical confidence in the truth of their theories, an abhorrence of bureaucratic "red tape," an inability to accept the status quo, and a reluctance to put others at risk prior to experimenting on themselves. There also seems to be some sort of triggering event in at least some of these cases. Dr. Seth injected himself with the HIV vaccine when the government cogs stalled; Dr. Forssman gained inspiration from drawings of horses; Dr. Simpson witnessed too many painful labors and wanted to change things for the better; Dr. Hunter wanted to eradicate gonorrhea (his motivation remains unclear).

Dr. William J. Harrington, the physician who elucidated the nature of an autoimmune type of anemia called idiopathic thrombocytopenic purpura (ITP) was motivated by the tragic death of one of his patients. In 1945, a 17-year-old girl presented with severe vaginal bleeding to the Emergency Room of Cambridge City Hospital in Boston. Although she was initially thought to be aborting a pregnancy, eventually the doctors correctly diagnosed her with ITP, a disease characterized by diffuse bleeding into the skin and other organs. The only successful cure at that time was splenectomy. Tragically, the patient died following a surgical mishap leading Dr. Harrington to swear to himself that he would find the cause of this mysterious disease. He keenly noted that infants born to mothers with ITP developed a temporary anemia and theorized that this might be due to a factor transmitted from the mother's blood through the placenta and into the baby. With only that observation to go on, he injected himself intravenously with about 8 ounces of blood from a patient with ITP and succeeded in developing a temporary anemia. He survived and his experiment set the foundation for further research, which led to the recognition of ITP as an autoimmune blood disorder – a disease in which the body tries to destroy its own blood cells.

The story of Dr. Wolfgang Krause illustrates well the aggregate of factors that may prompt a physician to engage in risky self-experimentation. Krause was an orthopedic surgeon in Kassel, West Germany, a hard working practitioner with little interest in research. As an adolescent he was amongst the top 50 skiers in Germany and most likely would have chosen an athletic career but for an accidental back injury that thwarted his dreams. Having come from a family of physicians, he easily converted from skier to orthopedic surgeon ("the jocks of docs"). In 1968, Dr. Krause was greatly dismayed when a dozen of his hip repair surgery patients developed progressively increasing fevers and died within 10 days in spite of intense efforts to maintain a totally sterile environment during surgery. Paradoxically, the administration of strong antibiotics (which treat even most virulent bacteria) worsened the condition of his patients, so it was initially believed that they might have succumbed to a viral infection. Much to their surprise, autopsies demonstrated that all of the patients had died of a widespread fungal infection due to Monilia (*Candida albicans*). Dr. Krause plunged into the literature of Moniliasis and surmised that the fungus was able to pass through the bowel wall and into the patient's blood during or just after this highly invasive surgery. He decided to test his hypothesis but first he needed an experimental human subject.

The relatively fresh memory of the horrific Nazi atrocities performed in the name of Science was a clear barrier to any risky experimentation on human volunteers. Dr. Krause said, "In Germany doctors would have considered this experiment on another man a moral crime. Perhaps doctors of another nationality might have had a different attitude but not in Germany." Clearly, Dr. Krause was unwilling to test a potentially dangerous hypothesis on human volunteers and later stated, "I could have asked a patient but I did not believe anyone would be willing. Man is not an (experimental) animal. The patient could have died." In the end there was only a single suitable candidate left – Wolfgang Krause.

Dr. Krause believed that given his youth and excellent health the intended experiment was not likely to be dangerous. The German experts that he consulted prior to the trial were much more sanguine and feared that a massive, intentional fungal exposure could lead to a lethal, systemic infection. To cover his bases and to minimize the economic loss to his family if things were to go awry, Dr. Krause prudently purchased a large life insurance policy before initiating the experiment. In spite of last minute second thoughts, he decided to cross the experimental Rubicon and ingested two steins of a concoction containing millions of fungal organism followed by another stein of mineral water "to clean the palate." Krause was able to rapidly quaff three steins of fluid with no difficulty, reportedly saying that such drinking could not possibly be a problem for a former German medical student.

Only 2 hours after swallowing the fungal concoction he became ill and in the next 7 hours his temperature climbed to 101°F. Although he felt horrible physically, his spirits remained high. Cultures of both his blood and urine confirmed that the fungus had breached his bowel wall and spread throughout his body in a matter of hours. Krause fully recovered in less than 2 days following two doses of Epsom salts to purge his intestines and intravenous and oral Nystatin, an antifungal medication. After publishing the results of his study, Dr. Krause ended his foray into experimental research and happily returned to his beloved orthopedic practice. We would imagine that he has since put his steins to better use.

Altman perhaps provided the best argument for self-experimentation in his book "Who Goes First." He boldly states, "Why call self-experimentation foolish when we climb mountains, become test pilots, build bridges and skyscrapers? In any experiment, the outcome is not known ahead of time. If the researcher claims there is no risk, why is the researcher unwilling to try it? Doctors' lives are no more valuable than those of the other members of society whom they ask to volunteer for their research." Physicians may be motivated by compassion, fame, financial gain, professional prestige, or mental illness to experiment on themselves. Many researchers will spend decades trying to prove their theories and die with their pens clutched in their hands (or slumped over their laptops), never knowing if their convictions held true. Others will put their money where their mouths are and find out once and for all if they were right or terribly wrong.

Physicians and Suicide

Just like other animals, humankind has a strong ancestral instinct for self-preservation, in most cases choosing to avoid danger and delay, as much as possible, the inevitability of death. Physicians, by virtue of their profession, know better than anyone the manifold manifestations of death and are committed professionally to combat it, day in and day out. As they are so familiar with our common enemy, The Grim Reaper, one would think that it would inspire less dread in them than in their patients. In fact, quite the opposite is true is some cases. Many physicians who become sick are closet hypochondriacs to the extreme and seriously contemplate their impending doom whenever they fall ill. Their medical knowledge works against them: every headache becomes meningitis, backaches become pancreatic cancer, and indigestion must be a heart attack. In short, physicians share a fear of the great unknown with their patients. Doctors are, in fact, human and are born with a will to survive; most will run from death as fast as they can.

On the other hand, the Freudian school of psychology contends that the instinct for self-preservation is balanced by an innate drive towards death, destruction and non-existence. This theory claims that an ingrained "death drive" is responsible for widely prevalent subconscious or conscious aggression and violent behavior towards others, culminating in homicide, as well as for compulsive self destructive behavior leading to premature death. The manifestations of the latter such as drug and alcohol abuse, self-neglect, avoidance of proper medical care, and risk taking behavior keep medical examiners in business. Without the Freudian death drive, there would be a glut of unemployed forensic pathologists writing books.

Conscious self-destructive behavior may result in self-centered acts such as suicide or in heroic efforts by channeling the death drive toward actions that save the lives of others. The latter, positive use of the psyche must be employed by military medics in the field in combat situations. Some physicians also display this type of heroic behavior to a somewhat lesser degree in that they are willing to forego sleep, food, and sex to treat perfect strangers in emergency rooms and operating suites for hours on end. We have discussed in depth what happens when doctors direct their inner hostilities toward their patients and experimental subjects throughout this book. Now let us consider what happens when physicians unleash the primitive drive back to inorganic matter on themselves.

An increased tendency for physicians to commit suicide was noted as early as the 1860s but it took about a hundred years until scientific research provided concrete data to verify this trend. Most studies have documented an increased frequency of suicides in physicians, particularly female physicians, as compared to their counterparts in the general population and other professional groups. Between 250 and 400 physicians, the size of a couple of medical school graduating classes, lose their lives to suicide every year in the United States. Like the rest of society, the most common means involve drug overdose, hanging, or firearms. There are no striking differences in the choice of suicidal methods between the various medical specialties except for anesthesiologists. Half of the time, they kill themselves with drugs including anesthetic agents.

A 2004 compilation of studies done over the past 50 years disclosed that male physicians were at a 1.4 times risk to kill themselves compared to their patients. More startling is that women physicians were 2.3 times more likely to commit suicide that the general population. A National Occupational Mortality Survey of a database of physicians classified by race and gender between 1984 and 1995 confirmed this worrisome pattern. White male physicians showed a higher risk rate of 2.9 times that of the general male population while white female physicians carried a 3.6 times greater risk for suicide than the rest of society. Whereas black male physicians showed a 2.3 times higher risk than the general population, there were no reported suicides among black female physicians. Other studies have reported that the relative frequency of suicide for male physicians was as much as three times higher than that of the general male population; there was a six times larger frequency for female physicians compared to women in general and to other professionals. Medical students and residents show a comparable but even worse pattern with suicide being the most common cause of death after accidental fatalities. In fact, a study by Dyrbe of 4,300 of medical students from seven medical schools between 2006 and 2007 revealed that 30% of them experienced burnout and 10% had suicidal ideation. Chances are many of your doctors feel worse about themselves than you do.

The increased tendency of physicians to commit suicide has been attributed to a conglomerate of genetic and developmental factors, medical culture stressors and professional circumstances. It has been suggested that some of the suicide completers are so-called "wounded healers," attracted to the medical field as a moth is to a flame. These doctors may have entered medicine following traumatic family experiences including abuse, episodes of psychiatric illness, or to overcompensate for parental or peer belittling. Once the physician has entered practice, the stress of the job can magnify any simmering, underlying mental illness. Dealing with terminal illnesses, death, and suffering can also weigh heavily on the practitioner. Studies have shown that 75% of healthcare providers experience severe emotional stress or depression upon learning of the death of one of their patients. Throw on top of that governmental regulation of healthcare, the constant fear of malpractice litigation, and increasing insurance premiums with diminished reimbursement for services and you have a recipe for disaster in predisposed individuals.

Physicians are, by and large, perfectionists – this is a good thing if you are a patient. In order to provide quality care to patients, they often sacrifice their own well-being. In fact, some physicians have a well-developed "martyr complex." They will not sleep and live off of coffee and candy bars to monitor a patient on the brink of death. When and if they go home, some require drugs or alcohol to forget their day. Their work may consume them; many have lost their families while tending to their charges. In the end, Medicine has become their spouse – and she/he can be an unpredictable lover.

Unfortunately, a good part of the medical establishment still sees suicide as carrying a repulsive stigma. Colleagues attempting or completing suicide may be considered weak-willed or virtual traitors in Medicine's war against disease and death. Physicians choose to see themselves as the cure rather than part of the problem. To acknowledge the overwhelming pain and despair of a suicidal compatriot may entail a deep gaze into a mirror. And many doctors don't want to see a flawed human being staring back at them. Doctors must compartmentalize in order to function – the frailty of others cannot be allowed to permeate their shell. When the seal corrodes, however, and the human within the healer is exposed the shell often doesn't crack; it explodes.

Studies have shown that 12% of all male physicians and 18% of all female physicians suffer from depression. In recent years, local medical societies and the National Psychiatric Association have initiated educational programs and seminars directed at recognizing the signs of depression and changes in behavior that often lead up to physician suicides. Efforts are also being made to remove the stigma of suicide as it should be viewed as the ultimate symptom of a fatal disease rather than a character flaw. The importance of prompt treatment of depressed doctors and other caregivers is being stressed at a national level. These all appear to be steps in the right direction. On the other hand, statutory provisions in over 30 states subject physicians to possible penalties if they report mental diseases, such as depression, on medical license applications. This is hardly incentive for the physician applicant to disclose this serious medical condition and seek appropriate treatment. Similarly, if a physician voluntarily admits that they have a substance abuse problem (and we have all heard that admitting that you have a problem is the first step toward a cure) they may face restrictions on their license. Some doctors have the courage to address these problems, even at the risk of forfeiting their livelihood. Others do not and risk forfeiting their lives.

To sum it up, doctors face all of the usual stressors that lead other people in all walks of life to kill themselves. They have financial troubles, broken relationships, personal losses, and problems on the job. To compound this, they are in the business of making life and death decisions, some right, some wrong, which can save or cost lives. They are surrounded by a world of illness, suffering, and, sometimes, death. Following 4 years of college, 4 years of medical school, and additional years of indentured servitude called residency, they get to try to start-up a practice while paying off hundreds of thousands of dollars of debt. Many work to the point of physical exhaustion, others give in to physical addictions. Malpractice lawyers see them as "cash cows;" their families see them hardly at all. It is no wonder that many of us physicians know someone who has committed suicide; those of us who don't probably one day will.

Section 4
Politics and Medicine

Chapter 12
Libel Plots Against Physicians (Who Killed Dr. Zhivago?)

> *The death of a man is a tragedy; the death of millions is a statistic.*
>
> – Josef Stalin

In the freezing, early morning hours of March 13, 1953 *Pravda*, the official newspaper of the Communist Party of the Soviet Union, greeted its readers with strident, bold headlines of a murderous plot against the highest levels of the communist leadership. The would-be killers were none other than a band of malevolent doctors. Western observers, who wryly noted that *Pravda* (ironically meaning "truth" in Russian) and its sister paper *Izvestia* rarely reported unadulterated news, eyed the dramatic account with a healthy dose of skepticism. The average Russian, however, bombarded with sophisticated and perennial communist propaganda most likely viewed the news as equivalent to the Gospel. Communist parties throughout the world generally toed the Soviet line and turned governmental fiction into reality. Strangely enough, Russian physicians were more frightened by these headlines than the allegedly targeted leaders. And they had reason to be. This tune had been played before by the leader of Russia.

Plots and Purges

Josef Stalin, the cruel and undisputed dictator of the Soviet Union for more than 30 years, had a habit of periodically uncovering plots to overthrow his regime that had to be countered by "cleansing" blood baths. In fact, a few of them may actually have been based in reality. The others were created to allow Stalin to reach some sort of political end and the means to get there were often gruesome.

In the early 1930s, millions of Russian peasants contemptuously labeled by Stalin as "kulaks" were accused of being anti-revolutionary rural capitalists and exploiters. The eradication of several million of these insurgents was required to thwart this coup. Many, many thousands more were sent to concentrations camps to work as unpaid serfs, the menial cogs in the State's rapidly industrializing Communist machine. In 1931, when this murderous campaign was in full swing, *Time* published an interview of Stalin by Lady Astor, the first woman to be seated in the British

J.A. Perper and S.J. Cina, *When Doctors Kill: Who, Why, and How*,
DOI 10.1007/978-1-4419-1369-2_12, © Springer Science+Business Media, LLC 2010

House of Commons and George Bernard Shaw, the famous playwright. When Lady Astor boldly asked Stalin: "When are you going to stop killing people?" Stalin coolly replied: "When it is no longer necessary. Soon I hope." He was a refreshingly honest politician. Years later, in the midst of World War II, Sir Winston Churchill visited Russia for talks with Stalin who was his ally against Nazi Germany at the time. On the last night before Churchill's departure, Stalin invited the Englishman to his quarters for drinks (an offer Churchill could not refuse). After a few drinks and an improvised dinner, when the ice was finally broken, Churchill casually asked Stalin about the bloody liquidation of the kulaks 11 years before. Although Western Europeans had heard rumors of the slaughter, no one knew the full scale of the murders. According to *Time*, Stalin replied, "Ten millions," and holding up his hands with stubby fingers extended he added, "It was fearful. Four years it lasted." Clearly, Stalin was peeved at the inefficiency of the operation.

A second wave of major killings engineered by Stalin known as "The Great Purge" (Bolshaya Chistka) in Russia and "The Great Terror" in the West occurred between 1936 and 1938. It was a conglomerate of campaigns of political repression and persecution against allegedly unfaithful members of the Communist Party and others groups branded as spies, saboteurs, opponents of Stalinist policies, anti-revolutionaries, and enemies of the people. It started with three high-profile trials in Moscow ending in the execution of almost all senior Communist Party leaders from the old guard; Stalin perceived them all to be potential competitors or adversaries. The Salem witches probably had more unbiased juries.

The movement expanded to the rank and file of the party and to specific social groups viewed by Stalin as undesirable or threatening to his power base. Secret mass executions were carried out in style and patterns eerily resembling those carried out by Hitler and his henchmen. Assassinations, deportations to Siberia and internment in Gulags (Russian concentration camps) were carried out mercilessly on an unprecedented scale. In 1937 an increasingly paranoid Stalin started a purge of the Red Army, accusing its leaders of treason and collusion with Nazi Germany. By 1939, he had successfully liquidated most of the Soviet Army's top staff, including the majority of the generals and other high-ranking officers. Though bad for the morale of the troops, he had successfully eliminated any possible risk that the military might attempt to remove him from power.

The estimated number of killings of the Soviet citizenry in the Great Purge ranges from the official figure of 681,692 to nearly two million throughout all of the Soviet Republic. That's about 1,000 people a day for 3 years give or take a few hundred thousand. Unfortunately for physicians, they were on Stalin's hit list.

Stalin and the Doctors

The complete details of Stalin's plot against the physicians are difficult to ascertain even now, partially due to the insular nature of the Soviet Union. Russian society under Stalin was so tightly self-policed that it remains impossible to clearly identify the major players in this scheme which included spies, counterspies and double agents. Historical documentation of this chapter of Stalin's reign is exceedingly skimpy. It's almost like Stalin didn't want anyone to know that he was killing millions of people.

In 1948, Andrei Zhdanov, one of the major Communist Soviet leaders, died of heart disease at a Moscow health resort reserved for the Soviet elite. A heavy drinker, Zhdanov rarely followed his doctor's advice and his health deteriorated significantly in the weeks prior to his demise. Days before Zhdanov's death, Dr. Lidia Timashuk, a junior physician assigned to read Zhdanov's electrocardiograms, accused the senior treating physicians of criminal negligence for failing to diagnose an obvious heart attack. The chief doctor dismissed her complaints after meeting with multiple senior specialists; a ploy likely intended to neutralize Timashuk's accusations rather than to actually assist the dying patient. However Timashuk, who apparently was a part-time agent of the Soviet secret police (as many Soviet citizens were at the time), persisted in her complaints. After Zhdanov's death her accusatory letters reached Stalin's desk. The dictator read the letter, placed on it a note for "Into the archives" and did not act upon it until years later. Stalin knew how to conserve ammunition.

It is unclear whether Stalin began to plan the purge of the Soviet doctors at that time or if he retrieved this letter years later to justify a new, brutal, political campaign. We do know that the letter contained the fuel which could be used to burn a group Stalin had come to despise: doctors. Stalin's anti-Semitic feelings are well known but his grudge against physicians has received far less notoriety. Even before reaching his 70's Stalin clearly did not like or trust doctors. As a matter of fact, he refused to be treated by doctors and chose to consult only veterinarians for his health. His mistrust ran so deep that he chose to self-treat his hypertension with iodine drops. This is not effective; don't try this at home.

In the Stalinist system of Justice if the facts were insufficient to convict someone then they were skillfully fabricated and confessions were coerced. This served to ensure that Stalin's modus operandi, "Sentence first – verdict afterward," had an air of "legitimacy." Between October 1952 and February 1953 hundred of doctors were arrested after rumors were started by the government that they had been killing newborns in maternity wards and were poisoning Russian children and infecting them with Diphtheria. The jailed doctors were submitted to lengthy, exhausting and threatening interrogations. Some were beaten and a number of them died in jail. Stalin was personally involved in the interrogation of some of the Kremlin doctors. In November 1952, Semyon Ignatiev, the head of the Secret Police, relayed a directive from Stalin to his interrogators: "Beat them! You work like waiters in white gloves. If you want to be Chekists (secret police officers), take off your gloves!" Another interrogator is reported to have stated to a jailed doctor in November 1952: "We will beat you every day, we will tear out your arms and legs, but we will learn ... the truth." In March 1953, another police officer reported to the Chief of Soviet Security: "Comrade Stalin as a rule spoke with great anger, continually expressing dissatisfaction with the course of the investigation, he cursed, threatened and, as a rule demanded that the prisoners be beaten: "Beat them, beat them, beat them with death blows" he said."

By mid-January 1953, Stalin concluded that he had manufactured sufficient evidence to commence with trials for treason involving hundreds of physicians. He authorized the publication of the results of the investigation of the doctors by *Tass*, the Soviet News agency, and *Pravda*. Some of the most prestigious and prominent doctors in the USSR were formally charged with taking part in a vast plot to poison members of the top Soviet political and military leadership. *Pravda* reported the accusations under the headline "*Vicious Spies and Killers under the Mask of Academic Physicians*." All but two of the doctors accused were Jewish. The major points of the article, written with the usual virulence reserved for targets of the Communist Party, were the following:

– State security agencies had been tracking a group of "saboteur doctors" planning to kill the leaders of Soviet Union by "medical sabotage" for an unspecified period of time
– The "medical sabotage" consisted of intentional and vicious, incorrect diagnoses and inappropriate medical treatments using "very powerful medicines" and "harmful regimens"
– The accused were branded as "fiends and killers", "terrorists" and "inhuman beasts" who dishonored "the holy banner of science" and committed "monstrous crimes" by killing high rank Soviet leaders
– The accused were paid agents of "American intelligence," or of a spying "international Jewish Zionist organization" or part of a terrorist organization masquerading as a charitable philanthropic organization
– A number of physicians were long-term agents of the British secret intelligence agency
– "Big-wig" American and English partners preparing for a new World War against the Soviet Union used several doctors as spies; and, as a public service reminder to the readers, and
– The Soviet people must be mindful and highly vigilant of the subversive schemes of warmongers and their agents and everyone must play their part in strengthening the Soviet Armed Forces and intelligence agencies

On January 20, 1953, Dr. Timashuk was summoned to the Kremlin and Georgi Malenkov, a powerful member of the Politburo, praised her "patriotism" in unmasking the "criminal activity of professor doctors" and informed her that Stalin himself had investigated her complaints from 1948. Shortly thereafter she was awarded the Order of Lenin, the highest decoration of the Soviet Union for "unmasking doctors-killers." Furthermore the Soviet press showered her with high praise for her vigilance, comparing her with the French heroine Joan of Arc. This meeting marked a further intensification of the campaign against "the killers in white coats" as the press had branded them. The grave accusations against doctors engendered deep resentment by average citizens against all physicians and, by extension, against intellectuals in general. Yaakov Rapoport, a Russian researcher, wrote in his book "The doctors' plot of 1953:"

> Every physician was regarded as a potential murderer. I shall never forget the face of my laboratory assistant, distorted with fury and hatred, as she hissed through clenched teeth: "Damn intellectuals, they all deserve to be cudgeled." ... Meetings were held at all factories

and offices, some organized, some spontaneous, and almost all openly anti-Semitic. Speakers would vehemently demand that the criminals should be put to a terrible death. Many went so far as to offer their services in carrying out the actual executions.

At the start of Stalin's libelous plot against physicians 37 doctors were arrested, but hundreds more incarcerations followed. Many doctors were fired from their jobs, imprisoned, and sent to gulags or executed. Outside of Moscow, similar plots were allegedly discovered. In Ukraine, Dr. Victor Kogan-Yasny, the first physician in the USSR to treat diabetes with insulin and the savior of thousands of lives, was accused of engineering a plot against the government. He was arrested along with 35 other "plotters." While *Pravda* was preparing to publish a letter signed by many Soviet notables severely condemning all of the accused physicians and asking for maximum punishment for those already sentenced, it was never published because the incendiary campaign ended abruptly and unexpectedly in March 1953. If this vicious and contrived campaign against the doctors would have been a Greek tragedy, its dramatic and sudden collapse would be called a Deus ex machine, a totally surprising turn of events. In the case of the campaign against the doctors, many people of faith believed that their survival may have been the work of Deus ex Caelum, God in Heaven, with divine intervention coming in the form of a stroke.

On the night of February 28 or in the early morning of March 1, 1953, Stalin suffered a hemorrhagic stroke perhaps related to poisoning. Allegedly warfarin, a flavorless and powerful blood thinner (ironically also a rat poison), may have caused Stalin to bleed into his brain due to his high blood pressure. Perhaps his iodine drops weren't working or he wasn't listening to his veterinarian. He was found at midday on March 1 by a chambermaid who entered his room when he failed to get up as expected. Initially, his political "friends" denied him treatment but eventually he received some medical care. Comatose, he clung to life until March 5 or 6 when his death was officially announced. The Lord works in mysterious ways. After Stalin's death, the new leadership admitted that the charges against the persecuted physicians and other intellectuals had been entirely invented under the direction of Stalin and acknowledged that all confessions had been extracted by torture. Nevertheless, the careers of most of the doctors involved effectively ended and they were forced to leave their practices in many of the larger cities such as Moscow and Leningrad. When an average person is besmirched and then exonerated, a return to normalcy may be difficult. When the allegations have been made against a person that you have to trust your life to, reparations are impossible. The case against the doctors was officially dismissed on March 31, 1953 by the newly appointed Minister of Internal Affairs Lavrenty Beria.

Several days later the Presidium of the Central Committee of the Communist Party officially arrested the Chief Investigator of the Secret Police and the Deputy Minister of State Security for their roles in the fabrication of the plot; the latter was eventually executed. On April 4 *Pravda* carried a statement by Lavrenty Beria exonerating nine Soviet doctors (seven of them Jews) who had previously been accused of "wrecking, espionage and terrorist activities" against the Soviet Government. Seven of the doctors were immediately released – but two had already died at the hands of their jailers. After ordering the release of the doctors Beria revoked Timashuk's Order of Lenin award. Weeks later, he boasted that he had poisoned Stalin saying: "I did him in! I saved you all." As poetic Justice would have it Beria, who also participated in carrying out the campaign against the doctors, was eventually executed in December 1953 for complicity in the same criminal purge he claimed to have thwarted.

Three years later in a secret speech at the 20th Soviet Communist Party Congress Nikita Khrushchev asserted that Stalin had personally ordered that the cases against physicians be developed and confessions elicited. He went on to state that the "doctors' plot" was to be the first stage of a new "Great Purge." Khrushchev revealed that Stalin had intended to include members of the Politburo in the list of victims after the doctors and other intellectuals had been taken care of. It is fortunate for them that politicians were not considered intellectuals to Stalin. No comment.

Many scholars researching the libelous plot against doctors agree with Khrushchev's report. It seems likely that an aging, paranoid Stalin felt a campaign was necessary to purge the Soviet leadership in order to unify the country and prepare it for an anticipated new World War against the West. "Hardening of the arteries" of the brain may also have played a role in his twisted reasoning. A year before he died Stalin reluctantly saw a doctor who told the dictator he had cerebral arteriosclerosis and that he could have a stroke if he didn't rest. Stalin responded by having him arrested, dissolving his family, and decimating a thriving career. A dictator can choose to ruin one life or eradicate an entire social class based on some innate prejudice, paranoia or simply on a whim. Several million graves attest to Stalin's fickle nature.

Chapter 13
Judge, Jury, Executioner, and Doctor

> *The benevolent despot who sees himself as a shepherd of the*
> *people still demands from others the submissiveness of sheep.*
>
> – Eric Hoffer

Power, particularly political power giving control of the few over the many, may be a very intoxicating draught. There is much truth in the adage coined by Lord Acton more than a century ago that "power corrupts and absolute power corrupts absolutely." Less known but just as true is his adjacent pronouncement that "great men are almost always bad men."

Nowadays most physicians, at least in Western countries and in the United States of America in particular, shy away from politics. Many physicians see in political life a descent from the high social standing of medicine to a much less respected and highly time-consuming social obligation. Another likely reason is that physicians can act autonomously as demigods, making life and death decisions without having to endure the media scrutiny inherent in politics. Aside from being monitored by insurance companies, state medical Boards, the federal government, and a slew of malpractice attorneys, physicians can basically do what they want without having to answer to anyone. Further, the physician of today has to try to pay off massive student loans by cramming as many patients into a day as possible effectively eliminating the time and energy required for successful public service. It is no wonder that political involvement by physicians has substantially diminished both in United States and abroad in recent decades (Howard Dean, the "yelping doctor," being a notable exception).

An interesting question is whether the few physicians who choose to enter political life and walk the corridors of power are more compassionate than the average politician. At first glance, one may believe that the physicians' creed of "above all do no harm" would encourage a physician-politician to do what is best for the people whenever possible. Unfortunately, successful politics is rather like the proverbial Bluebeard's Castle with many sumptuous halls and elegant banquet rooms arrayed above a lattice of bloody secret rooms that few people see. It seems that the rare doctors who have become very powerful or autocratic leaders have had no reluctance to leave the ballroom, walk down the stairs and turn the key to enter the chamber of horrors. The following physician-politicians have distinguished themselves by an unusual disregard for human life. Their life and death decisions were made on a grand scale.

J.A. Perper and S.J. Cina, *When Doctors Kill: Who, Why, and How*,   121
DOI 10.1007/978-1-4419-1369-2_13, © Springer Science+Business Media, LLC 2010

Dr. Ernesto "Che" Guevara: A Physician in Search of a Revolution

Che Guevara, the romantic revolutionary hero still depicted on t-shirts, was a trained healer. The many facets of his life can be compared to an Indian idol sprouting many arms, the multiplicity of hands holding the books of the Greek classical philosophers, the works of Marx and Lenin, the blazing pens of a fiery writer, grenades, machine guns, and a variety of executioner's tools. In spite of a brilliant mind, Guevara's compassion was very selective and selective compassion is not true compassion at all (sort of like unconditional love with a few strings attached). His fanatical devotees purged themselves of any humane feelings toward disobedient followers, dissidents, political opponents, their own families and people at large.

Guevara was born in Argentina in 1928 to a family with very strong leftist beliefs. His nickname "Che" was an affectionate term for "hey man" an early indicator of his endearing, charismatic way with people. He completed his medical studies at the University of Buenos Aires and after graduation worked for a short time as a physician. But he had more important things to do than to save lives.

In a 1960 speech, he readily confessed: "When I began to study medicine, most of the concepts that I now have as a revolutionary were absent from my store of ideals. I wanted to succeed just as everyone wants to succeed. I dreamed of becoming a famous researcher; I dreamed of working tirelessly to aid humanity, but this was conceived as personal achievement. I was – as we all are – a product of my environment." Not long after finishing his studies, Guevara's adventurous nature prevailed and the prospective medical researcher left his practice to tour South America. The striking poverty he encountered during his travels boosted his revolutionary beliefs and zeal and he became enthralled with the activities of the Bolivian socialist government of Jacobo Arbenz. Guevara recorded his South American road trip experience in a book the "Motorcycle Diaries" (made into a fine film in 2004) in which he reveals the first inklings of his burgeoning communist beliefs. He wrote:

> To be a revolutionary doctor or to be a revolutionary at all, there must first be a revolution. The isolated effort of one man, regardless of its purity of ideals, is worthless. If one works alone in some isolated corner of Latin America because of a desire to sacrifice one's entire life to noble ideals, it makes no difference because one fights against adverse governments and social conditions that prevent progress. To be useful it is essential to make a revolution. So today one has the right and the duty of being, above everything else, a revolutionary doctor, that is, a man who uses his professional knowledge to serve the Revolution and the people.

Dr. Guevara decided to pursue his revolutionary fantasies by joining forces with a young rebel named Fidel Castro. Che soon proved himself to be a very competent and creative commander and he became one of Castro's closest associates. In 1956 Guevara, Castro and 80 other men and women arrived in Cuba in an attempt to overthrow the government of General Fulgencio Batista. This group later became known as the "July 26 Movement." They planned to set up their base in the Sierra Maestra mountains but were attacked by government troops prior to their arrival. They quickly rebounded from this defeat and enlisted local support by redistributing lands to the poor peasants ("share the wealth!") eventually overcoming Batista's forces in spite of the American government's opposition to this revolt. For his service to the revolution, Guevara was appointed by Castro as the Commander of the Rebel Army Column. In this capacity, Guevara was given the task of purging the military and the government of undesirable and anti-revolutionary elements. Castro also put Che in charge of San Carlos de la Cabaña prison, a stone fortress that had defended Havana against English pirates in the eighteenth century. He would put this piece of real estate to good use.

During the first half of 1959, Dr. Guevara acted both as a judge and executioner of people accused of being contra-revolutionaries in a manner chillingly reminiscent of the Stalinist secret trials. He took to this task with relish and ordered the killing of many hundreds if not thousands of Cubans. Reliable reports indicate that Che was personally involved in torturing and killing his political opponents. He also occasionally psychologically tortured the relatives of his victims by having them beg for the lives of relatives who were already dead.

In a number of books and articles, Guevara expressed his radical revolutionary and communist philosophy by advocating guerilla warfare as the most desirable mechanism for social and political change. As a matter of fact, his beliefs were perhaps to the left of both Castro and the rulers of Russia. His contributions to Western communism cannot be underestimated. A cover story in *Time* magazine in August 1960 described the anatomy of the Cuban Revolution's leadership as Che Guevara's "brain", Fidel Castro's "heart" and Raúl Castro's "fist." The U.S.-backed Bay of Pigs invasion in April 1961 offered Castro a perfect opportunity to further solidify his power and eliminate any perceived political threats. Tens of thousands of Cubans alleged to support the invasion were imprisoned leading to a new series of executions. As Guevara himself told the Soviet ambassador Sergei Kudriavtsev, the contra-revolutionaries were never "to raise their heads again."

According to one biography, Guevara irresponsibly bragged in 1961 that, "this country (Cuba) is willing to risk everything in an atomic war of unimaginable destructiveness to defend a principle." Just after the Cuban missile crisis ended – with Russia's Nikita Khrushchev negotiating a deal with the United States behind Castro's back – Guevara told a British periodical: "If the rockets had remained, we would have used them all and directed them against the very heart of the United States, including New York, in our defense against aggression." A couple of years later, at the United Nations, he reiterated: "As Marxists we have maintained that peaceful coexistence among nations does not include coexistence between exploiters and the exploited." Apparently the Soviets were saner than Guevara, as they were not in a hurry to rush into a mutually annihilating nuclear war. Perhaps Guevera and Dr. Strangelove could have formed their own nuclear medical society.

In April 1965, after less than 4 years of working as an Economic Minister for Cuba, Guevara apparently became fed up with bureaucratic work. Energized by his restless spirit and revolutionary zeal, Guevara jumped at the chance to lead a group of Cuban soldiers to the Central African Republic of Congo in late 1965. Their plan was to spark a revolt by mobilizing the people against the pro-Western government, a perfect job for our doctor-rebel. His plan was simple – have a group of 100 Cubans set up camp in the lake-side mountains and start a grassroots revolution. This mission was an abject failure. Che himself admitted that his 7-month stay in the Fizi-Barak Mountains was an "unmitigated disaster". He returned to Cuba, never to see the African continent again. Undiscouraged he decided to try his luck again, this time in Bolivia. He hoped he could repeat his success in Cuba by mobilizing the poor Bolivian tin-miners to form a revolutionary army. Unfortunately for Che, in trying to obtain manpower and resources for his intended army he oppressed and terrorized the local peasants and Indians, the very people he had hoped to recruit. Apparently, Guevara forgot his own teachings that a rebel guerilla army cannot survive without a supporting local population into which it can smoothly blend. The locals had no sympathy for Che and had no qualms in assisting Bolivian government agents and the CIA in tracking and capturing Dr. Guevara. In 1967 he was executed without a trial and his body was burned on site.

Following his death Guevara became an icon of the extreme left and of the young and empowered. He has been immortalized not as a physician but as a romantic rebel, motorcyclist and revolutionary who showed no hesitation to die for his ideals and beliefs. His many critics, however, see him as a communist soldier of fortune and quasi-mercenary globetrotter who believed that the proper lubricant for the wheels of social progress was the blood of his enemies and the tears of widows and children. Maybe he should have stayed in medicine.

Psychiatrists and Genocide

Two Serbian psychiatrists carry major responsibility for the genocidal killing of more than 100,000 people during the military conflicts of the 1990s associated with the breakup of the Yugoslavian Republic. After the disintegration of the Ottoman Empire following the First World War, Yugoslavia was formed from the merger of a number of southern Slavic states including Slovenia, Croatia, Bosnia–Herzegovina, Serbia and Macedonia. Despite this forced geopolitical melding centuries-old conflicts between Roman Catholics and Eastern Orthodox Christians and between Christian and Muslims frustrated attempts for true national unity. After World War II, Josip Broz Tito, a national hero, recreated Yugoslavia as a multi-national communist State made up of six republics: Croatia, Slovenia, Macedonia, Bosnia, Herzegovina and Montenegro. Under the strong dictatorship of Tito, the simmering mutual resentments between the various ethnic and religious groups were largely kept in check under an official program of Brotherhood and Unity.

With the death of Tito in 1994, the Yugoslavian Federation started to unravel at the seams and the various Republics split apart along religious and ethnic lines. Conflicts soon broke out, the most highly publicized and lethal arising between Serbia and the Muslims in Bosnia and Kosovo, a southern province within Serbia that was seeking independence. The ensuing war claimed tens of thousands of lives and resulted in the massive displacement and flight of Bosnian and Kosovoan

Muslims creating more than a million refugees. Acts of genocide have been well documented and the Serbian leader Slobodan Milosevic became a regular feature on the nightly news. Less well known are the actions of two psychiatrists pulling the strings behind the genocide.

Dr. Jovan Rascovic laid the ideological groundwork for the genocide. In the 1980s and 1990s Raskovic, a Croatian-born Serbian psychiatrist, practiced at the Neuropsychiatric Clinic in Sibenik near the southern border of Bosnia–Herzegovina. In his clinic he was known to prefer to treat depression with electroshock therapy, particularly if the patients were Croatian women and children. He was a member of the Communist Party (renamed the Serbian Socialist party) and earlier in his career had publicly supported Soviet dictator Joseph Stalin against Tito. Raskovic was also an ardent Serbian Nationalist and he helped draft a document entitled *The Memorandum* in 1986. This publication described in detail how a greater Serbia was to be carved out from portions of Yugoslavia. In 1990, Raskovic published a manifesto entitled *Luda Zemlja* (A Mad Country). The book opens with a description of the genocide campaign carried out against the Serbs during the Second World War and tries to explain its roots based on psychiatric findings. Raskovic expounds upon his psychoanalytical theories pertaining to the different ethnic groups in Yugoslavia, theories he claimed were based on his psychiatric practice (but which could not be supported by any objective or credible scientific proof). "Serbs by nature possess the qualities of authority with certain aggressive and open elements ... Muslims are fixated on the anal phase ... Their character tends to appropriate things, dominate like a boss, value people by their possessions, their money, their social position, etc.... [Croats] are fixated on the castration complex ... under perpetual fear of castration, losing something that belongs only to himself." It follows that given their fear of castration the Croats would be afraid of everything, and therefore could not assert themselves or exercise authority or leadership. They must therefore be "guided" and he knew just who should be leading them.

Raskovic claimed that the Serbs "by nature possess the qualities of authority with certain aggressive and open elements" dictating that they were best suited to rule and dominate the other Yugoslavian people. He further asserted that the Serbs are the only people ever to overcome the Oedipus Complex and dare to stand up to and "kill" the father (the Oedipus Complex is, according to Freud's theory, a deeply repressed sexual urge of a son to kill his father and marry his mother). Raskovic heavily advertised his unproven and inflammatory psychiatric theories throughout the country in newspapers and on television as part of a media campaign in which he presented himself as a psychiatrist of worldwide stature. His propagandistic activities solidified and legitimized the Croatian Serbs' support of secession into a Greater Serbia and further enflamed the hatred toward non-Serbians. His thoughts and actions created the backdrop against which the horrors of the Yugoslavian wars were soon to occur.

In January 1992, a few months prior to his death and only 2 months before the start of the Bosnian–Herzegovinian conflict, Rascovic had an apparent change of heart. In a public television interview he recognized his nefarious role in fanning the flames of ethnic and religious hatred that had facilitated the burgeoning genocidal wars. He stated,

I feel responsible because I made the preparations for this war, even if not the military preparations. If I hadn't created this emotional strain in the Serbian people, nothing would have happened ... My party and I lit the fuse of Serbian nationalism not only in Croatia but everywhere else in Bosnia–Herzegovina. It's impossible to imagine an SDP (Serbian Democratic Party) in Bosnia–Herzegovina or a Mr. Karadzic in power without our influence.

Of course, you have to remember that doctors have an overinflated sense of importance. While Raskovic certainly played a role in this tragedy, it also would have likely played out without him.

Dr. Radovan Karadzic was a much more interesting and multifaceted personality than Rascovic. He was not only a medical doctor but also a dark and nationalistic poet, ecologist, soccer coach, businessman, chicken farmer, genocidal activist, and, finally, a War Crimes fugitive who spent several years avoiding justice. Dr. Karadzic was born in a stable in the village of Petnijca in the mountains of Montenegro during the last days of the Second World War. He was the son of a Chetnik, the Serbian nationalist guerrillas who fought both the Nazi occupiers and Tito. When he was 15-years old, Karadzic moved to Sarajevo, a major Bosnian city, where he eventually graduated as a medical doctor and specialized in psychiatry with a special interest in the treatment of depression. He also studied abroad researching neurotic disorders and depression at Næstved Hospital in Denmark in 1970; in 1974–1975 he spent a year pursuing further training at Columbia University in New York. During the 1970s and 1980s Karadzic worked at various medical posts including the Zagreb Centre for Mental Health in Croatia, the Health Centre in Belgrade, and as official psychiatrist for the Sarajevo national soccer team. Who knew that soccer could be so stressful? Although not particularly active in politics during the days of the Yugoslavian State, Karadzic was nevertheless an ardent Serbian nationalist. He wrote numerous dark, enigmatic poems calling for violence and evoking graphic images of cruelty, destruction and war. He later claimed his writing foretold of the debacles in Bosnia and Kosovo. We forgot to mention that physicians are prophets as well as demigods.

With the impending breakup of Yugoslavia, Karadzic's political activities intensified and he rapidly climbed the pyramid of political power. He spoke eloquently on numerous occasions on the rights of the Bosnian Serbs to independence using his poems as a tool to agitate and motivate his audiences. In March 1992 Dr. Karadzic declared the formation of the Serbian Bosnian secessionist state of Republika Srpska and he was "elected" its president. His party, supported by Serbian leader Slobodan Milosevic, created a genocidal military machine to fight against the Bosniaks (Bosnian Muslims) and Croats. Karadzic's military was behind the infamous siege of Sarajevo that lasted for almost 2 years. Thousands of civilians died, many of them deliberately targeted by bombs or sniper fire. In fighting Kosovo's Muslims, Karadzic attempted to cement the support of Christian Serbs by emphasizing repeatedly that "our faith is present in all our thinking and decision, and the voice of the Church is obeyed as the voice of supreme authority." He essentially created a Holy War.

Hundreds of thousands of Bosniaks and Croats were driven from their homes in a brutal campaign of "ethnic cleansing." Numerous atrocities were documented, including the widespread rape of thousands of Bosniak women and girls. This was all done under orders by a physician. The Bosnian Serb forces also operated "punishment camps" where prisoners-of-war were starved and tortured. The European Union, United States and NATO eventually attempted to stop the hostilities and find a political solution but they dragged their feet. It took almost 3 years of genocide prior to direct military intervention by the West before the combatants were effectively separated. The carnage claimed the lives of more than a hundred thousand people and the displacement of more than 1.7 million others.

By 1995, The Hague International Tribunal of Justice had issued an arrest warrant for both Dr. Karadzic and Ratko Mladic, his Bosnian Serb military commander, for genocide and war crimes. In 1996, Karadzic resigned under pressure from his post in Republika Srpska and in 1997 he went into hiding with a $5 million bounty on his head. Dr. Karadzic assumed the identity of Dragan Dabic, a Serb killed in battle near Sarajevo, and started to work in a private clinic in New Belgrade as a practitioner of alternative medicine. He presented himself as a "human quantum energy" expert and alternative medicine guru. He wrote for a local health magazine and gave many lectures but he never got his own cable television show. He was able to evade capture for over a decade in spite of his fairly numerous public appearances. When he was finally arrested in July 2008 while getting out of a city bus, he was virtually unrecognizable with a head crowned with long white hair fashioned in a top-knot and a long bushy white beard. He looked more like a refugee wizard from the *Lord of the Rings* than a fugitive from The Hague.

He was charged by the UN war crimes tribunal with six counts of genocide and complicity in genocide, two counts of crimes against humanity, and violating the laws of war. His breaches of the Geneva Convention included setting up concentration camps and organizing the torture, rape and massacre of civilians; desecrating places of worship; and taking UN peacekeepers hostage and using them as human shields. As of 2008, his trial had not started. It should be noted that in spite of the very serious criminal charges brought against Karadzic, many Serbs still remain his ardent supporters and have publicly protested his detention and pending trial.

A number of physician-politicians who initially appeared to be honest and caring were elected democratically according to due process of law. Unfortunately, they later turned into cruel dictators who ordered the death of thousands and lined their pockets with money robbed from their country's treasuries. It is uncertain whether they were corrupt from the very beginning or became so as a result of the inexorable temptation of power. Perhaps some insights can be gleaned from the reigns of Papa Doc Duvalier, the former dictator of Haiti, and Dr. Hastings Kamuzu Banda, the President of Malawi.

"Papa Doc"

Dr. François Duvalier, known as "Papa Doc" (1907–1971), was the President of Haiti from 1957 until his death. He was born in Port-au-Prince, the capital and the largest city on the island, the son of a teacher, journalist and Justice of the Peace. His mother was a mentally unstable woman who worked in a bakery and eventually had to be hospitalized in an asylum where she died in 1921. The invasion of Haiti in 1915 by the United States Marines followed by the ruthless repression of any political dissent by the ruling class significantly impacted upon the political views of young Duvalier. He was also acutely aware of the deep resentment that the poor Black majority bore towards the small but powerful Haitian elite, a class composed predominantly of mulattos.

He studied medicine at the University of Haiti and graduated in 1934 with his M.D. degree. After completing his training he worked in several local hospitals as a staff physician. His adoring patients called him "Papa Doc," a nickname he liked and continued to use in later years when he saw himself as the father of his nation. By 1938, Dr. Duvalier had developed a deep interest in the African roots of Haitian culture, even helping to found "Le Groupe des Griots," an enclave of writers committed to Black Nationalism (negritude) and religious mysticism. Duvalier became involved in both activities and personally conducted an ethnological study of Vodou (a mixture of West African beliefs and Roman Catholicism), Haiti's native religion. Negritude and Vodou (anglicized to Voodoo) would eventually become the horses that would carry his chariot of ambition to ultimate political victory.

In the early 1940s, Dr. Duvalier became involved in a U.S.-sponsored campaign to control the spread of contagious tropical diseases in Haiti. He even spent a year in training at the University of Michigan studying public health. He was praised for his commitment to reducing the human devastation caused by a variety of infections among Haiti's poor including malaria and yaws. Yaws is an infectious disease of the skin, bones, and joints caused by a bacterium related to the micro-organism that causes syphilis; it is not sexually transmitted. Later in his political career, he was quick to bring up his selfless dedication to his poor and sick patients. Though he was prone to exaggerating his contribution to public health, at least this was not a bald-faced lie (as many of his later pronouncements turned out to be). In 1946, Duvalier joined the government of President Dumarsais Estimé becoming Director General of the National Public Health Service. Two years later he was promoted to Minister of Public Health and Labor. However, in May 1950 President Estimé was overthrown in a military coup and Paul Magloire became President of Haiti. Dr. Duvalier left the government and returned to medical practice but behind the scenes he became very politically active and by 1954 he was the leader of the opposition faction. Pursued by the military-sponsored government for his defiance Duvalier went underground, hiding in the interior of the island and practicing medicine.

In December 1956 the military relinquished power, President Magloire resigned, and a general political amnesty allowed Duvalier to come out of hiding. Haiti's political instability persisted unabated and no less than six provisional governments succeeded each other in the following 10 months. With army backing, in a shameless, rigged election, Duvalier was elected president for a 6-year term in September 1957. He promised to fulfill his populist vision to end the domination of the mulatto elite and bring political and economic power to the black Haitian majority. Shortly after being sworn into office, Duvalier revived the traditions of Vodou which he then uses to strengthen his political control. The principal belief in Haitian Vodou is that there are various deities, or Loa, who are subordinate to a greater God, known as Bon Dyè (a vitiation of the French words Bon Dieu – the Good Lord). The Loa may reward, harm, abduct or enter the soul of believers and possess them. Papa Doc claimed to be a Vodou priest and among the masses of Haiti's superstitious poor he was greatly feared as a practitioner of black magic. Over his career he certainly amassed a number of souls.

After a botched attempt to overthrow him in 1958, Duvalier rapidly moved to consolidate his power. Believing that the army was planning to depose him (as it had done to previous leaders) he disbanded all law enforcement agencies in Haiti, executed all high-ranking generals, reduced and crippled the military forces, and closed the military academy. For good measure, he also banned all political parties and night curfews were ordered. To keep law enforcement completely loyal to his own ruling family he created his own private security force in 1959. With his chief aide Clément Barbot, Papa Doc organized the Milice Volontaires de la Sécurité Nationale or VMSN (Volunteers' Militia for National Security), a private militia consisting of 9,000–15,000 recruits from the slums of Port-au-Prince. This militia, popularly known as Tonton Macoutes, was ruthlessly used to smother dissent and terrorize and murder opponents. The Tonton Macoutes were granted automatic amnesty through Duvalier's powers for any crime they committed. The name Tonton Macoute (literally translated as "Uncle Gunnysack") originated from Haitian Creole folklore. It was the name of a bogeyman that walked the streets after dark kidnapping children who stayed out too late and stowing them away in his burlap sack never to be seen again. Similar to the climate of Stalinist Russia, those who dared to speak out against Duvalier would disappear in the night and would never be seen or heard from again. Anyone who mentioned the MSVN risked their own abduction. The Macoutes had no official salary and made their living through protection rackets, crime and extortion schemes.

On May 24, 1959 Duvalier, a diabetic since early childhood, suffered a massive heart attack and was subsequently unconscious for 9 hours. There has been some speculation that his may have been brought on by either an accidental or intentional insulin overdose. Many believed that some brain damage received during this episode affected his mental health and made him paranoid and irrational or, to be perfectly accurate, more paranoid and irrational than he had been. While incapacitated, Duvalier's presidential powers were delegated to Clement Barbot, his chief aide and leader of the Tonton Macoutes. Upon his recovery, Duvalier accused Barbot of trying to replace him as president and threw him in jail. In 1961, Duvalier manipulated the elections to have his term extended to 1967 and, not-surprisingly, "won" decisively with an official tally of 1,320,748 votes to zero. "Latin America has witnessed many fraudulent elections," the *New York Times* reported the day following the election, "but none will have been more outrageous than the one which has just taken place in Haiti."

Skillfully using mystic populism and terror, Duvalier overcame all of Haiti's main power brokers – the military, the mulatto business community, and the Catholic Church. Human rights abuses were commonplace under Papa Doc and up to 30,000 of his enemies were repeatedly tortured and murdered. Haiti, already the poorest country in the Americas, became poorer still under his leadership. Paradoxically, the poorer the country became the richer Duvalier and his acolytes came to be as attested to by their bloated Swiss bank accounts. Duvalier knew well how to sell the misery of his people abroad attracting millions of dollars in aid from both the United States and the European Community. As is true of most dictatorships, the funds never reached their intended destination flowing instead into the private coffers of Duvalier and his friends. Following the re-election, America raised concerns about the misappropriation of aid money by Duvalier and all aid from the United States was suspended in 1962. The following year diplomatic relations were also suspended and the US ambassador was withdrawn.

In 1963 Barbot was released from prison. He promptly began plotting to overthrow Duvalier (for real, this time) and kidnap his children. However, the coup which was to take place in July 1963 was uncovered at the last moment and Duvalier subsequently ordered a massive search for Barbot and his fellow conspirators. During the search, Duvalier received information that Barbot had transformed himself into a black dog. Duvalier then ordered that all black dogs in Haiti be put to death (which should have been called the "Labrador Retriever massacre of '63"). Barbot was later captured (in human form) and was shot. In another quelling of insurrection, Duvalier ordered the head of an executed rebel to be packed in ice and brought to him to allow him to commune with the dead man's spirit. Maybe that heart attack did result in a bit of brain damage.

Duvalier's dictatorship became more extreme and irrational. He assiduously cultivated his personality cult, portraying himself as a powerful Vodou sorcerer and as the Loa Baron Samedi, a magical Vodou spirit. In the pantheon of loas, Baron Samedi is a god of the dead often portrayed as wearing a white top hat, black tuxedo, dark glasses, and cotton plugs in the nostrils, as if to resemble a corpse dressed and prepared for burial in Haitian style. He has a white, skull-like face and basically resembles the bad guy in one of the old James Bond movies. If that wasn't enough, Duvalier's aids drafted an alternative Lord's Prayer, modified to accommodate the greatness of Papa Doc:

> Our Doc, who art in the National Palace for life, hallowed be Thy name by present and future generations. Thy will be done in Port-au-Prince as it is in the provinces. Give us this day our new Haiti and forgive not the trespasses of those anti-patriots who daily spit upon our country …

Papa Doc extended his dominance over the Catholic clergy by expelling almost all of Haiti's foreign-born bishops in the name of nationalism and replacing them with his political allies. In response the Vatican excommunicated him from the Church but reinstated him a year later. At least Dr. Duvalier wasn't trying to play God-he was only playing Pope.

The elite got richer and the poor got poorer. The per capita annual income sank to $80, the lowest in the Western hemisphere and the illiteracy rate remained the highest at about 90%. Eventually, mass media support in Haiti began to drift away from Papa Doc. In response to this affront, Duvalier had no qualms in sending his enemies in the media to the ghastly Fort Dimanche to be tortured to death. The country's leading newspaper editors and radio station owners were jailed for false sedition charges and many Haitians fled to exile in the United States and Canada, especially French-speaking Quebec. Nevertheless, Duvalier continued to have significant support among Haiti's black rural population who still saw in him a champion of their claims against the dominant mulatto élite. In 1971, with death knocking at his door, Duvalier had the Haitian constitution amended so that he could be succeeded by his young son, Jean-Claude, who came to be known as "Baby Doc." He was not a doctor; actually, he studied law. Power was transferred to Jean-Claude, who at the age of 19, became the youngest president in the world. He was ousted from power in February 1986 and he and his wife fled to a villa in France near Cannes.

Dr. François "Papa Doc" Duvalier died on April 21, 1971 in Port-au-Prince. After 30 years of dictatorial rule the Duvalier dynasty left behind an impoverished and ruined country, with well over half of Haiti's workers unemployed, over 80% of Haitians illiterate, almost a third of Haitian children dying before their fifth birthday, and the lowest per capita annual income in the Caribbean.

"The Great Lion"

Another interesting example of homicidal politics and personal greed is Dr. Hastings Kamuzu Banda, the now deceased dictator of Malawi, who died at the (very) ripe age of 99 years (more or less). It is unclear when he was conceived as no birth registrations were done in rural Africa at that time. Most estimates suggest he was born between 1886 and 1906. He was born to the Chewa tribe in rural Africa and worked several menial jobs prior to moving to America in 1925. After graduating from Central State University in Ohio he studied medicine at Meharry Medical College in Tennessee graduating in 1937. He received a second medical degree from the School of Medicine of the Royal College of Physicians and Surgeons of the University of Edinburgh in 1941. His life was a true "rags to riches" story.

Malawi is a landlocked country in Southeast Africa bounded by Zambia, Tanzania and Mozambique. It is one of the world's least developed countries with a population close to 14 million. Although it has developed something of an agricultural economy over the past several decades, the country depends heavily on outside aid to meet the needs of its many people and support its government. Malawi was first populated during the tenth century by Bantu tribes and remained under native rule until 1891 when it was colonized by the British under the name

Nyasaland. In 1953, Britain merged Nyasaland with Northern and Southern Rhodesia in what was known as the Central African Federation (CAF). This linkage triggered opposition from Africans nationalists including Dr. Hastings Banda who was practicing in Ghana. Despite living abroad for decades, Banda was elected president of the NAC (Nyasaland African Congress) shortly after his return to his homeland. He worked tirelessly to mobilize nationalist sentiment before being jailed by colonial authorities in 1959. He was released in 1960 and subsequently asked to help draft a new Constitution for Nyasaland with a clause granting Africans the majority in the colony's Legislative Counsel. His activism had greatly paid off for his people.

In 1961, Banda's Malawi Congress Party (MCP) gained the majority in the Legislative Counsel and he was elected Prime Minister in 1963. On July 6, 1964, Nyasaland gained independence from British rule and renamed itself Malawi. It was Banda himself who chose the name "Malawi" for the former Nyasaland; he had seen it on an old French map and liked the sound of it. Under a new constitution, Malawi became a single-party state and Banda declared himself president-for-life in 1970. His official title was "His Excellency the Life President of the Republic of Malawi, Ngwazi Dr. Hastings Kamuzu Banda." The title Ngwazi means "Chief of Chiefs" in the Chichewa language or "The Great Lion." Banda became a leader of the pro-Western bloc in Africa and he received support from the West during the Cold War. He generally supported women's rights, improved the country's infrastructure, and maintained a good educational system relative to other African countries. Clearly, he had a lot of potential to be a force for good in the region. He was criticized, however, for maintaining full diplomatic relations with South Africa during Apartheid and he was condemned for his highly repressive regime.

For almost 30 years Banda ruled autocratically, mercilessly suppressing opposition to his party and ensuring that he had no living personal enemies. Malawi became eventually a police state. Mail was opened and often edited. Telephones were tapped and conversations were cut off if anyone said a critical word about the government. Needless to say, overt opposition was not tolerated. Banda actively encouraged the people to report those who criticized him, even if they were relatives. Thousands of Malawians were victimized by being thrown in jail for harboring different political views from the ruling class. Many were confined to detention camps for years on end without being charged or tried in a court of law. Many politicians who fled into exile were pursued by Banda's secret agents, mostly by the notorious Malawi Young Pioneers, and assassinated.

In 1983, a major political activist who opposed Dr. Banda, Attati Mpakati, was killed by a letter bomb in Zimbabwe. Four years earlier Banda had admitted that he had tried to have him killed. That same year, the "Mwanza Four" consisting of three cabinet ministers and a member of Parliament were murdered; officially, they all died in a car accident. Apparently the air bags didn't stop the bullets that, according to witnesses, caused the wounds on their bodies. Not surprisingly, an inquiry was not conducted to establish the circumstances leading to their deaths and no one, not even relatives, was allowed to formally mourn their deaths. The most prominent dissident who perished abroad at the hands of Dr. Banda was journalist and politician Mkwapatira Mhango. He was firebombed together with two of his wives and five of his children in Zambia in 1989. Human rights websites list other instances of imprisonment, repetitive torture, abduction, and murder of Dr. Banda's political enemies.

It was impossible to avoid or ignore Banda during his reign in Malawi. Every business building was required to have an official picture of Banda hanging on the wall, and no poster, clock, or picture could be higher than his image. Before every movie shown in every theater, a video of Banda waving to the people was played with the national anthem streaming in the background. When Banda visited a city, a bevy of women were expected to greet him at the airport and dance for him. A special garment, bearing the president's picture, was the required attire for these performances. Churches were government sanctioned. All movies were first viewed by the Malawi Censorship Board and edited for content as were videotapes (DVDs didn't exist yet for any young readers). Once edited, the movie was given a sticker stating that it was now suitable for viewing and sent back to the owner. Books and magazines were also reviewed. Pages, or parts of pages, were cut out of magazines like *Newsweek* and *Time*. Newspapers and radio broadcasts were tightly controlled and mainly served as outlets for government propaganda. Television was banned. His picture adorned the national currency. If you bought a stamp in Malawi, you were licking the side opposite his head.

Banda's 30 years of leadership were also marked by episodes of extreme, intolerant behavior. For example, after visiting swinging London at the end of the 1960s he decreed that no women in his country should wear mini or even midi skirts nor should they appear in public wearing trousers. Men were forbidden to grow their hair long or sprout beards or moustaches which were seen as signs of rebellious behavior. Men could be seized and forced to have a haircut at the discretion of border officials or the police. Kissing in public was not allowed and movies which contained kissing scenes were censored. Foreigners who broke any of these rules were often "PI'ed" (declared Prohibited Immigrants and deported). In many ways, he created an ultraconservative utopia. His regime also strongly discouraged the teaching of pre-Banda history and many books on these subjects were burned. Dr. Banda also attempted to eradicate the culture of Northern African tribes such as the Tumbuka.

All adult citizens were required to be members of the MCP. Party cards had to be carried at all times and had to be presented at random police inspections. The cards were sold to the citizens at substantial profits by Banda's Malawi Youth Pioneers. In some cases, these youths even sold cards for unborn children and pocketed the cash. When the good doctor travelled around the country he did so in full presidential style with a cavalcade of cars with sirens, flashing lights and motorcycle escorts. All other commuters were supposed to stop their cars immediately, get out, and wave. Anyone who failed to stop before the first of the motorcyclists reached them had to answer charges of contempt and breach of security. The penalties ranged from a fine of 10 shillings to 10,000 pounds with jail sentences for locals and deportation for foreigners. The official tourist guide included a warning that if anyone ·entered the country with the purpose of overthrowing his regime, they would be "cut to ribbons and fed to the crocodiles." Tourism was not a major source of revenue for Malawi.

Under international pressure Banda agreed to a referendum in 1993 resulting in the formation of multiparty democracy and free elections in 1994. A new Constitution was written and Banda's "life presidency" came to an end when he lost his bid for re-election by a landslide. On November 25, 1997, Dr. Hastings Banda died in a Johannesburg clinic.

Dr. Banda legacy's includes several bright spots in spite of his dictatorial style and ruthless conduct. He created academic and economic opportunities for women and encouraged them to participate in all aspects of public life. Banda also did much for the country's infrastructure including the construction of major roads, airports, hospitals and schools. He founded Kamuzu Academy, a school modeled on Eton, at which Malawian children were taught Latin and Classical Greek. The country also made great economic strides during his term of office and its agricultural exports blossomed. While in office, Banda created a business empire that eventually produced one-third of the country's gross domestic product and employed 10% of the wage-earning workforce. He also accumulated at least $320 million in personal assets. Not bad, even for a doctor.

Chapter 14
Trading Treatment for Terror

Everybody hates death, fears death. But only those, the believers
who know the life after death and the reward after death,
would be the ones who will be seeking death.

– British terrorist Dr. Mohamed Atta

There are actually hundreds of definitions of terrorism and cynics have claimed that "one man's terrorist is another man's hero." Terrorists seem particularly fond of this definition. However, it seems more reasonable to rely on the 2004 definition of terrorism adopted by the United Nations Security Council: "Criminal acts, including against civilians, committed with the intent to cause death or serious bodily injury, or taking of hostages, with the purpose to provoke a state of terror in the general public or in a group of persons or particular persons, intimidate a population or compel a government or an international organization to do or to abstain from doing any act." Similarly, on March 17, 2005 a UN panel defined terrorism as any act: "Intended to cause death or serious bodily harm to civilians or non-combatants with the purpose of intimidating a population or compelling a government or an international organization to do or abstain from doing any act." These definitions make it fairly clear that terrorists are not heroes.

Intense nationalism and religious extremism, alone or in combination, have engendered terrorism in many corners of the modern world. Organizations such as the Irish Republican Army (IRA), the Basque separatists in Spain, Jewish groups such as the Irgun and Lehi in pre-Israeli Palestine, Palestinian Arab groups such as Hamas, and various extremist Islamic groups, particularly Hizballah and al-Qaeda, are considered terrorist groups (except, of course, by their members). In the past two decades, however, extremist Islamic groups have unquestionably become the dominant organizations behind terroristic attacks both in terms of the number of people murdered and frequency of incidents. Furthermore, they have been virtually the only organizations in which physicians have played a prominent role both directly and indirectly in terroristic activities. It is legitimate to ask, "Why are the majority of terrorists currently of the Islamic faith and why are some physicians of this faith attracted to terrorism?"

Some have argued that Islam is inherently violent and that it aspires to conquer and dominate the entire world. Others have denied such a negative viewpoint pointing out that hundreds of millions of Muslims throughout the world are peaceful and are not involved in terrorism or violence. The truth is that most Muslims are peaceful, law-abiding citizens and that Muslim extremists have a tendency to be intolerant of other religions or cultures and may resort to terrorism. They likely see the excesses of Western society ("sex, drugs, and rock and roll") as an affront to Allah and the eradication of this plague is a service to the remainder of humanity. Also, from a historical perspective, maybe it's just their turn to be the bad guys. The behavior of Christians during the Crusades and Jews in portions of the Old Testament seems just as intolerant and barbaric as the crimes of modern day Muslim extremists. And remember that Muslims are not always the murderers; thousands of Muslims in Serbia/Croatia were the victims of ethnic cleansing just a few years ago. Only the Buddhists seem to really get along with everybody and everything.

Islamic terrorists, at least the ones involved in major attacks, are generally well-educated. Unfortunately for us, anti-Western philosophy and religious extremism are built into the curriculum of select Muslim schools. From an early age, bright children are taught to read, write, memorize the Koran, pray, and hate Americans. Following this sound fundamental training, many of the gifted students attend college, either at home or abroad, and may progress to graduate school. Resultantly, the Islamic education system creates very sophisticated individuals who have been brainwashed since kindergarten. No other religion, at present, stresses the importance of education combined with intolerance as Islam. It should then serve as no surprise that college graduates, including physicians, have served as suicide-bombers, cyber-terrorists, masterminds, organizers, and fundraisers in extremist terrorist organizations. Despite years of training designed to alleviate suffering and heal the sick, Muslim physicians are not immune from radical Islamic beliefs and all that goes with them.

Physicians on the Front Lines

It is quite rare to find physicians who directly perform terrorist acts. Nevertheless, in 2007 Great Britain was greatly dismayed when it uncovered an alleged eight-member Islamic terror group consisting of four physicians, a Ph.D. in mechanical engineering, two medical students, and a medical technician. Several of the suspects were related to each other and most were employed in hospitals run by Britain's National Health Service. The Service did (and still does) rely on foreign doctors to meet staffing shortfalls. In fact, of the almost 240,000 British doctors registered with the General Medical Council, more than a third of them trained in countries other than England including many thousands from Islamic countries.

Dr. Bilal Talal Abdulla, a 27-year-old British physician, was at the center of the alleged conspiracy. He was born in Aylesbury, a pleasant city in Buckinghamshire not far from London. He spent his formative years, however, in the swarming streets of Baghdad where he was taught to intensely hate the West. He came from an ultra-conservative Muslim family that practiced Sharia law, the stringent

Islamic rules dating back to the sixth century. Abdulla's views were so extreme that his mother did not dare to take her scarf off in his presence even when he was just a schoolboy. By the time he had graduated from medical school in 2004, his extremist views had sharpened considerably. He was incensed by the U.S. and British invasion of Iraq and the subsequent Western occupation of his country. One of his professors, Ahmed Ali, of the University of Baghdad College of Medicine said that Abdulla was one of his most vociferous students. "He didn't care about his studies. He only cared about the resistance," he recalled, "many times in class he interrupted to talk about the Mujahedeen. I thought he was crazy. But we couldn't do anything in 2003 and 2004 because the resistance was controlling everything, including the university." Abdulla graduated as a physician in Iraq in 2004 and qualified to work in Britain in August 2006. As he had extended family members in Cambridge, Abdulla completed part of his training at the city's renowned Addenbrooke Hospital.

Abdulla was a "strictly observant Muslim" known for being knowledgeable about the Koran and his ability to read Arabic. During his time in Cambridge he was also linked to the radical Muslim group Hizb ut-Tahir. Shiraz Maher, a former member of the group, said: "He was certainly very angry about what was happening in Iraq. He supported the insurgency. He loudly cheered the deaths of British and American troops. But to say it was just all about Iraq or foreign policy is mistaken. It feeds off a much wider ideological infrastructure." Abdulla reportedly once berated a Muslim roommate for not being devout enough and allegedly showed him a gruesome video of a beheading, warning him that the same fate could befall him if he was not more committed to his faith. He allegedly had a number of videos of Abu Musab al Zarqawi, al-Qaeda's leader in Iraq, who recently was killed in a gunfight with American troops.

Years earlier in Jordan, the young Abdulla had met Mohammed Asha, a Saudi Arabian national, who was to become a skilled brain surgeon and his closest friend. When recruited into the terrorist plot, Asha allegedly joined Abdulla's group. Abdulla had also become close to Dr. Kafeel Ahmed, an Indian physician who willingly joined the conspiracy. A few other extremists rounded out the cadre. The attack plan was developed by Dr. Abdulla, Dr. Kafeel Ahmed, and mechanical engineer Mohammed Asha in 2004–2005 at the Islamic Academy Charitable Trust in Cambridge. The three decided to carry out terror attacks out of revenge and as a "punishment" for the British Middle East policy of "persecution of Muslims" and for Britain's role in the war in Iraq. Abdulla and Ahmed rented a house in Houston, a pretty village in Renfrewshire, 5 minutes from the Glasgow airport which was to be one of their targets. On May 28, 2007 Abdulla traveled to Heathrow Airport to meet Ahmed, who had flown in from Mumbai (former Bombay), India. The two men drove in a rental car to Asha's home in Newcastle-under-Lyme for further discussion and refinement of their plans. Potential targets in London included the Old Bailey, the center of town, and the West End. On June 2–3, the conspirators bought three Mercedes, a BMW and a Jeep via Auto Trader magazine from different sellers in five different cities in order to avoid raising suspicions. A few days later Abdulla and Ahmed bought gas canisters, nails, gas cans and mobile phones to use in car bombs from several different shops in Glasgow, Leeds, Preston, Dunfermline, Edinburgh and Blackburn.

On June 28, 2007, Abdulla and Ahmed drove to London in two brand new Mercedes sedans armed with car bombs consisting of gas cylinders and nails concealed under duvets and pillows. They parked the cars, one blue the other green, near the "Tiger Tiger" nightclub in the West End of London. The club was packed at the time with more than 500 people, mostly young revelers. The two men, who had stopped to fill their cars with "as much fuel as possible" on the way, opened the valves on the gas cylinders and retreated to "a safe distance." Although this was a well thought out plan, as everyone knows, perfect planning does not always result in perfect execution (literally). At around 1:30 AM on June 29, 2007 the two men tried to detonate the car bombs by calling the mobile phones inside the cars which had been rigged up to home-made detonators. Fortunately for the intended victims, the car bombs failed to detonate and the two terrorists decided to abandon their non-cooperative vehicles. After dumping the cars the two men fled by catching separate rickshaws before rendezvousing and returning to Scotland. The car bombs were discovered smoking but intact several hours after the botched attempt. A responding fireman, Andrew Shaw, unlocked the driver's door and put his head inside and saw a large gas canister wedged behind a seat. "The bottom of it was facing me and the nozzle and valve would be in the middle of the car," he testified later, "I tried to get it out but I couldn't." He eventually yanked it out with brute force only then discovering a mass of nails and other shrapnel in the bottom of the car. "It was one of those moments when everything falls in to place in a matter of seconds," he stated, "I was a little bit annoyed with myself that it didn't occur to me sooner … On the centre console there was at least one, possibly two, mobile phones and wires coming from the phone and at that point it doesn't take long for the penny to drop." The device was soon defused by a Metropolitan Police explosives officers and an intense investigation was immediately started.

It was clear to the conspirators that they had little time left before the police would be able to trace the cars back to them but they were deeply committed not to fail again. On June 30 Abdulla and Ahmed drove back to Glasgow and attempted to carry out a car bomb suicide attack on Glasgow Airport by ramming their Jeep Cherokee into the main doors of the terminal building. The vehicle was later described as a "mobile fire bomb" packed with ten gas containers, four oil containers and a number of glass bottles, some with wicks attached to create "Molotov cocktails." True to form for the amateur terrorists, the Jeep got stuck in the door of the airport prior to causing any significant damage. Undeterred, Kafeel Ahmed then reversed the car and with the engine revving and tires screeching made a number of further attempts to crash through the doors. He repeatedly struck the pillars or door frame until the vehicle became inextricably trapped. These guys may have been brain surgeons but they weren't rocket scientists.

Despite their entrapment, the men continued to shout "Allahu Akbar" ("God is great") throughout the assault. They smashed the gas-filled bottles in the vehicle in an effort to detonate the mobile bomb to no avail. The car did eventually burst into flames but did not explode. Ahmed got out of the vehicle but was immediately engulfed in flames. Police and members of the public tried to extinguish the fire but Ahmed, though himself alight, tried to obstruct them by punching and kicking at them. He was eventually handcuffed and arrested after being tear-gassed. He died days later with burns over 90% of his head and body at the Royal Alexandra Hospital where he had worked for the prior 3 months. Abdulla survived with no serious injuries. When police later searched the home of Mohammed Asha they reportedly found a poem written in the first person amounting to a pledge of allegiance to "Osama", presumably bin Laden.

The surviving alleged ringleaders of the conspiracy, Abdulla and Asha, were arrested and put on trial but plead not guilty. Abdulla claimed he never intended to kill or injure anyone but was simply taking part in a protest, a defense dismissed as "ludicrous" by the prosecution. Asha, a senior house officer in the neurology department of University Hospital of North Staffordshire, was not accused of being directly involved in either attack but was indicted for supplying money to buy the cars and bomb components and providing "spiritual and ideological guidance." After describing in great detail the unfolding of the attacks, the prosecutor, Jonathan Laidlaw QC (Queen's Counsel) stated at the trial that "these men were intent on committing murder on an indiscriminate and a whole scale level." Laidlaw emphasized that the most shocking aspect of the case was that the plot was carried out by two physicians. "Apart from the shocking nature of the activity these two defendants were engaged in, the extraordinary thing about this case is that both men are doctors," Mr. Laidlaw said. He continued, that these two well trained practitioners had "… turned their attention away from the treating of illness to the planning of murder." On December 16, 2008, Abdulla was sentenced to at least 32 years of imprisonment. Asha was found "not guilty" on all counts.

The British experience with terrorist doctors was not an isolated event. In September 2005, Coalition forces in Iraq captured Anis 'Abd-al-Razaq' Ali Muhammad, also known as Dr. Sa'ad or Dr. Anis. Dr. Sa'ad was a senior member of al-Qaeda in Baghdad as well as one of the terrorist organization's key "physicians." He was a pharmacist by training who was also acting as a medical doctor, treating wounded terrorists in and around the Baghdad area. Coalition forces also captured Mazen Mahdi Salih Mahdi Khudayr, also known as Dr. Mazen or Dr. Layth. In addition to being a leading arms dealer for the terrorist group, this physician was also attempting to open a clinic to treat wounded terrorists in Iraq. Additional doctors are still working for al-Qaeda.

The Fort Hood Massacre

In the early afternoon of November 5, 2009, Dr. Nidal Hasan, a 39 year-old psychiatrist and active duty major in the U.S. Army, conducted a terrorist attack on Fort Hood, Texas. Unprovoked and shouting in Arabic "Allahu Akbar" ("God is Great"), he began shooting fellow soldiers in a crowded medical processing center with two concealed guns which he had smuggled on post. Before being wounded by two brave, civilian police officers, he succeeded in killing 13 people and wounding another 29 innocent souls. This terrorist attack shocked the nation; the crime was committed on U.S. soil (a major Army post no less!) by an Army officer. And a doctor.

Government officials, including President Obama and the high brass of the Army, worried about a possible backlash against American Muslims and Army personnel who practiced Islam. They advised the stunned American public not to jump to conclusions about what may have prompted the cowardly attack. Initially such caution was clearly understandable, but as additional information started to flow in about the assassin, his background and behavior, and the detailed circumstances of the massacre, the motivation of the attacks became quite clear. He was an Islamic extremist who had been in contact with al-Qaeda operatives. And the government may have been aware of this prior to the attack. Let the Senate Hearings begin!

Nidal Malik Hasan was born in Arlington, Virginia on September 8, 1970, the oldest son of a Palestinian immigrant couple who had moved to America from a small West Bank Palestinian town, near Jerusalem. Hasan graduated from Roanoke's William Fleming High School in 1988 and, soon thereafter enlisted in the U.S. Army over his parents' objections. The Army subsequently covered the expenses of his college education and he graduated with honors from Virginia Tech with a bachelor's degree in biochemistry.

After graduation, he entered the officer basic training program at Fort Sam Houston in Texas then went on to medical school at the Uniformed Services University of Health Sciences with taxpayers footing all the bills. He earned an M.D. degree then completed his internship and residency in psychiatry at Walter Reed Hospital in Washington, DC. In 2007 he began a 2-year fellowship in preventive and disaster psychiatry in Bethesda, Maryland, while earning a master's degree in public health. His teachers described him as being beset with personal and professional problems and requiring quite intensive help. Nevertheless in May 2009, after completing his training, he was promoted from captain to major. Two months later he was transferred to Fort Hood, the Army's largest active duty military post in the United States, home to more than 50,000 military personnel and another 150,000 family members and other civilians. It is a city unto itself.

Unlike many physicians completing their training, Hasan was not in financial straits when he arrived at Fort Hood. His college and medical school had been paid for by the Army and, rather than earning the pittance offered to residents in civilian training programs, Hasan was paid well as an Army officer while in residency. Though he did not owe anyone any money for his training, he owed the Army an active duty commitment as payback. It is a very fair deal. Military scholarships allow many people of limited financial means the opportunity to become physicians – one of the authors of this work can attest to that.

Nonetheless, Hassan wanted out of the Army badly. His motivations to leave the service included his firsthand experience with war casualties as a resident at Walter Reed Hospital, the horror stories he heard from veterans with post-traumatic stress disorder (PTSD) that he treated, his opposition to the wars in Iraq and Afghanistan, his uneasiness about fighting his Muslim brethren, and feelings that he was being harassed by other military members for his religion. As if he wasn't miserable enough, he was about to enter his personal version of Hell as he was scheduled to deploy to the Middle East in the near future.

Many physicians who serve in the military wish they were civilians. Countless appeals have been made to Congress, the President and God himself to spare physicians of their active duty commitments. Although some military doctors have pulled some outlandish, unethical stunts to get out of the service, none had chosen mass murder as a means of escape. There had to be something different about Nidal that led him to act the way he did. That something may well be Islamic extremism.

Nidal immersed himself in Islam after the death of his parents (his father died in 1998, his mother in 2001). His religious intensity markedly increased and he was a regular in the local mosque. According to his uncle, he spent much of his free time absorbed in the reading of Islamic texts. Hasan was particularly attentive not to miss any of the five daily required Islamic prayers and devotedly attended Mosque services as early as 5:00 in the morning, often in military uniform. When off duty he used to be dressed either in military clothing or in a white Arabic aba, a loose sleeveless outer garment. None of this is a crime and, in fact, this type of devotion to God is admirable.

Hasan sought to meet a mate who shared his religious beliefs, but met with no success. In a form that Nidal filled out in an attempt to find a match, he identified himself as a Palestinian (although he was a born American) and in his list of pre-ferred nationalities for a possible match he listed in descending order a Palestinian Muslim woman, an Arabic one, an Indian or Pakistani lady, a European Muslim and, at the very end of the list, an American woman. This rank order may be indica-tive of a deep bias against Americanized Islam. Although there was no lack of interested Muslim women willing to meet and marry a doctor, Nabil failed in his quest as none met his exacting religious specifications. In parallel with his deep devotion to Islamic religious practices, Hasan apparently drifted toward militant Islamic beliefs and religious extremism.

A former classmate in the master's degree program recalled that in 2008, Major Hasan gave a rather inappropriate political presentation at Walter Reed Medical Center entitled "Why the War on Terror is a War on Islam." To say that this was contrary to the official position of the U.S. Army is an understatement. In this lec-ture he reportedly stated: "It's getting harder and harder for Muslims in the service to morally justify being in a military that seems constantly engaged against fellow Muslims." In the lecture he also warned the audience of senior Army physicians that in order to avoid "adverse events," the military should allow Muslim soldiers to be released as conscientious objectors instead of compelling them to fight in wars against other Muslims. A number of students complained to their professors about Nidal's behavior, including blatantly anti-American statements and his obvious admiration of suicide bombers, but no action was ever taken against him. We now tragically know what Dr. Hasan considers an adverse event.

In late July 2009, Major Hasan moved into a small, run-down, scantily furnished, one-bedroom apartment in a poor section of Killeen, Texas adjacent to Fort Hood. This part of Texas is great for performing maneuvers in tanks and exploding ordnance – it is not a great vacation destination. His neighbors described him as being a friendly but rather lonely man who kept very much to himself. Major Hasan's duties at Fort Hood included the psychiatric assessment of soldiers before deployment.

A few days after renting his apartment, Major Hasan bought an FN Herstal 5.7-mm pistol at a popular local weapons store for more than a thousand dollars. Guns Galore, was conveniently located midway between the base and the Islamic Community of Greater Killeen mosque, which he began attending in early September 2009. Osman Danquah, the co-founder of the mosque, recalled that Nidal had asked him how he should counsel young Muslim soldiers who object to the war. Danquah, a retired sergeant and a veteran of Persian Gulf War, told him that unless they were applying for discharge as conscious objectors, voluntary soldiers must honor their obligation and do their job. Danquah also told Dr, Hasan that there was something wrong with him, though he could not quite put his finger on it.

In late October 2009, less than 2 weeks before his murderous rampage, Major Hasan took leave of Syed Ahmed Ali, the imam of the Greater Killeen mosque, deceptively stating that he was leaving for Virginia to be with his family. On Wednesday, November 4, the day before the shooting, Major Hasan gave a neighbor all of his belongings including a Koran, bags of vegetables, a mattress, clothing, and odds and ends from his almost bare one-room flat. He told her that he will not need them as he was to be deployed to Iraq or Afghanistan. On the eve of the shooting he had dinner with Duane Reasoner, an 18-year-old Muslim who prayed at his mosque and whom he befriended, at the Golden Corral, their favorite restaurant. Reasoner said that this was the first time that their discussion veered away from the religious discussions that they usually had into politics. Mr. Reasoner recalled that Major Hasan was visibly upset and "he didn't want to go to Afghanistan. He felt he was supposed to quit (the military). In the Koran, it says you are not supposed to have alliances with Jews or Christians, and if you are killed in the military fighting against Muslims, you will go to Hell."

In the early morning of the next day, Dr. Nidal Malik Hasan left his apartment at 6:00 AM to attend prayers at the brick mosque near Fort Hood. After the prayers, he said goodbye to his friends and asked forgiveness from one man for any past offenses. "I'm going traveling," he reportedly told a fellow worshiper, giving him a hug. "I won't be here tomorrow." He then went to buy some things at a nearby convenience store where a security camera captured him wearing traditional, white, Arab clothing and a white cap at the counter at about 6:20.

Around 1:00 PM Major Hasan walked into a processing center at Fort Hood where soldiers were getting medical attention before being deployed overseas. He had shed his Arab garb and was now wearing his camouflage battle dress uniform. According to witnesses, at first he sat quietly at an empty table. At about 1:20 PM he bowed his head for several seconds, as if in prayer, stood up, and drew a firearm while shouting "Allahu Akbar." He then opened fire on the unarmed crowd.

He systematically circled the room, sparing some people while firing point blank on others several times. In all, he fired more than 100 rounds. The room became a chamber of horrors with the floor soaked with blood, survivors hiding behind flimsy tables and chairs, and dead or wounded victims slumped over chairs or lying motionless on the floor. All but one of the dead were soldiers.

Two responding civilian police officers, Sgt. Kimberly D. Munley and Senior Sgt. Mark Todd, arrived at the scene and found Major Hasan chasing a wounded soldier outside the building. They engaged the assailant and in the exchange of fire, Hasan received multiple gunshot wounds and was disabled. Munley was also hit several times. There is some controversy as to which officer felled the assailant, but this is largely academic (except for the fact that this must be figured out prior to the made-for-television movie). The fact is both are heroes and their quick actions saved additional lives. The incident was over at 1:27 PM. The entire carnage took only 7 minutes.

Hasan was transported to a local hospital where he was placed on life support apparatus. Eventually he recovered consciousness, but was left paralyzed from the waist down from his wounds. In this particular case, being wheelchair bound will likely not engender much sympathy from a jury when he goes to trial.

The military authorities and the FBI started an immediate investigation into the horrendous attack. On November 12, 2009, 1 week after the killings, Major Hasan was charged by the Army with 13 counts of premeditated murder of 12 military personnel and one civilian. He can face the death penalty on each count. The mass media conducted its own investigation into the background of the accused and the circumstances leading up to the attack, producing a wealth of mostly accurate information. Although some stations offered a "fair and balanced" assessment of the situation, other agencies appeared to tow a more politically correct line. At the risk of upsetting some readers, we have placed Dr. Hasan in the chapter on terrorists and we believe our position is very defensible. Like other terrorists in this chapter, he fits the profile of an Islamic extremist.

Consider the fact that he identified himself as a Palestinian rather than as an American, though he was born here. His bitter complaints to other worshippers at his mosque about the "oppression" of Muslims in America speak volumes about his ideological and religious identity. Hasan also allegedly placed militant Islamic messages on the Internet. In one posting ascribed to the physician, he compared the heroism of a soldier who throws himself on a grenade to protect fellow soldiers to the suicide bombers who sacrifice themselves to protect Islam. In addition, allegedly Hasan "once gave a lecture to other doctors in which he said non-believers should be beheaded and have boiling oil poured down their throats" and actually "was attempting to make contact with people associated with al Qaeda." Interestingly, a search of Hasan's apartment several days after the shootings found a box of his business cards that bore Hasan's full name, his medical specialty (psychiatry), and the initials SoA. Several sources have suggested that this may signify "Soldier of Allah," a name that prominent al-Qaeda recruiter Anwar Awlaki uses to address his disciples. Of note, Hasan allegedly had emailed Awlaki at least 20 times. Alternatively, he may have placed SoA on his card because he was a fan of the Muslim rap group Soldiers of Allah out of Los Angeles. We just report, you decide.

One obvious question is: "How could the military have ignored all of these red flags?" One possibility is that, based on personal experience, there is a tendency for senior military officers to overlook the flaws of personnel under their supervision if disciplinary procedures may make their own lives more difficult. Colonels in particular do not like to "rock the boat" by launching investigations into the behavior of their junior officers. Doing so can adversely affect their chances of becoming generals or coasting into a smooth, honorable retirement. So if a senior officer can look the other way when an Army resident states that he admires the "single mind-edness of purpose" of the shooters at Columbine High School or a junior officer can get away with giving forensic pathology lectures while wearing a butcher's apron over his uniform, are we really surprised that Hasan's disturbing activities were brushed under the rug?

Granted, Dr. Hasan's situation was more grave than the ones described above and it defies logic that something was not done. Recently NPR (National Public Radio) reported that two psychiatrists who had worked closely with the gunman at Walter Reed stated that he could be belligerent and belittle colleagues without provocation. "When I heard the news about Hasan, honestly, my first thought was, 'That makes a lot of sense. That completely fits the person I knew.'" Another individual familiar with Major Hasan emphatically stated that he would not trust Hasan to be in a war in the same foxhole with him. Clearly there was something the matter with the doctor that was bad for morale.

Let's assume for a moment that Dr. Hasan was just unpleasant to work with and the aforementioned statements merely represent the subjective impressions of two colleagues. Is there anything more concrete that should have been acted on? Well, there were the email exchanges with Anwar Awlaki, the al Qaeda recruiter. These associations were apparently explained away as necessary for Hasan's psychiatric research on the attitudes of Muslim soldiers at war with other Muslims. Interestingly, days after Major Hasan's murders Awlaki praised him as a "hero" and a "man of conscience" stating: " The only way a Muslim could Islamically justify serving as a soldier in the U.S. Army is if his intention is to follow the footsteps of men like Nidal." Sort of sounds like they were on the same page.

There was also Hasan's attendance at the Dar Al-Hijrah Islamic Center in Falls Church, Virginia in 1991, a mosque which had been the haven of three of the 9/11 bombers. Granted, attending this mosque is not a crime and many devout Muslims worship there. But given the circumstances in this case, one must wonder who Dr. Hasan chose to lay his mat next to.

The Massacre at Fort Hood may have significant implications for Muslims serving in the military. Dr. Hasan's rampage may well incite harassment against Muslims serving in the armed forces and increase the stress they are already under. It may also result in subtle racial profiling manifested by covert background checks and invasions of the privacy of certain racial and religious groups serving in the Army, Navy, Air Force and Marines. It will be a great misfortune if innocent soldiers, air-men, sailors, and officers are marginalized because of the extremism of this one disgruntled, disillusioned, and misguided psychiatrist. On the other hand, one must wonder if there are other terrorists serving in the armed forces at home or abroad willing to commit treason for their religious beliefs. If this one doctor killed or wounded over 40 people in 7 minutes with a couple of handguns; what could a sleeper terrorist cell of four or five of our own soldiers do to the rest of their unit during a battle against al-Qaeda warriors?

Doctors as Terrorist Leaders

Some physicians have traded the gratitude of patients, financial well-being, and preferential social standing for leadership positions in terrorist groups. Dr. Ayman Muhammad Rabaie al-Zawahiri (1951–), an Egyptian surgeon by training, is unquestionably the foremost figure among doctor-terrorists. As a leading member of al-Qaeda (the number two man, after Osama bin Laden) he has masterminded many of its terror operations. He has been referred to as the "real brains" of al-Qaeda by bin Laden's biographer no less! Dr. al-Zawahiri enrolled in his first fanatical group, the Muslim Brotherhood in Egypt, when he was only 14. This is not surprising as racial, ethnic, and religious hatred is virtually always a home-grown product and al-Zawahiri's father, Dr. Mohammad Rabi al-Zawahiri, was also a Muslim Brotherhood enthusiastic follower. The younger al-Zawahiri managed to complete medical school in between episodes of terrorist attacks and prison.

In his elective time, he directed a number of rebellions designed to overthrow the secular Egyptian government. He eventually joined Islamic Jihad, which assassinated Egyptian president Anwar Sadat in 1981, and he spent time in prison on charges related to that murder. After Sadat's death, Islamic Jihad split and Dr. al-Zawahiri became the leader of one of the splinter groups. Hard pressure from the Egyptian government forced him to seek refuge in Afghanistan where he met and worked closely with his future commander and friend Osama bin Laden. In the early 1990s al-Zawahiri was smuggled into United Stated under a false name and succeeded in raising more than half a million dollars for his terror organization. In 1998, the doctor engineered the simultaneous bombings of U.S. embassies in the East African capitals of Dar es Salaam (Tanzania) and Nairobi (Kenya) in which hundreds of people were killed. Zawahiri was sentenced to death in absentia by an Egyptian military tribunal in 1999 for his role in the 1997 "Luxor Massacre" in which 58 foreign tourists and four Egyptians were gunned down or hacked to death. The United States is currently offering a reward of $25 million for information leading to his arrest.

There are other physicians, including many Palestinians, who occupy important positions of leadership in terror organizations including:

- Dr. Abu Hafiza is another high-level al-Qaeda operative. A Moroccan psychiatrist, he was the mastermind behind al-Qaeda's devastating terror attacks in Spain in that left 191 dead and almost 2,000 injured on March 11, 2004. He was hoping that this attack would be such a blow to the European psyche that a "domino effect" would ensue leading to the removal of several Western leaders including

Britain's Tony Blair. Although this phase of his plan didn't quite work out, 3 days after the bombings Spain elected a new Prime Minister and all of their troops were removed from Iraq within 3 months. He also provided "counseling" to the 9/11 killers.

- Dr. Abdel Aziz al-Rantisi, a Palestinian pediatrician, was the co-founder and spiritual leader of the militant Palestinian organization, Hamas. He was targeted and killed by an air-to-ground Israeli missile.
- Dr. Mahmoud al-Zahar, an Egyptian-trained surgeon born to an Egyptian mother and a Palestinian father, is also a Hamas co-founder and leader. He was appointed Foreign Minister of the Gaza strip region controlled by Hamas in 2006 by Prime Minister Ismail Haniyeh. He has stated in the past that he would like to see the Gaza strip become "Hamaston." Some sources suggest he became the leader of Hamas after Ahmed Yassin was assassinated in 2004 but the organization would not confirm this rumor out of fear of Israeli reprisals. He also teaches medical students.
- Dr. Fathi Abd al-Aziz Shiqaqi (1951–1995), co-founded the Palestinian Islamic Jihad (PIJ) faction in the early 1970s, was also a pediatrician. He was an early advocate of and creative genius behind suicide bombings. In the 1990s he repetitively visited Libyan leader Muammar al-Gaddafi who promised to help finance Shaqaqi's group. He was also financially supported by Iraq and Hizballah. In 1995, a lone man (probably an agent of Mossad, Israel's Secret Service) walked up to Shaqaqi as he was returning to his hotel in Malta and shot him with a gun equipped with a silencer. Over 40,000 people attended his funeral.
- Dr. George Habash, a pediatrician and Christian Palestinian, founded and served as chief of the Popular Front for the Liberation of Palestine (PFLP), an influential group second only to Yassar Arafat's Fattah movement. His group created and mastered the tactic of skyjacking for political gains. The PFLP's first major success was the hijacking of an El Al plane in 1968. Two years later, he masterminded the hijackings of four Western airliners over the United States, Europe, the Far East and the Persian Gulf. The aircraft were blown up after the passengers and crews were forced to disembark. Perhaps his medical training resulted in this unusual act of compassion for a terrorist. Dr. Habash was also behind the hijacking of an Air France plane to Uganda which was resolved after Israeli commandos stormed the airport in Entebbe. Fortunately, he died of a heart attack in 2008 in Amman, Jordan and is no longer practicing.
- Dr. Wadih Haddad was second-in command to Dr. Habash in the PFLP and worked out many of the details of its terrorist operations. Little is known about his background. The famed assassin and terrorist "Carlos the Jackal" worked closely with Haddad and the PFLP to perpetrate skyjackings and other terrorist attacks. The 1968 skyjacking of the El Al flight by PFLP was Haddad's debut on the terrorist scene. Haddad also planned the assassinations of several of the Arab world's oil ministers including the Saudi Arabian Oil Minister. He died of cancer in East Berlin in 1978.

The world is apparently fated to suffer the scourges of terrorism for many years to come. We do not have and we cannot devise a reasonable way to deal with the terrorist problem because with extremists *their way is the only way*. Negotiations and diplomacy simply don't work with people who are committed to killing you even if it means killing themselves. This does not mean that we cannot take measures to protect ourselves. Western governments can make determined efforts to uproot centers of hateful indoctrination, punish their proponents, deny any funding to terror organizations or countries, and dedicate staff and money to developing means of detecting terroristic activities. Weakness is not an option against these folks. Doctor-terrorists will continue to surface, particularly in countries that combine education with religious fanaticism. These physicians will kill more people in a fraction of a second than any other doctor will save in a lifetime.

Chapter 15
Guilty Until Proven Innocent

> *Saints should always be judged guilty until they are proved*
> *innocent.*
>
> – George Orwell

The Sam Sheppard case may never be resolved. Based solely on the final outcome of his appeal, however, it would appear that he may have been unjustly accused of murder. He was not the first nor will he be the last physician to suffer this ignominy. As recently as 2005 one such case caught the national spotlight.

Katrina and Dr. Pou

Hurricane Katrina was the costliest and one of the top five most devastating storms in the history of the United States. After crossing Florida as a category 1 hurricane, the newly christened Katrina gained strength over the waters of the Gulf of Mexico and then slightly weakened before making a second landfall in Southeast Louisiana. The most severe loss of life and property damage occurred in New Orleans, Louisiana which was extensively flooded after the levee system catastrophically failed. Eventually 80% of the city and much of the neighboring parishes were inundated with floodwaters that lingered for weeks. At least 1,836 people lost their lives during the hurricane and in the subsequent floods making it the deadliest U.S. hurricane since the unnamed 1928 Okeechobee Hurricane. The storm was estimated to have caused damages exceeding $81 billion dollars. All levels of government, federal, state, and local, inexcusably failed to provide effective and prompt help. For days dead bodies were decomposing in the infested waters, residents were trapped in their flooded homes, and hospital patients had to wait for a belated evacuation in sweltering heat, without electricity and with little drinkable water. This is the background against which homicide charges were brought against Dr. Marie Anne Pou, a respected ear, nose, and throat surgeon, and two hospital nurses.

Born in 1956 into a family that included a number of physicians, Marie Anne Pou was exposed early to the challenges of medical practice. She and her siblings often accompanied their father on weekend house calls and were impressed by his skills and sensitive contact with patients. It is not difficult to understand why Pou decided quite early in her life to be a doctor. Her Katrina saga started as a routine weekend with Anna heading to work at New Orleans Memorial Hospital. Hurricane Katrina appeared heading for Florida and although warnings were issued for New Orleans there did not appear to be a real threat. Dr. Pou decided to stay with her patients and ride out the storm if it reached them. It did and the rest is history.

After the storm had passed on Monday August 29, 2005 the hospital administration prematurely congratulated itself on not having had the hospital evacuated. While they celebrated, the levees were collapsing. By Tuesday, water was rising in the streets eventually reaching a depth of 10 ft. The hospital basement flooded and the generators failed. When nightfall came, the hospital and the city were enveloped in darkness. Water pressure dropped, toilets backed up and the temperature began to rise. The deteriorating situation had dire consequences. Pou later said the hospital staff struggled to climb stairwells, carry supplies, and spent 2-hour shifts squeezing ventilators to keep patients alive. "The heat was so terrible, it wore you down," Pou said. "We were trying to keep the patients comfortable. The 9 year-old daughter of one of the nurses even took shifts fanning them." Airboats evacuated some patients and babies from the nursery but most remained. About seven medical staffers, including Dr. Pou, stayed with the patients. "Tuesday night was when we realized we were going to be there for a while," Pou said. All she could do was to keep critically ill patients comfortable. The staff gathered supplies, rationed food and water, and prayed. Under the military's orders, the staff initiated reverse triage. Instead of addressing the needs of the sickest patients, the healthiest ones were taken out first in an effort to save the greatest number of people. Many had to be carried to the roof. It was slow, backbreaking work with as many as ten people struggling up the dark stairs with a stretcher. At least 34 people died waiting for rescuers. Pou was one of the last to leave Memorial Hospital. She returned to New Orleans – her house had not been flooded – from Baton Rouge a few months later at Thanksgiving. In January 2006 she started working at a Baton Rouge hospital, trying to put Katrina behind her. Many felt she was a heroine.

In July 2006, she was greeted by four police officers upon her arrival home from a 13-hour day of surgery. They handcuffed her, still in her scrubs, and drove her to jail. She was booked on four counts of second-degree murder together with two of the hospital nurses. Attorney General Charles Foti accused Dr. Pou and the nurses of using a "lethal cocktail" of prescription drugs to kill four elderly patients at Memorial Hospital 3 days after Hurricane Katrina. Pou strongly contended that she killed no one during those desperate days, although she acknowledges patients were sedated for their comfort. She unequivocally stated, "I did not murder those patients. . . . I do not believe in euthanasia. I don't think it's anyone's decision to make when a patient dies. However, what I do believe in is comfort care, and that means that we ensure that they do not suffer pain." She was then released on bond. A year after her arrest, charges were still not filed by then New Orleans Parish District Attorney Eddie Jordan, and a Grand Jury that investigated the case declined to issue indictments against Dr. Pou. Two civil lawsuits related to the deaths are pending.

While a number of details surrounding the circumstances of the deaths were murky and of a subjective nature, others were crystal clear:

- New Orleans' Memorial Hospital, where Dr. Pou worked, had a capacity of only 200 beds. But on the eve of the storm the facility accommodated a total of 2,000 people, including medical and supportive staff, their families and neighbors who sought refuge
- Dr. Pou and the remaining medical staff had to work in extremely trying conditions
- The hospital was hit hard by the storm and lost all electrical power as the basement generators became flooded
- With the power loss the air conditioning system broke down and the health workers had to break the windows to get some relief from temperatures reaching more than 110°F
- The toilets had backed up and the air was so rancid that it was burning the throat
- The evacuation of most of the patients from the hospital was delayed for almost 4 days
- The priority order of patient to be evacuated was changed by military order from evacuating the most sickly patients first to evacuating the patients who had the best chance of survival
- Most of the physicians have been evacuated but Dr. Pou and a small number of nursing personnel chose to stay on and care for the patients
- The patients on the seventh floor which included the four alleged murder victims were the most severely ill patients in the hospital. In fact, some had DNR (do not resuscitate) orders issued prior to the storm, and
- Stories of murders, robbery, and gang rape circulated through Memorial Hospital where the people trapped inside, including more than 200 patients, feared for their lives.

Second hand information, however, and a few facts suggested that Dr. Pou may have been involved in accelerating the final hours of some patients:

- A nurse reported hearing Dr. Pou state that one of the patients on the seventh floor could not be evacuated and that no living patient was to be left behind
- A fellow physician, Dr. King, reported that before he was evacuated he observed a nervous Dr. Pou holding many syringes in her hands at the entry to the seventh floor in the company of two nurses. Dr. King stated that according to the hospital's protocol and custom physicians never administered injections to patients (of course, customarily they didn't work under these conditions, either)
- Nine severely ill patients on the seventh floor all died at about the same time on the fourth day after the hurricane shortly before help finally arrived
- In all nine the postmortem toxicological analysis showed elevated levels of morphine and midazolam (a sedative like Valium but stronger) even though most of them were not prescribed morphine or midazolam, and

– Autopsies of the deceased listed the cause of death as combined drug intoxication, although the manner of death was listed by the Coroner as undetermined (i.e. impossible to determine whether the death was natural, suicide, accident or homicide).

Based on the suspicious circumstances surrounding these clustered deaths, Attorney General Charles Foti, a former sheriff of the Orleans Parish, decided to arrest Dr. Pou and the two nurses on charges of homicide. Foti allegedly made his decision based on his interpretation of the facts of the case and also relied on the opinion of Dr. Cyril Wecht, a forensic pathologist recommended by the Coroner, Dr. Maynard. Foti, who was in the process of running for re-election ordered the arrest and turned it into a media event. In 2006, during an internationally televised news conference debating the Memorial Hospital investigation, Foti categorically stated "This is a homicide; it is not euthanasia."

By trying Dr. Pou in the media rather than Court, the Attorney General made a series of basic tactical errors which were to haunt him and, in conjunction with insufficient evidence, bring the case ignominiously down. The first error was making strident public accusations against a reputable physician with no record of supporting euthanasia, no known "God complex," and who was one of the few doctors who chose to stay with and treat her patients while most other healthcare providers basically fled. The public often frowns upon charging a hero or a heroine with murder especially if it seems to be politically motivated. Further, the alleged crimes occurred during a time in which the government failed to address the suffering of thousands of Katrina's victims, yet the same government now wanted to prosecute a doctor who was doing her job. It was no wonder that hundreds of Louisiana residents supported Dr. Pou and contributed to her defense fund.

The prosecution's case lingered for more than 2 years, raising further questions about the reliability and sufficiency of the accusatory evidence before it totally collapsed. In the aftermath of the Pou arrest, Charles Foti lost his bid for re-election and a new Attorney General was elected. The new Attorney General asked additional forensic experts (well-known forensic pathologists Drs. Cyril Wecht and Michael Baden and Dr. Steven Karch, a well-respected forensic pathologist with expertise in toxicology) as well as an ethicist (Dr. Kaplan) for their opinions. The forensic consultants, except Dr. Karch, were of the opinion that there was sufficient credible evidence to conclude that the deaths of the involved patients were homicide by drugs. For unknown reasons these experts were never called to testify before the Grand Jury which ultimately dismissed the case. Several years later, Dr. Karch stated unequivocally: "There was no evidence to take before a Grand Jury (against Pou)." As a forensic specialist grounded in both pathology and toxicology the opinion of Dr. Karch should have carried particular weight since these cases were thought to be the result of a drug overdose.

Dr. Pou is still working as a doctor but she has also found also a new vocation, advocating laws to protect physicians and other healthcare specialists from being sued for the altruistic rendering of care during dire emergencies. She had been successful in promoting such legislation both at the federal and state levels. On July 8,

2008 Governor Bobby Jindal of Louisiana signed the last bill in a three-piece legislation package designed to protect medical personnel and patients during future disasters. Two of the new laws limit civil lawsuits against medical professionals who work during a declared disaster. The third directs prosecutors to use a medical panel to review evidence when a doctor or nurse is suspected of euthanasia or other criminal medical actions during a disaster. These measures extend the so-called "Good Samaritan law" which protects ordinary citizens who render emergency assistance from lawsuits to health care professionals who are working during a disaster. The Pou case proves at least one thing-truly no good deed goes unpunished.

The Benghazi Six

In another less publicized case, groundless accusations of intentionally killing more than 450 children by infecting them with AIDS kept a Palestinian doctor and five Bulgarian nurses imprisoned for 8 years in Libya. They were ultimately released after widespread international outrage, diplomatic pressure, and the payment of $400 million to the families of the victims (after filtration through the Libyan government, of course) by Western countries. It is somewhat hard to understand why the free world had to pay for the mistakes and incompetency of the Libyan medical system but free nations have repeatedly made clandestine agreements with terrorists and terrorist states that often reward rather than punish them for their crimes. In this case, the freedom of the Benghazi Six was bought for about $65 million each.

The AIDS epidemic among Libyan children in Benghazi started to slowly unfold in the mid 1990s. Dr. Achris Ahmed, who headed the Benghazi HIV Committee, stated that the first case of AIDS at the Al Fateh Children's Hospital was diagnosed in June 1997, a year before a group of Bulgarian nurses even began working at the Libyan hospital. Several months later, doctors diagnosed a second AIDS case. "But we knew little about the virus because there is no HIV in Libya," Dr. Ahmed was quoted to have said. Dris Lagha's 8-year-old daughter, Rokaya Lagha, was the seventh case to be diagnosed back in September 1998. "The doctor was confused," Lagha is reported to have said, recalling the day he learned the devastating news. "He didn't seem to know much about the virus, and we didn't know what to do." Some parents were told they could do nothing. Others were told, "This is from God." By December 1998, the epidemic had become a social issue. "Because AIDS is a sexually transmitted disease, many of our kids were mocked and ostracized. Many stopped going to school," said one concerned parent. Some children were treated like animals by their own families, "We isolated our kids, thinking they might infect their sisters and brothers or us." Some were locked away and thrown food like dogs. "We were afraid to touch or hold them," said another parent.

In November 1998, the Libyan "Le magazine" published an expose about the spread of AIDS at El-Fatih Children's Hospital in Benghazi, the second largest city in Libya. Investigation by the Libyan police revealed that over 400 children at the hospital had been diagnosed with HIV infection and 56 of them had died of AIDS. The

Libyan public was enraged by this report and, even in a dictatorship, a leader has to pay attention to deep feelings that could undermine the ruler's authority. Since admitting that its healthcare system was subpar and its knowledge of AIDS was pathetic was not an option, placing the blame on others was the self-evident solution. In February 1999, the Bulgarian embassy in Libya announced that 23 Bulgarians had gone missing and were apparently abducted by unidentified armed men. A week later the Embassy was informed by the Libyan authorities that "precautionary measures" had been taken against a doctor and nurses working at the Benghazi Children's Hospital. These measures consisted of arrest warrants for intentionally infecting Benghazi children with the HIV. The accused consisted of Dr. Ashraf al-Hajuj, a Palestinian physician, and five Bulgarian nurses who became widely known as "the Benghazi Six". The murder conspiracy theory soon had a powerful champion in Libya's ruler, the "brother-leader" himself, Colonel Muammar Gadhafi. He declared that either America's CIA or the Mossad (Israel's "CIA") had developed a unique strain of the killer virus and given it to the suspects to experiment on Libya's children. Several years later, Saif al-Islam, Gadhafi's son, challenged his father's argument that the outbreak was a foreign plot and publicly asserted: "There is no conspiracy. There is no hand of Mossad or the CIA. This was a question of mismanagement, or negligence, or bad luck, or maybe all three." Nonetheless, popular belief in the foreigners' guilt remained unshaken even when it was disclosed that their confessions followed intense torture.

The first case against the Six was brought in the People's Court (Mahkamat al-Sha`b), a body convened for crimes against the state. The trial began on February 7, 2000. The charges were intentionally "murdering with a lethal substance (Article 371 of the Penal Code), randomly killing with the aim of attacking the security of the State (Article 202), and causing an epidemic through spreading harmful virus, leading to the death of persons (Article 305)." In addition, the Bulgarians were accused of violating Libyan customs and traditions by engaging in non-marital sexual relations and drinking alcohol in public places, distilling alcohol, and illegally transacting in foreign currency. All defendants plead not guilty to all charges. The prosecutors submitted confessions of the defendants into evidence but during the trial every one of them was recanted; the defendants maintained that they were coerced to confess by torture. Supporting this claim, the nurses had filed civil suits against ten Libyan police officers accusing them of physical abuse. The methods of interrogation employed by the authorities included forcing the nurses to undress before them, putting insects on their bodies, setting dogs on them, hanging them by their hands until the wrists and shoulders became dislocated, thrashing their feet with cables, beating them with electrical prods over the breast and genitalia, and sexual abuse. The women were also deprived of water and denied sleep in a tiny cell without a toilet and were threatened with death if they did not confess.

The prosecution asserted that the prisoners were part of a plot to subvert Libya by foreign secret service agencies stating, "To those services, child killing is nothing new. In this way they want to prevent Libya from playing an important role in the Arab World and to disturb calm in the country. The killing of the children by that virus is a means by which those secret services achieve their ends."

In calling for the death penalty, the prosecutor said, "These people have no moral human feelings once they have killed those children. They have sold themselves to the devil." The defendants denied being part of any conspiracy, disclosed that some of them had never met prior to their arrest, and refuted the accusation that they had been paid to infect the children. Their defense lawyers argued that no incriminating physical evidence was submitted such as blood bottles alleged to contain contaminated plasma, syringes used to infect the children, distilling apparatus for alcohol production, or sexually compromising photographs of the Bulgarian defendants. One of the lawyers argued that four of the defendants had been very recently hired and did not have the time or opportunity to infect the children even if they wanted to. The employment records of the nurses supported this claim. A year after the trial began the People's Court ruled that it did not have jurisdiction in the matter. The case was then bound over to ordinary criminal court.

The second trial took place in the Benghazi Appeals Court beginning in July 2003. Tight security measures were in place to protect the defendants from mobs outside of the courthouse. Police officers with submachine guns guarded the venue as relatives of the children gathered in front of the building. The prosecutor began by saying that the charges did not reflect the real number of children infected by the suspects – the real number of children infected was 429. The defense countered with testimony from Professor Luc Montagnier, the co-discoverer of the HIV, who testified that the virus infecting 393 Libyan children was a rare strain found mostly in Western Africa but also throughout the continent – but not in America, Bulgaria, or Israel. Montagnier told the court that an infected child admitted for treatment at the hospital probably started the outbreak. He said that injection was not the only possible means of infection and that any medical or surgical procedure involving penetration of the skin could have transmitted the virus unless sterilization practices were followed. These revelations prompted the Court to order a new expert study of the case records by a panel of appointed Libyan physicians. After an exhaustive, "unbiased" review, the panel concluded that the mass infections were more likely due to deliberate actions because the viral load in the blood of the infected children was too high, an indication that the infection was intentional. Not a real surprising result coming from a group of puppets who probably couldn't spell HIV. Dr. Montagnier commented later that the report of the Libyan doctors "contained many mistakes showing that they didn't understand much about HIV." On May 6, 2004, the Criminal Court in Benghazi sentenced all of the Six to death by firing squad for intentionally infecting 426 Libyan children with AIDS. "The hospital," Montagnier said, "needed a scapegoat."

The convictions were appealed to the Libyan Supreme Court which heard the case in 2005. Eventually the Supreme Court revoked the death sentences and ordered a new trial. During the retrial some 50 relatives of the infected children demonstrated outside the court, holding poster-sized pictures of their children and wielding placards that read "Death for the children killers" and "HIV made in Bulgaria." In December 2006, the court once again found all six defendants guilty and sentenced them to death in spite of scientific evidence that the youngsters likely had the virus before the medical workers had come to Libya.

The United States and Europe reacted with justifiable outrage to the unreasonable verdict issued against the six co-defendants who had already had served 7 years in jail. In contrast, the Libyan public celebrated as if their team had just won the Superbowl. After the sentence was pronounced, dozens of relatives outside the Tripoli court chanted "Execution! Execution!" Ibrahim Mohammed al-Aurabi, the father of an infected child, shouted, "God is great! Long live the Libyan judiciary!" Surprisingly, several months later it was announced that the sentences would be commuted to life imprisonment. Coincidentally, earlier that same day the Libyan government had negotiated a $400 million settlement with the families of the 426 HIV "victims." It also turns out, by sheer coincidence, that the European Commission committed $461 million to the Benghazi International Fund that morning. Coincidentally, earlier that same day the Libyan government had negotiated a $400 million settlement with the families of the 426 HIV "victims". It also turns out, by sheer coincidence, that the European Commission committed $461 million to the Benghazi International Fund that morning.

On July 24, 2007 Nicolas Sarkozy, the President of France, officially announced that European negotiators had obtained the extradition of the prisoners, including the Palestinian doctor, who had been granted Bulgarian citizenship a month earlier. The released prisoners left Libya on a French government plane accompanied by the European Union's External Affairs Commissioner and the wife of the French President, Cécilia Sarkozy. Technically Libya did not free the Six but rather allowed them to serve their sentences in Bulgaria. Upon landing in Europe, however, they were immediately pardoned by the Bulgarian President, Georgi Parvanov, to the great dismay of the Libyan public. The Libyan episode dramatically emphasized the risks to life and limb encountered by foreign medical workers in non-democratic countries.

The American legal system is founded on the premise that a person is innocent until proven guilty. In fact, it has been said that it is better to let 99 guilty people go free than to convict one innocent person. Although our system doesn't always work perfectly it is better than most other judicial options. The tribulations of Dr. Pou and the Benghazi Six have something in common; these doctors and nurses were likely trying their best to help their patients but ended up fighting for their lives and freedom. Both cases are similar in that they became national media events but at that point the paths diverged. In New Orleans, public sentiment was behind the accused and the protestors were anti-government. In Libya, the population rallied behind their dictator and completely bought the story sold by the political machine. The former case ended up with an appropriate outcome based on the available facts and a victory for the judicial system; the latter almost ended up in the death of six innocent health care practitioners following a legal farce. While anyone can fall victim to unfair accusations, citizens in countries with an open legal system have a better chance of seeing justice served than those who are targeted by the very government responsible for conducting a fair trial.

Section 5
What Now?

Chapter 16
Euthanasia, and Assisted Suicide: What Would Hippocrates Do?

The road to Hell is paved with good intentions.

– Unknown (originally attributed to Samuel Johnson)

Suicide, the killing of oneself, wastes countless lives and robs society of many gifted individuals. In addition to the average person beset with depression over a broken relationship, financial troubles, or the loss of a job, extremely creative people have also taken their own lives while in the throes of depression. Both Vincent van Gogh, the post-impressionist painter, and author Ernest Hemingway died by gunshot wounds; British novelist Virginia Woolf filled her pockets with stones and walked into a river near her home; and Kurt Cobain, lead singer of Nirvana, killed himself with a shotgun. There about one million suicides occur every year in addition to 20 million suicide attempts throughout the world. The National Institutes of Health (NIH) sees suicide as a major preventable health problem in America and for good reason. More than 32,000 successful suicides are registered every year in the United States with many of the victims being healthy, young adults. Teen suicide has also become an escalating tragedy and occasional pre-teen suicides are reported. There has been religious, ethical, and social opposition to suicide for millennia. It has been characterized as an affront to a life-giving God and a usurpation of the divine power over life and death. It has been widely perceived as the ultimate selfish act. In some locales, suicide has been considered a crime; botched attempts have led to the confiscation of the property of survivors in some cases and imprisonment or fines in others. It does not carry the death penalty.

A Short History of Suicide

Suicide is as old as humankind. In describing the tragic death of King Saul, the Bible mentions both attempted suicide and assisted suicide:

"The battle became fierce against Saul. The archers hit him and he was severely wounded by the archers. Then Saul said to his armor bearer, "Draw your sword, and thrust me through with it, lest these uncircumcised men come and thrust me through and abuse me." However, his armor bearer would not, for he was greatly afraid.

J.A. Perper and S.J. Cina, *When Doctors Kill: Who, Why, and How*,
DOI 10.1007/978-1-4419-1369-2_16, © Springer Science+Business Media, LLC 2010

Therefore Saul took a sword and fell on it", but he did not die. Saul then begged an Amalekite to take his life: "Stand beside me and slay me for anguish has seized me and yet my life still lingers." The bible quotes the Amalekite as saying: "So I stood beside him and slew him because I was sure that he could not live after he had fallen" (II Samuel 1:1–10). When the Amalekite reported his actions to King David, perhaps expecting a reward, he was immediately executed.

In ancient Rome free citizens who wanted to commit suicide could do so legally if they formally applied for permission from the Senate. If their petition was approved they were given hemlock free of charge (the Roman version of a medical entitlement). However, Roman law specifically forbade the suicide of certain groups. Romans scheduled to stand trial for capital offenses could not legally kill themselves. If they did so prior to trial and conviction the state lost the right to seize their property. The suicide of a soldier was considered desertion from the army and was also illegal. If a slave committed suicide within 6 months of purchase, the master could claim a full refund from the former owner. Suicides committed for personal reasons were frowned upon, as in the case of Mark Antony who committed suicide by stabbing himself with his sword when he mistakenly believed that his lover Cleopatra, Queen of Egypt, had killed herself. On the other hand, suicides committed for reasons of honor, such as after losing a decisive battle, were considered virtuous. This concept of virtuous suicide has lingered into modern times. The Japanese practice of "heroic" suicide continued until the end of the Second World War both in the form of the Kamikaze suicidal bombings by aviators and of harakiri, suicide committed by leaders who have failed in an assigned task. Sporadically, harakiri case reports are still published.

Ritualized suicides (sepukku) such as harakiri have been performed in Japan for centuries. Indeed it was an integral part of the code of the samurais. Dressed in a ceremonial kimono and often seated on sumptuous cushions, the warrior would place his sword in front of him and prepare for death by writing a stylized poem. With his selected attendant standing by, he would then open his kimono, take up his wakizashi (short sword) or a tanto (knife), and plunge it into his abdomen, making first a left-to-right cut and then a second slightly upward stroke. On the second stroke, the assistant would perform the daki-kubi ritual by decapitating the noble victim with a single sword stroke that left the head still attached to the body by a thin strip of flesh. This tradition encompassed both honorable suicide and legal assisted suicide. In modern America, suicide is no longer considered noble and assisted suicide can land you in jail.

The Physician and Suicide

Most of us are afraid of death. Even those who are believers in a better world to come are not usually in a hurry to experience this inevitable encounter. Physicians generally function as brakes on the wheels of a train which is speeding down tracks inevitably leading to either nothingness or the afterlife depending on your beliefs.

When well-intentioned, merciful doctors hit the accelerator instead of the brakes and assist patients to their final resting place serious ethical, religious, and legal issues surface. Certainly doctors make mistakes of various magnitudes, as all humans do, and some of these errors can unintentionally lead to a patient's death. In the vast majority of these instances, even if the mistakes were reckless and grave, the physician may well be subject to civil litigation but usually not criminal prosecution. However, when a physician intentionally acts in a sporadic or systematic fashion to enable or assist suicide or hasten death through euthanasia there is substantial exposure to criminal charges including accusations of manslaughter or murder.

A distinction should be made between assisting in suicide and enabling suicide. Enablement is a passive process whereas assisted suicide requires action. To assist someone who wishes to commit suicide, the doctor must do something which intentionally helps the patient to die. The physician's actions may consist of providing information on how to end one's life, giving depressed patients pills with dosage instructions that will lead to death, or designing equipment that can be used by a patient to take his or her own life. Physician-assisted suicide cases are the ones that make the headlines. Conversely, a physician may enable suicide by allowing a patient to forego life-saving treatment or by irresponsibly (or intentionally) prescribing powerful medications which can be misused by some patients. Physicians who run so-called "pills mills" may be unwitting enablers of suicide; at the least they significantly contribute to the current epidemic of accidental prescription drug overdoses. Upon request, even by telephone, their patients can receive narcotics and sedatives by fabricating the appropriate symptoms (which are easy to find on the internet) and answering a few quick questions.

It can be extremely difficult to prosecute a doctor for enabling suicide or facilitating an accidental overdose secondary to the unethical or semi-ethical practice of medicine. Law enforcement agencies occasionally use officers to play the role of requesting patients in "sting" operations in order to document the excessive amounts of medications being prescribed by some doctors. The premise for the subsequent arrests is that these physicians have essentially become drug dealers and are partially responsible for the overdose deaths some of their patients. They may also theoretically be held liable for other deaths outside of their patient pool if their overprescribed medications are sold on the street and used recreationally with fatal results. However, even when physicians have been brought to trial for these crimes, conviction proves to be very problematic and two or three retrials are not uncommon. The arguments made by the defense teams for the accused physicians consistently include one or more of the following valid points:

- Pain medications or sedatives are often requested by patients who can successfully fake their symptoms. You can create any virtual disease you want if you have an hour of Web access and a marginal ability to act. Studies have shown that doctors are not good at detecting deception even when forewarned. In fact, physicians were able to identify deception under experimental conditions only 10% of the time
- Large doses of medications are justified in some cases including medical conditions resulting in intractable pain. The savvy defense attorney may leave out the part that the oxycodone dosage that is appropriate for a person riddled with

metastatic cancer differs from the pain management needs of someone who calls
their physician for drugs to relieve the excruciating pain of a hangnail, and
– Physicians simply can't control their patients and force them to act responsibly

There are likely thousands of physicians across the country and far more scattered
throughout the world who have built thriving practices based on prescription drug
peddling. It is highly unlikely that any of them will be sent to prison for enabling
suicide though it is certain that some have done so on occasion.

Physician-Assisted Suicide

Physician-assisted suicide is a situation in which a physician provides information
and/or the means of committing suicide to requesting patients so they can painlessly terminate their own lives. In these cases, the patient always initiates the final
action leading to death. The doctor may actively participate by writing a prescription
for a lethal dose of pills for his suffering patient or by suggesting that the patient
consult a "how to do it" suicide guide such as "*Final Exit*" by Derek Humphry. A few
physicians have gone beyond the call of duty and aggressively assisted their
patients who wanted to die. In fact, in a few cases it seems that the patient may not
have wanted to "end it all" after all.

The doctor who popularized assisted suicide in the twentieth century was
Dr. Jack Kevorkian (a.k.a. "Dr. Death"). Kevorkian was born in 1928 in Pontiac,
Michigan to Armenian immigrants. A very gifted student he taught himself German
and Japanese during World War II while still in high school-it is unclear if he was
hedging his bets pending the outcome of the war. Kevorkian graduated from the
University of Michigan Medical School in 1952. Even in his student years, he
expressed an unusual interest in death. His beliefs about death and euthanasia
apparently crystallized when, as a medical intern, he witnessed the suffering of a
woman dying from cancer. Kevorkian went on to specialize in pathology and in this
capacity obtained a number of hospital positions including Chief of Pathology at
Saratoga General Hospital in Detroit. He published more than 30 professional
articles and booklets including one entitled "*Prescription Medicine: The Goodness
of Planned Death*" in which he defended the patient's right to suicide and euthanasia. He also advocated for the right of death row inmates to donate their organs for
transplantation or experimentation. Kevorkian's morbid interest in death also
spilled over to his recreational activities. A gifted painter, he created several very
depressing and scary paintings all with morbid themes. He also was a jazz musician
and composer of a musical piece entitled "*The Kevorkian Suite: A Very Still Life*."

After living in California for about a decade where he worked in a number of
hospitals, he returned to Michigan where he earned a living, in part, by publishing
articles on euthanasia in European journals. In 1989 after reading about a patient
who had asked for euthanasia, he developed a highly publicized lethal-injection
machine (the "Thanatron") that delivered intravenous toxic medications at the push

of a button. Later, he developed a variant of this death machine, the "Mercitron," that delivered fatal concentrations of carbon monoxide through a facemask. Both of these devices were operated by the patients requesting Dr. Kevorkian's "house call." On June 4, 1990 he performed his first physician-assisted suicide on a 54 year-old woman suffering from Alzheimer disease who had contacted him after reading his ad in the newspaper. The procedure was performed in the back of his Volkswagen van and consisted of an intravenous infusion of sodium pentothal (a short acting anesthetic) and potassium chloride (a chemical that stops the heart). Ostensibly, the patient injected her own medications into the intravenous catheter. After his third "medicide" (as Kevorkian preferred to label his actions) in 1991, his medical license was revoked for violating Michigan state laws regarding euthanasia. Undeterred, he continued to perform his medicides by providing his clients lethal carbon monoxide gas. A mounting debate was brewing: when does assisted suicide cross the line and become homicide?

On August 17, 1993 after helping 20 people to end their lives he was formally charged with violating Michigan law. He was jailed twice, first in November 1993 and then a month later. After his incarceration, Kevorkian went on a liquid-only hunger strike for 18 days and was released from prison in May 1994. By this time, he had gained a number of supporters in the general community and had obtained significant media exposure. Between 1990 and 1998, he carried out approximately 100 medicides. The relatives of some of his patients claimed that he had continued his procedures even after some of his victims had asked him to stop. Further, at least one of his patients had no significant or life-threatening pathological findings at autopsy and may have suffered from a mental or psychological disease. Even if you support the concept of physician-assisted suicide, this is not the type of patient suitable for this procedure.

During the 1990s Kevorkian dubbed himself a "death consultant" and continued his activities while successfully publicizing the issues of assisted suicide and euthanasia through TV talk shows and other media outlets. His "medical" exploits resulted in national and international notoriety. Kevorkian was even featured on the cover of *Time* magazine in 1993. Over the course of his consulting career Dr. Kevorkian became increasingly bold. He taunted the local Medical Examiner after several medicides and in some cases dropped the bodies (literally) at the Medical Examiner's Office. "Dr. Death", as he widely became known, conducted an aggressive publicity campaign for the legal recognition of assisted suicides. His continuous struggle was punctuated by intermittent prosecutions by the local State Attorney and short imprisonment terms. Kevorkian was tried three times for manslaughter or murder but was found not guilty each time because the final act triggering death was done by the victim and not by him (or at least no one had seen him push the plunger on the syringes). Also there was no specific Michigan law prohibiting assisted suicide.

Apparently, those failures of the State prosecution emboldened Kevorkian to further defy the authorities and under the light of television cameras, he publicly performed the medicide of Thomas Youk, a 52 year-old man with terminal Lou Gehrig disease. On the videotape, Kevorkian challenged the authorities to convict him or to make him stop assisting suicides. The gruesome show was broadcast the following month in November 1998 on the CBS television program *Sixty Minutes*.

This time, however, Kevorkian had administered the fatal injection of potassium chloride himself. As this action clearly crossed the line from assisted suicide into illegal voluntary euthanasia, he was successfully prosecuted in 1999 for murder and the illegal delivery of a controlled substance. He was found guilty of second-degree homicide and sentenced to 15–25 years of prison.

Kevorkian, in failing health, was granted parole in late 2006 and released in 2007 after promising not to perform any additional procedures. After his release from prison, he moved to the Detroit suburbs and in 2008 announced his intention to run for a seat in the U.S. House of Representatives. He received 2.6% of the vote. On January 15, 2008, Kevorkian gave his largest public lecture since his parole speaking to a crowd of nearly 5,000 people at the University of Florida. *The St. Petersburg Times* reported that Kevorkian expressed strong support for physician-assisted suicide and voluntary euthanasia for willing patients. In explaining his own involvement, Kevorkian said "My aim in helping the patient was not to cause death, I mean that's crazy," the paper quoted him, "My aim was to end the suffering." He concluded stating "I am a physician. I knew how to do it ... I did it humanely." He is still lecturing though his focus has shifted to tyranny in America. In February 2009 he ended his speech at Nova Southeastern University by displaying an American flag with a swastika replacing the field of stars. He has apparently stopped killing people and helping people to kill themselves. As far as we know.

Legal Assisted-Suicide

In 1994 Oregon became the first state in the Union to legalize physician-assisted suicide when 51% of the voters supported the Death with Dignity Act. The Act became effective in 1997 after several legal maneuvers aimed at its repeal failed. In 1999 there were only 27 applications for permits to commit assisted-suicide; by 2006 this number had increased to 46 in and to 49 in 2007. The voters of Washington State have approved the enactment of a similar law which became effective in March 2009. Both laws, in effect, actually authorize physician-enabled suicide rather than the type of aggressive assistance offered by Dr. Kevorkian. In these states doctors may legally prescribe lethal doses of medications to terminally ill patients. Physicians are not compelled to enable a patient's suicide, however, if it conflicts with their religious, ethical or personal beliefs. These laws specify in great detail when assisted-suicide is permissible and the state closely monitors practitioners to make sure this practice doesn't get out of hand.

"Excursional" Suicide

A company by the name of Dignitas legally helps gravely ill foreign nationals to commit suicide in Switzerland where this type of assistance is permissible (provided that the doctor is not killing the patient out of his own self-interest).

Dignitas' clients fly to Zurich where they are examined by a doctor to confirm their terminal illness and certify a sound state of mind. Patients eligible for assisted-suicide include those with cancer, quadriplegia, multiple sclerosis, and severe mental illnesses such as incurable bipolar disorder and schitzophrenia. Many patients are evaluated at Dignitas as a precaution; they want to have a means to end their suffering should it become intolerable. In fact, 70% of the visitors to Dignitas never are "treated" at the facility. If the patient decides that Dignitas offers them a viable solution to their problem, they are provided an apartment and a glass of water or juice containing sodium pentobarbital, a powerful sedative. After drinking the mixture, the patient becomes sleepy, falls into a coma, and dies of respiratory arrest in about 30 minutes.

In 2008, Dignitas assisted in the performance of 840 suicides at a charge of about $6,000 per case. For an extra couple of thousand dollars, the company would handle all funeral arrangements and registration fees. The clients predominantly came from Germany, Switzerland, and Britain but many other countries were represented. Although this company appears to be providing a service which is sought after and which people are willing to pay for (Capitalism 101) a number of former employees quit the company over ethical concerns. Some have even suggested that the corporation is simply a death mill existing solely to make a profit. Although the conservative Swiss politicians have recently proposed laws to regulate "suicide tourism" to date none of these laws have been enacted and it is business as usual at Dignitas. This lucrative business gives new meaning to the term "dying for a vacation."

Euthanasia

Euthanasia ("Good death" in Greek from "eu" meaning good and "thanatos" meaning death) is an action by a doctor, with presumed benevolent intentions, which causes the death of a patient having a terminal or irreversibly painful condition or who is in a state of hopeless and irreversible coma. Most cases of euthanasia are of a voluntary nature; other chapters in this book address the more nefarious "involuntary euthanasia" imposed upon groups of people who are considered "unfit to live" for eugenic reasons. The difference between assisted suicide and euthanasia is that the patient is not an active participant in euthanasia, except perhaps for expressing a wish to end his or her life. Voluntary euthanasia is performed by a doctor at the request of a conscious and mentally competent adult patient or at the behest of the legal next-of-kin if the patient cannot communicate his or her wishes. It amounts to what could be defined as "suicide by proxy." Dr. Kevorkian went to prison for an extended period of time when he crossed the line between physician-assisted suicide and voluntary euthanasia.

Euthanasia may be classified by the role or activity of the involved physician into active euthanasia and passive euthanasia. Active euthanasia most often occurs when a doctor directly causes the death of a patient by injecting fatal doses of a substance into the person. Passive euthanasia occurs when the doctor abstains from providing the patient with life saving medications, the administration of food and liquids, or from providing cardiopulmonary resuscitation. The latter situation is extremely common. Today patients can preemptively issue directives to their healthcare providers to refrain from starting resuscitation in the event that a cardiac arrest occurs (a "DNR" – do not resuscitate order). Patients can also restrict doctors from employing extraordinary means of keeping them alive in the setting of severe, irreversible injuries or terminal disease. Such directives can be accomplished either by drafting a Living Will, a formal declaration recognized by law, or upon admission to many hospitals. Other people choose to draft a Durable Power of Attorney for Health Care that assigns someone else the power to make health care decisions if the patient becomes unable to do so. This power should be delegated to someone who likes you. This representative can then tell the doctor what he or she can and cannot do to save or prolong the patient's life. Failure to respect the choices made by the patient or designee can result in civil actions and even criminal charges.

A doctor may participate in active euthanasia based on personal beliefs, humanitarian feelings, or for professional reasons. Regardless of the motivation, the physician has performed a felonious act in most countries, including the United States, and may be prosecuted for murder. Despite these serious charges, the Courts have been lenient with most physicians accused of voluntary euthanasia. Less than two dozen doctors have been prosecuted in the United States and the convicted doctors have usually received light sentences. The only notable exception was Dr. Kevorkian's stiff sentence but his crime was the culmination of a pattern of behavior, not a sporadic event. Furthermore, in spite of his crystal clear premeditation and public display of intentionality, "Dr. Death" was only convicted of second degree manslaughter and not of murder and served only a relatively short, 8-year sentence. The reason for this consistent and unusual leniency of American juries and Courts is the pervasive belief that when voluntary euthanasia is committed with the clear consent or at the request of a terminal patient for credible humanitarian reasons, there is little or no moral blame attached to the act. To frame it in religious terms, although the law may have been broken no sin was committed.

A case in point is the prosecution of Dr. Peter Rosier in 1986. Dr. Rosier, a prominent physician in Fort Meyers, Florida, was indicted by a Lee County Grand Jury for the first degree murder of his 43 year-old wife Patricia, a capital offense. Patricia had been diagnosed with lung cancer in 1985 and by 1986 the cancer had spread to her brain. Assuming that he would not be prosecuted for obeying his wife's final wish, Dr. Rosier freely and publicly admitted that he had given his wife a lethal injection at her request in order to relieve her suffering. Rosier also described his actions in great detail in the manuscript of a book he was writing about the incident. By the time his confession caught public notice, the body had long been cremated with a death certificate listing the cause of death as cancer. The local media quickly branded Dr. Rosier a "wife killer" and accused him of trying to draw interest to his intended book by bragging about his crime. The media coverage became so intense and excessive that the Court moved the trial up the Florida coast to St. Petersburg in order to find unbiased jurors. The prosecution's case was based on Dr. Rosier's televised confession, a confession to a reporter, accounts of the murder in the manuscript, a friend's testimony, and the testimony of Patricia's family members who were understandably upset with Rosier. The case was presented and the jury deliberated for only 3 hours prior to finding the defendant not guilty on all counts. The Court erupted in pandemonium when the verdict was read, "bedlam" according to the official transcript. If the prosecution could not prevail in this airtight case, how can it ever expect to win in trials in which the facts are not so clear cut?

There is another common medical practice that may also constitute a form of voluntary euthanasia, namely the administration of excessive medications to keep a dying patient comfortable. When a patient or family has requested "comfort care only" or "comfort measures" physicians will prescribe high doses of pain killers and sedatives which will be administered over a fairly short time interval. The patient's goal is met-there is no suffering-but death is an acceptable "side effect" of this treatment plan. These cases cannot be definitively identified as voluntary euthanasia for two main reasons. First, it cannot be proven that the intention of the physician was to end the patient's life rather than to ease suffering. Second, because of the phenomenon of drug tolerance patients receiving chronic pain medications can withstand very high doses of painkillers that would be lethal to most people. Even in the setting of fatal drug levels in these patients, death will likely be attributed to the underlying disease process or injury that necessitated the administration of the drugs in the first place. In truth, these doctors are acting in accordance with the Hippocratic Oath in that they relieve suffering. In contrast, physicians who assist in suicides or practice active euthanasia are violating the principle of "above all do no harm."

Karen and Terri

The deaths of Karen Ann Quinlan and Terri Schiavo illustrate vividly the conflicts inherent in discontinuing life support and the involvement of outside parties in the fray. They also serve to point out the variety of roles that physicians may play in these controversial cases. In the Quinlan case, expert medical opinions helped to clarify her diagnosis. Doctors ultimately hastened her death by first removing her from a ventilator and, years later, removing her feeding tube. The Schiavo case was even more explosive. In this case, physicians offered medical opinions which may have been partially or wholly politically motivated. While some doctors strove to meet her husband's wishes and discontinued the means by which she could continue to "live", other caregivers violated Terri's rights and body by forcing her to undergo invasive procedures that her legal guardian had adamantly refused. These two cases brought up issues in medical ethics that have not yet been resolved and likely never will be. As long as physicians continue to act like other humans, with their own emotions, biases, religious beliefs, and personal philosophies, there will be doctors sitting on both sides of the fence. For some, respect for the patient's wishes will be paramount; for others, the sacred nature of life itself will win out.

Karen Ann Quinlan

On April 15, 1975, 21 year-old Karen Ann Quinlan collapsed for unknown reasons at a party apparently after consuming alcohol and drugs. She stopped breathing at least two times each lasting about 15 minutes. She was brought unconscious to a hospital emergency room where she slipped into coma. After her condition stabilized, she had to be fed through a nasogastric tube and breathing required a respirator. She was diagnosed as being in a permanent vegetative state (i.e. having irreversible brain injury). Tests showed that she had no awareness of anything or anyone around her.

Her movements were limited to those at a primitive reflex level with some brain stem functions such as involuntary chewing motions, disjointed movements of the extremities, blinking of the eyes, grimacing, and making stereotypical cries and moans. As time progressed she became severely emaciated having lost at least 40 pounds and was contorted into a distorted fetal posture. Karen's father requested to be her Court appointed guardian for the express purpose of authorizing removal of her respirator. He was opposed not only by Karen's physicians who wished to prolong her life but by the local Prosecutor and the State Attorney General. Quinlan's physician argued that, in his opinion, Karen was not brain dead and that both medical standards and ethics required him to continue treating her by all means available. The government also intervened, arguing that the state's interest in protecting the sanctity of life must be protected and that removing her from a ventilator was tantamount to criminal homicide.

The New Jersey trial court denied Mr. Quinlan's request for guardianship and also rejected his request to terminate the use of the respirator, deciding that medical decisions pertaining to Karen rested solely with the attending physicians. The Court also discounted the argument that there is a legitimate legal distinction between ordinary and extraordinary means to sustain life. In 1976, however, the New Jersey Supreme Court reversed the decision and granted Mr. Quinlan's request. The New Jersey Supreme Court's ruling was based on Karen Quinlan's right to privacy, protected by the Constitution, which was violated when her physician and the hospital refused to remove the respirator. Although the Court recognized that the state had an interest in preserving life, it found that "the individual's right to privacy grows as the degree of bodily invasion increases and the prognosis dims." The Court also dismissed the idea that the medical profession was required to use all means at its disposal to keep patients alive. Rather, the "focal point of the decision [to terminate treatment] was whether the patient would return to a 'cognitive and sapient life' or remain in a 'biological vegetative existence.'"

Following this ruling, Karen Ann's father had the option to remove her from life support. According to the Court, Quinlan's right to privacy would be rendered meaningless unless her father could exercise it on her behalf. Central to the Court's decision was its belief that Quinlan's father was of "high character" and very "sincere, moral, ethical, and religious." The Court rejected the defense team's argument that a father's grief and anguish would render him unable to make life-and-death decisions concerning his daughter. Karen's physicians gradually weaned her from the respirator during May of 1976. Surprisingly, she continued to breathe on her own. Given this surprise her father chose not to terminate artificial nutrition and hydration. Karen lived another 9 years in a coma prior to her death in 1985. As a result of this case, ethics committees proliferated and a debate arose as to what should be the physician's role in the discontinuation of life support. As we shall see, this issue had not been resolved even two decades later.

Terri Schiavo

While Karen Quinlan's case engendered a great deal of public interest, it did not reach the mass media magnitude of the Terri Schiavo case. Beginning as the personal choice of a single family, it became a polarizing event involving the American public, the state of Florida, the United States Congress and Supreme Court, and the President himself. Theresa (Terri) Marie Schiavo was a 27 year-old Florida woman who collapsed in the hallway of her St. Petersburg apartment in the early morning of February 25, 1990. Her husband, Michael Schiavo, was with her when the incident occurred and he promptly dialed 911. By the time paramedics and firefighters arrived at the scene Terri was not breathing and had no pulse. The emergency medical team attempted to revive her and defibrillated her several times while transporting her to a local hospital. On admission, the medical examination and radiological studies did not reveal any trauma but she was comatose and her blood potassium level was very low at 2.0 mEq/L (the normal range for adults is 3.5–5.0 mEq/L). Potassium is an element found in human cells which is essential to life. Low levels can cause sudden collapse and death due to an irregular heart rhythm or cardiac arrest. Schiavo remained comatose for 2½ months. When she emerged from the coma, Schiavo regained a sleep-wake cycle, but did not show awareness of herself or her surroundings. The sleep/wake cycle is an automatic function of the brain controlled by a light-sensitive biological "master clock" located in the hypothalamus, a structure near the center of the brain. She was diagnosed as being in a persistent vegetative state with extensive damage to the higher brain structures (the parts of the mind that make us think and define "who we are") due to a loss of oxygen to the brain during her cardiac arrest episodes.

Although the cause of Terri's collapse was never definitively determined, a likely explanation was a severe electrolyte imbalance, namely hypokalemia. Hypokalemia (low levels of serum potassium) can be induced by starvation diets as a result of poor food intake or by medications or drugs such as diuretics or caffeine that increase the elimination of potassium from the body. Published excerpts of Terri's medical chart noted that "she apparently has been trying to keep her weight down with dieting by herself, drinking liquids most of the time during the day and drinking about 10–15 glasses of iced tea." Iced tea is a mild diuretic that causes fluid loss. Some have suggested that the low potassium level detected upon her admission to the hospital could have been a spurious result caused by the intravascular administration of fluids during the attempt to resuscitate her resulting in dilution of her blood. This is very unlikely because the concentrations of other chemicals in her blood, such as sodium and chloride, would also have been lowered and this was not the case.

It is uncertain whether Terri had bulimia. Bulimia nervosa is an eating disorder predominantly seen in young women consisting of cycles of eating large amounts of food in a short time followed by episodes of "purging." The most common form of the disease practiced by more than 75% of people afflicted is self-induced vomiting although fasting, the use of laxatives, enemas, diuretics, and over-exercising are also common. Hypokalemia and other electrolyte abnormalities have been reported in association with bulimia. It should be noted that Terri Schiavo's husband filed and won a malpractice suit against her obstetrician, Dr. Stephen Igel, on the basis that the physician failed to recognize and diagnose her with this eating disorder. In November 1992, a jury awarded Mr. Schiavo one million dollars.

For years after the collapse, Schiavo remained in a persistent comatose state. She was initially fed by a nasogastric tube (a tube inserted in the stomach through one of the nostrils) and later on by a PEG tube (a tube entering the stomach directly through an incision in the abdominal wall). For the first 3 years after this tragedy her husband Michael and her parents, Robert and Mary Schindler, enjoyed an amicable relationship. That ended in 1993 and the parties literally stopped speaking to each other. In 1994, Michael Schiavo consulted with doctors and concluded that his wife would not recover and opted to authorize a "do-not-resuscitate (DNR) order" in case of a cardiac arrest. In 1998, 8 years after Terri's collapse and several years after he had received the settlement money, Michael Schiavo petitioned the Pinellas County Circuit Court to remove her feeding tube. Terri's parents opposed this arguing that she was still conscious. For the next 5 years a complex array of legal and political battles were to be fought between the husband and parents simply due to the absence of a Living Will which could have specified Terri's wishes prior to her collapse. By March 2005, the Schiavo case had generated no less than 14 appeals and numerous motions, petitions, and hearings in the Florida courts; five suits in Federal District Court; and four denials of *certiorari* (to take the case for review from the lower courts) by the Supreme Court of the United States.

In 2001, the Court of Appeals appointed five board-certified neurologists to evaluate the case. Two were chosen by Schiavo's parents, two by her husband, and one was to be selected by mutual agreement of the parties. The Schindler family selected Dr. William Maxfield (a radiologist) and Dr. William Hammesfahr (a neurologist); Michael Schiavo selected Dr. Ronald Cranford and Dr. Melvin Greer (both neurologists); and, because the parties failed to agree on a fifth, the court selected Dr. Peter Bambakidis (a neurologist). These five doctors examined Schiavo's medical records, brain scans, videos, and Schiavo herself. Drs. Cranford,

Greer, and Bambakidis testified that Schiavo was in a persistent vegetative based on imaging studies of her brain which showed massive loss of cerebral tissue and an EEG showing no cerebral cortical activity. In short, there was no evidence that she could think or that she ever would be able to again. Drs. Maxfield and Hammesfahr (selected by the Schindlers) testified that Terri was in a minimally conscious state and claimed that their personal methods of treatment might help the patient. Both PVS (persistent vegetative stress) and minimal consciousness are a result of severe brain injury but as the name indicates in the first there is no consciousness at all while in the latter there is a minimal degree of awareness. There is a slight difference in prognosis as well. Patients in a PVS almost never recover, while patients in a minimally conscious state have a very small chance of improvement but they never return to normal neurological function.

As part of the court-ordered medical examination of the patient, 6 hours of video of Terri Schiavo were taped and filed at the Pinellas County courthouse. The tape included Terri with her mother and neurologist William Hammesfahr. The entire tape was viewed by the Judge who wrote, [Terri Schiavo] "clearly does not consistently respond to her mother." From that 6 hours of video, the Schindlers and their supporters produced six clips totaling almost 6 minutes and released them to public websites. Although Terri's parents received a great deal of sympathy and backing from conservative political groups and large segments of the public, the Judge ruled that Terri was in a persistent vegetative state and was beyond hope of significant improvement. The Court was particularly critical of Dr. Hammesfahr's testimony that claimed positive results in similar cases following vasodilatation therapy, the efficacy of which could not be validated by scientific research. The Judge stated, "He [Dr. Hammesfahr] testified that he has treated about 50 patients in the same or worse condition than Terri Schiavo since 1994 but he offered no names, no case studies, no videos and no test results to support his claim that he had success in all but one of them. If his therapy is as effective as he would lead this Court to believe, it is inconceivable that he would not produce clinical results of these patients he has treated. And surely the medical literature would be replete with this new, now patented, procedure." Dr. Maxfield's hyperbaric oxygen therapy suggestion did not fare much better with the Judge who observed that, "It is interesting to note the absence of any case studies since this therapy is not new and this condition has long been in the medical arena." In short, the more credible medical evidence suggested that Terri would never recover and that her husband was free to have the feeding tube removed.

After another round of legal battles, Schiavo's feeding tube was removed on October 15, 2003. Within a week, when the Schindlers' final appeal was exhausted, the Florida Legislature hastily passed "Terri's Law" giving Governor Jeb Bush the authority to intervene in the case. Bush immediately ordered the feeding tube reinserted. Bush sent the Florida Department of Law Enforcement to remove Schiavo from hospice and transfer her to Morton Plant Rehabilitation Hospital in Clearwater where her feeding tube was surgically implanted by a physician. One could argue that the doctor committed battery when he touched the patient against her will and the wishes of her legal guardian. The emergency legislation also included the appointment of a guardian ad litem for Terri, Dr. Jay Wolfson, to "deduce and represent the best wishes and best interests" of Terri Schiavo and report them to Governor Bush. Michael Schiavo, backed by the American Civil Liberties Union (ACLU) and millions of others, opposed the Governor's intervention in the Schiavo case. On May 5, 2004 the Honorable W. Douglas Baird, a Circuit Court Judge in Florida's Sixth Circuit, found "Terri's Law" unconstitutional and struck it down. Governor Bush appealed this decision to the Second District Court of Appeals who sent it directly to Florida's Supreme Court who confirmed that this law violated Terri's Constitutional rights. Ultimately, the feeding tube was removed by a doctor in what can be construed as active euthanasia. Terri died at a Pinellas Park hospice facility on March 31, 2005 at the age of 41.

An autopsy performed by Dr. Jon R. Thogmartin substantiated the presence of severe brain atrophy. Her brain weighed half of what it should have and much of the cerebral cortex, the "thinking" part of the brain, had been destroyed. Dr. Thogmartin, the Medical Examiner, concluded that "Mrs. Schiavo suffered severe anoxic brain injury. The cause of which cannot be determined with reasonable medical certainty. The manner of death will therefore be certified as undetermined." Dr. Stephen J. Nelson, a neuropathology consultant and forensic pathologist, described microscopic changes in the brain consistent with a persistent vegetative state but warned that "neuropathology examination alone of the decedent's brain – or any brain for that matter – cannot prove or disprove a diagnosis of persistent vegetative state or minimally conscious state." We agree wholeheartedly. The only way a doctor can assess responsiveness is by observing the living patient.

What Is Right?

Like most people, physicians have strong opinions on assisted suicide and euthanasia. Some endorse it as a final service to a patient while others condemn it as an affront to everything a doctor has sworn to uphold. Legitimate arguments can be made for both sides. When faced with these situations, the physician must ask, "Should I trust in my own judgment and knowledge of medicine to prolong this life or must I relinquish my power over life and death to a mere patient and respect their 'free will'?" The answer should reflect how they would like to be treated if they were the patient.

Chapter 17
Malpractice or Murder?

> *Even top caliber hospitals cannot escape medical mistakes that*
> *sometimes result in irreparable damage to patients.*
>
> – Carl Levin

Seneca, a first century Roman philosopher, coined the popular adage, "To err is human (Errare humanum est)." Much lesser known is his follow-up sentence "to persist is diabolical (perseverare diabolicum)." Most if not all doctors make mistakes some of which result in frank malpractice and litigation. After a physician has gone through the time, money, guilt, and remorse associated with a malpractice suit, he is unlikely to make the same mistake again. Of course, some doctors never learn.

Physicians are inundated by a barrage of technical data, emotional issues, signs and symptoms, treatment options, and concerned family members whenever they are faced with diagnosing and curing a serious illness. Unlike other professions, doctors are expected to get the right answer all of the time. If a lawyer won 90% of his cases, he would probably make partner in his firm in short order. If a quarterback completed 80% of his passes, he would be in the Pro Bowl. If a weatherman made accurate predictions 50% of the time he would be, well, a weatherman. But if a doctor killed one patient out of 100 he could lose his license and livelihood. In medicine, a 99% batting average isn't good enough.

The Joint Commission on Accreditation of Health Care Organizations defines a medical error as "an unintended act, either of omission or commission, or an act that does not achieve its intended outcome." This definition and others do not take into consideration the fact that medical errors could be at times a reflection of the imperfection of medical science. The individual practitioner may not have made an error at all yet the desired outcome or cure was not attained. Therefore, from a practical standpoint it is more appropriate to consider a medical error a deviation from the current standard of care.

J.A. Perper and S.J. Cina, *When Doctors Kill: Who, Why, and How,*
DOI 10.1007/978-1-4419-1369-2_17, © Springer Science+Business Media, LLC 2010

The Current Problem

A 1984 Harvard study of more than 30,000 records from 51 randomly selected hospitals in New York found that adverse medical events occur in more than 3.7% of admissions and that more than a quarter of these were due to medical negligence. Close to 14% of the adverse medical events were fatal and 2.6% resulted in severe disability. When extrapolated to the 2.7 million patients discharged from New York hospitals that year about 13,450 people died and 2,550 were seriously injured. A 1992 Colorado and Utah study of almost 15,000 randomly selected patients from 28 hospitals suggested that more than 44,000 Americans were expected to die yearly from medical errors. This estimate was confirmed in 1999 when The Institute of Medicine published *"To Err is Human: Building a Safer Health Care System."* This study estimated that there are about 44,000–98,000 medical error-induced deaths per year in the United States, more than the number of fatalities resulting from traffic accidents, AIDS or breast cancer. It has been argued that most of the current estimates of adverse medical events are underestimations as they are based on reported or detected cases. In fact, deaths due to iatrogenic diseases (caused by doctors) may well reach a quarter of a million making them the third major cause of death in this country.

Medical Errors by Individual Physicians

Simply put, a doctor is a repairperson who fixes broken bodies and minds. The difference between physicians and other repair people is that the results of medical errors are more tragic and the likelihood of grave error is significantly higher. If a plumber incidentally blows out a pipe while repairing a septic tank, it is inconvenient and distasteful. If a surgeon blows out a body "pipe", it is fatal. Medical errors resulting in injury or death may be classified in two major groups, slips/lapses and mistakes. Slips and lapses are involuntary, skill-based errors in performance usually occurring when attention is diverted whereas mistakes are the result of deficient medical knowledge, errors in judgment or inadequate medical skill. In recent decades, the amount of medical knowledge has increased exponentially. Even specialists have a hard time keeping up with the avalanche of scientific literature pertaining to their specific facet of health care. It is inevitable that general doctors will not be able to meet the standard of care on occasion since they may not even know what it is. More disturbing than the doctor who harms a patient out of ignorance are the physicians who repeatedly fail to reach correct diagnoses or deliver adequate care with disastrous complications. These dangerous doctors may jump from state to state to avoid detection and prosecution.

A rather vivid example is that of Dr. Jose Efrain Veizaga-Mendez. Dr. Veizaga-Mendez, a native of Bolivia, graduated from San Simon's University School of Medicine in Cochabamba, Bolivia in 1965. He then emigrated to the United States and completed his internship and residency. By early 2000, a pattern of severe medical mistakes emerged among his patients and in 2006 he had to relinquish his Massachusetts medical license. Shortly thereafter, he applied and was hired on as a surgeon by the Veteran Administration (VA) Hospital in Marion, Illinois. One of his patients died in August 2007 because of uncontrolled bleeding within a day following a routine gallbladder removal. Three days after this tragic death, Dr. Veizaga-Mendez resigned from the hospital and applied for another medical license in North Dakota. Following his departure from the VA, a systematic review of all surgical cases found that between October 2006 and March 2007 there were that at least ten deaths "directly attributable" to substandard care by two surgeons, one being Dr. Veizaga-Mendez. During that time period, only two deaths would have been expected. In October 2007, Dr. Veizaga-Mendez's medical license was suspended in Illinois.

Dr. Veizaga-Mendez was penalized for allegedly committing a series of grievous mistakes leading to unnecessary surgeries and protracted pain. Unfortunately, Dr. Veizaga-Mendez's case is not isolated. Most of the 5,000 doctors who face disciplinary action in the United States have medical licenses in more than one state according to the Federation of State Medical Boards. Therefore, they have the option to jump from one state to another to continue to practice. Although communication between state medical boards has improved, some dysfunctional practitioners still slip through the cracks.

Medical errors are not limited to VA Hospitals or busy urban medical centers. Both the poor and the rich and famous may suffer the consequences of medical misadventures. For example, the 2-week old twin babies of Dennis Quaid, a well-known actor, almost died after inadvertently receiving a massive dose of heparin (a blood thinner), 1,000 times more than was prescribed. This adverse event occurred in spite of the fact that the hospital had been previously warned by the FDA (Federal Drug Administration) of the potential mix-up between these two concentrations of heparin because of the similarities of the appearance and labeling of the bottles. In March 2006, the wife and four children of the late actor John Ritter, beloved leading man of the "Three's Company" TV series, reached a settlement with the hospital and doctors they felt were responsible for his death. Ritter's family alleged that physicians misdiagnosed a tear in his aorta as a heart attack leading to inadequate treatment and his untimely death. In another instance, comedian Dana Carvey sued his heart surgeon for operating on the wrong artery when he underwent a double bypass in 1998. The case was settled for an undisclosed amount which Carvey donated to charity. Clearly, this funny man has a big heart. Carvey later said, "This lawsuit, from the beginning, was about accountability and doing everything I could to make sure that it wouldn't happen to someone else."

As a matter of fact some experts have pointed out that celebrities may receive a lesser quality of medical care than the average individual due to a number of factors including a reluctance by physicians to conduct some required tests that may be intrusive or very uncomfortable, performing an excessive number of tests (some which may result in serious side effects or generate confusing data), trying heroic therapies which are highly unlikely to succeed and result in more pain than relief, and disrupting "normal" treatment by introducing too many superspecialists. Some physicians, so-called "doctors to the stars," are willing to prescribe medications such as pain killers and sedatives indiscriminately to famous clients rather than addressing their underlying physical, mental, or emotional needs. On the plus side for superstars, we bet celebrities don't have to sit in waiting rooms for hours or haggle with insurance companies.

Murder Versus Malpractice

What penalty should be exacted from physicians who make grave or fatal mistakes? In the vast majority of cases in which a physician or a medical institution may be reasonably held responsible for malpractice it is clear that that there was no intention or plan for the adverse event to occur. This being the case, these wrongful deaths result in civil suits rather than criminal charges. When malpractice is proven, there is usually financial compensation paid to the patient (if living) or their family. Punishment for the doctor may also be imposed by the state's Board of Medicine. It is only when the doctor's recklessness in diagnosis or medical care reaches a very high degree that prosecutorial actions for assault, manslaughter or murder are contemplated or carried out.

Despite what you have read in this book, doctors are rarely charged with manslaughter and almost never for murder. A killing is considered manslaughter when there is no specific intent to cause fatal harm or death. A crime is considered murder when a person is killed with "malice aforethought" or premeditation. Both murder and manslaughter are considered homicides, defined as the act of taking away the life of another person. Some physicians found guilty of overprescribing painkillers or potentially addicting medications or exercising highly reckless medical care have been charged and convicted of manslaughter. Serial killers, on the other hand, are tried for murder.

In the late 1980s, Dr. Ricardo Samitier, a Miami plastic surgeon who routinely performed silicone lip enhancement, decided to apply his experience to penis enlargement. He performed penis-widening operation in which he injected fat extracted from the abdomen or other parts of the body into the penile shaft. His lucrative practice was cut short in 1992 after one of his patients, a 47 year-old lounge singer who had been on heparin, died of bleeding following the surgery. Dr. Samitier was convicted of manslaughter and sentenced to 5 years in prison. In 1989 Dr. Milos Klvana, a California obstetrician, was convicted on nine counts of second-degree murder. The trial testimony substantiated highly incompetent and negligent medical care including failure to monitor the medical condition of women during delivery, reckless disregard of fetal stress or shortness of breath in newborns, repeated absences during deliveries, and failure to perform high-risk deliveries in the hospital when they were indicated.

In 2002 Dr. James F. Graves, a Florida pain management specialist, became the first doctor found guilty by a jury on four counts of manslaughter, one count of racketeering and five counts of unlawful delivery of a controlled substance in connection with recklessly and indiscriminately over-prescribing OxyContin®. It was also alleged that he sold medications to known addicts and drug dealers. In May 2005 a Dallas County Grand Jury indicted Dr. Daniel Maynard, a Dallas physician, for operating a "pillmill" and allegedly over-prescribing narcotic medications to a number of patients who overdosed and died. Most recently, Dr. Sandeep Kapoor, a "doctor to the stars", and Dr. Khristine Eroshevich have been charged with conspiracy to provide vast amount of drugs to Anna Nicole Smith, a model who died of an overdose of prescription medications. Doctors who prescribe pills upon request can make a lot of money; they can also go to prison for a long time.

Complex medicolegal problems and the nuances of medical negligence may pose challenges to juries and to criminal courts. A rather famous case in point is that of Commander Donal M. Billig, the former chief heart surgeon at the Bethesda Naval Hospital. In 1986 he was convicted of involuntary manslaughter and negligent homicide in the deaths of three patients and sentenced to 4 years imprisonment. After serving 25 months of his sentence, however, the Navy/Marine Corps Court of Military Review reversed the conviction stating that Billig was convicted in a highly publicized trial in which he had been the victim of "a smear campaign." Prosecutors sought to portray him "as a bungling, one-eyed surgeon who should have known better than even to enter an operating room because of his past mistakes and poor eyesight." This contention was based on 20/400 vision in his right eye, the result of a horrendous tennis accident. He had also been dismissed at one hospital and stripped of operating privileges at another prior to assuming his post in the Navy. Nonetheless, the Appeals Court stated that the prosecution's tactics "…should not have been permitted by the military judge" because it forced Dr. Billig to defend himself not only against the charges involving patients at Bethesda but "to explain and account for virtually all of his mistakes, professional setbacks, or surgical misadventures during the previous 20 years." The prosecution stressed that this pattern of practice over two decades was exactly the reason to put him in prison. The Court didn't buy this very logical argument. In setting aside the conviction, the Appeals Court concluded that it was not satisfied beyond a reasonable doubt that Dr. Billig was guilty of any of the derelictions for which he was convicted. The court essentially found that the surgical procedures and techniques for which Dr. Billig had been condemned were consistent with medically accepted standards and that some of the adverse medical outcomes for which he had been blamed might have been due to other causes. In May 1988, the Navy announced that Dr. Billig would receive an honorable discharge and that it would not appeal the review panel's decision. In an interesting side note, allegations of juror bribery surfaced after the appeals court decision but the case had already been closed.

In some cases the legal pendulum seemed to have move excessively in the direction of prosecution of physicians who made only bona fide mistakes. Dr. Gerald Einaugler, a 49 year-old New York internist, was asked to assume the medical care of a 78 year-old woman transferred from a nearby hospital to a nursing home. The doctor erroneously believe that the catheter protruding from the patient's abdominal wall was a gastrostomy tube (i.e. a tube placed through the skin and into the stomach) and ordered that liquid feedings be administered through it. Unfortunately, it was actually a port used for peritoneal dialysis, a treatment for kidney failure. After 2 days of these feedings, the patient's belly began to swell and she became short of breath. A nurse discovered the mistake and notified Dr. Einaugler by telephone. He consulted a kidney specialist who advised him to admit the patient to a hospital for immediate care but he allegedly chose not to follow this advice. After examining the patient and finding her to be in what he thought was stable condition, he delayed the transfer for about 10 hours. The patient was then brought to the emergency room but died 4 days later.

Dr. Einaugler was eventually convicted of manslaughter and in 1997 sentenced to 52 years of prison. He served only six weekends prior to being pardoned by Governor George Pataki. The New York Medical Society saw this criminal prosecution as an unjustified attack on practicing physicians as a group and strongly argued that it "is a terrible policy to criminalize mistakes in professional judgment; it is just as inappropriate to criminalize a doctor's clinical judgment as it would be to criminalize a lawyer's tactical judgment." It would seem that criminal charges were improper in the Einaugler case; these lapses in medical judgment, however, lay the foundations for a solid case of negligence in civil court. Indeed a New York Medical Society leader implicitly agreed and stated, "Mistakes of judgment should not be liable to criminal prosecution. Traditionally errors in judgment are handled through peer review and malpractice (suits)."

Clearly serious mistakes in medical care should be subject to civil litigation and, very rarely, criminal proceedings. We all want our doctors practicing the highest standard of care possible. But also consider that the increase in the number of civil and criminal suits against physicians can and has resulted in a number of adverse outcomes for patients. Many physicians concerned with their legal liability related to prescribing narcotic medications for pain or other medications with abuse potential may prescribe medications in less than appropriate dosages to patients in real pain that clearly need them. Other physicians practicing today adhere to the doctrine of "self protective medicine." They order excessive or outlandish tests that not only significantly increase the cost of medical care but also can result in physical harm to some patients. While this practice philosophy may ensure that no diagnosis is missed, it also opens up the doctor to charges of Medicare fraud. Too few tests can lead to lawsuits – too many to Medicare audits. Either way, the doctor loses. So does the patient.

The pervasive fear of lawsuits and the associated astronomical malpractice insurance premiums has driven doctors out of several specialties, such as obstetrics, and left areas of the country badly underserved by qualified physicians. Over the next several decades, there will be a severe shortage of doctors in many parts of the Western world. Rather than facing economic devastation, humiliation, and imprisonment some of the best and brightest students are avoiding medicine and seeking out safer pastures. Most will find jobs where they are allowed to make mistakes once in a while.

Chapter 18
It's All Natural!

> *The market for alternative medicine is vast and growing ...*
> *This trend must be guided by scientific inquiry, clinical judgment,*
> *regulatory authority and shared decision-making.*
>
> – David Eisenburg

There are a number of healing practices that belong to the general group of alternative or complementary medicine. A 1990 survey published in the *New England Journal of Medicine* indicated that that there were 425 million visits to alternative or complementary medical practitioners compared to 388 million visits to traditional primary care doctors. Americans spent about $13.7 billion in 1 year alone on alternative medicine, only $3.4 billion of which was covered by insurance. Clearly, non-traditional medicine is big business and patients are willing to pay for these services out of their own pockets. Although some practitioners of unconventional medicine are trained physicians, many are not. Nonetheless, their patients treat them as doctors and, as we have seen, doctors are capable of killing.

Alternative and Complementary Medicine

Alternative medicine healers exclusively advocate for methods other than conventional medicine to treat illnesses while complementary medicine specialists provide treatments that work in conjunction with traditional medicine. Alternative medicine is not taught in most medical schools but some patients swear by it and are completely devoted to their "doctors" who practice it. In many cases, these treatments do relieve pain and suffering and improve quality of life. It is unclear, however, if the benefits are "real" (i.e. based on sound scientific principles of physiology and anatomy) or a placebo effect. There are more than 32 flavors of alternative and complementary medicine that may be used separately or in tandem. The most common include:

- *Acupuncture and acupressure techniques*, integral to traditional Chinese medicine, this art has been practiced for thousands of years. Acupuncture involves the insertion of fine, thin metal needles in predetermined skin areas called meridians that impact on sensory, motor or emotional functions. Acupressure involves the application of pressure to the same areas. This technique has provided relief to patients for millennia, however, as with any technique that involves piercing the skin there are risks for bleeding and infection

- *Ayurveda* is a 5,000 year-old form of Indian traditional medicine that represents the ancestry of several variants of the Chinese healing arts. It combines massage, aromatherapy, diet, meditation, and the use of herbs to restore balance to the body. Some of these techniques also fall under the heading of *Herbalism*. Though these medications have been used for hundreds of years and may be helpful to some people, seizures may develop in others as a reaction to rosemary, sage, fennel, hyssop, and other natural healing agents. This century, Dr. Deepak Chopra has been a leader in this field
- *Aroma therapy* is a form of therapy in which the scent of essential oils from flowers, herbs, and trees is inhaled to promote health and well-being. It is commonly used as an adjunct to massage at many high-end spas. Though it can be very relaxing, certain patients may be allergic to some of the compounds used, such as eucalyptus, and develop severe, life-threatening reactions
- *Chelation therapy* assumes that many diseases are due to poisoning by various heavy metals (such as lead, mercury, etc.) that have to be purged from the body by "detoxifying" medicines. This technique includes shooting a molecule, EDTA, into the blood to catch the wandering atoms. Though chelation does remove several heavy metals from the blood and may be useful when little kids have eaten lead paint, it is not without significant risks. EDTA can cause seizures, kidney failure, and other problems. On another down note it may make your lungs stop working
- *Chiropractic* involves manipulation of the spine to correct ubiquitous "subluxations" that may cause back pain, stress, or a variety of symptoms throughout the body. Chiropractors are divided into two groups, the conservative chiropractors or "straights" that use only traditional spine manipulations and "mixers" that also use many other modalities of alternative therapy. One of the authors has been manipulated by a chiropractor (as well as many other people resulting in severe "trust issues") and found temporary relief from back pain. We are also aware that manipulation of the neck by chiropractors has resulted in tears of the arteries supplying the base of the brain with resultant sudden death
- *Colonics* entails the instillation of a variety of oils, liquids, herbs and other natural substances into the rectum and beyond. The idea is to purge the body of all toxins and remove materials that have been spackled onto the bowel wall for years. This procedure is not without risks. People with colon tumors and diverticulosis may be prone to colonic rupture if fluid or gas is forced up the rectum whether recreationally or for medicinal purposes. And, for the record, the authors have collectively performed close to 20,000 autopsies and have yet to find 10 pounds of undigested red meat or chewing gum trapped in someone's colon

- *Dianetics* is a curative method created and popularized by L. Ron Hubbard, the science fiction writer who founded the Church of Scientology. Subscribers to this philosophical form of healing are taught that both physical and mental diseases are the result of forgotten "engrams" (traumatic life events) rather than viruses, bacteria, and malignant cells. Some cures can be achieved by taking "mind trips" back to the time of birth and in-utero enabling the engrams to be "cleared" by moving them from the "reactive (unconscious) mind" into the "memory bank" of the conscious mind. As we would one day like to meet Tom Cruise and John Travolta we will not elaborate further on the efficacy of this treatment plan
- *Faith Healing* is practiced by many religious groups. Studies have shown that while prayer can speed healing and improve a patient's outlook on life, medicine is also a good thing. *Faith healing* in and of itself doesn't kill anyone. People die, however, by relying on faith alone and not seeking proper medical care
- *Ear candling*, also called ear coning or thermal-auricular therapy, is a dangerous and ineffective practice intended to assist the natural clearing of earwax from a person's ear by lighting one end of a hollow candle and placing the other end in the ear canal. It should fall into the "don't try this at home" category of things
- *Homeopathy* is a form of alternative medicine devised by Dr. Samuel Hahnemann in the late 1700s. The theory goes that if a substance can kill you in large doses or cause symptoms similar to the ones you are suffering from, then that same substance can cure you when administered in sub-microscopically, diluted doses. Though it is unlikely to help a sick person it was less risky than blood-letting and blistering, treatments commonly employed by Dr. Hahnemann's colleagues back in the day
- *Hydrotherapy* is one of our personal favorites. Warm water jetted around the body is very relaxing and it can be a wonderful way to meet new friends. Immersion in hot water, however, can lead to hyperthermia, loss of consciousness, and death by drowning. People using drugs and alcohol in hot tubs are particularly at risk for bad outcomes. In particular, DO NOT take a wine enema while you are in a hot tub. Very bad things can happen (a real case!)
- *Hypnosis* can be a valuable technique when used by certified health care professionals. It can be extremely embarrassing if it is employed by a nightclub entertainer who makes you squat down and quack like a duck
- *Meditation techniques* can soothe the mind and relieve stress. Care should be taken to avoid malnutrition and dehydration since fasting often accompanies "hard-core" meditation therapy
- *Naturopathy* is an alternative type of medicine that recommends using only natural remedies such as herbs and healthy foods instead of synthetic drugs or surgery. In the United States naturopaths are formally trained in 16 states and entitled to use the title ND or NMD. One should remember that just because something is a natural product, such as a plant, doesn't mean it is good for you. Socrates, a very smart guy, went to meet Zeus after he ingested hemlock. Cocaine and heroin, which are bad for you, are derived from the coca plant and poppies, respectively. It is no wonder that Dorothy felt woozy and passed out

while crossing that field of poppies in the *Wizard of Oz*. Or perhaps Judy
Garland just thought it was a good place to crash for a while

– *Ozone therapy* involves the administration of ozone, oxygen or hydrogen peroxide
  by various means including blood treatments, ozone gas saunas, rectal and vaginal
  insufflation, and injection into the joints. It has some legitimate uses in modern
  medicine but other applications are likely quackery. The use of oxygen by inexperienced "healthcare providers" poses a risk of fire and incinerating patients. Also,
  hydrogen peroxide can be fatal if ingested in large quantities by producing bubbles
  that are absorbed through the stomach wall and into the bloodstream

– *Polarity therapy* is an untestable methodology developed by Randolph Stone in
  the late 1940s to early 1950s. It was claimed that healing could be achieved
  through manipulation of what was described as complementary (or polarized)
  forces within the body, similar or identical to the yin and yang spiritual forces
  described in Chinese philosophy. Since no one can find these forces or measure
  them, this theory cannot be proven wrong or right

– *Reflexology* is the practice of massaging, squeezing, or pushing on parts of the
  feet (and occasionally the hands or ears) to improve general health. The practice
  is based on the belief that certain areas of the foot are interconnected with
  different body organs

– *Reiki* is a type of therapeutic touch developed in 1922 by Mikao Usui. After 3
  weeks of fasting and meditating on Mount Kurama in Japan, Usui claimed to
  have received the ability of "healing without energy depletion." A portion of the
  practice, tenohira or palm healing, is a technique whereby practitioners believe
  they are moving "healing energy" through their palms and into the patient

– *Tai chi*, the traditional Chinese gymnastic movement technique is believed to
  decrease stress, reduce hypertension and improve the movement of individuals
  with Parkinson's disease. It also contributes to generalized health and gives you
  a cool Ninja look while you are doing it, and

– *Yoga*, a cluster of Indian healing techniques, involves transcendental meditation,
  control of posture and breathing, and stretching. It is designed to both improve
  health and purify the soul from our earthly constricting passions and urges.
  It also improves flexibility and strength

Increasingly, physicians who practice allopathic medicine (the traditional M.D.-type
of doctor) are recognizing the value of some of these techniques (such as yoga) and
have encouraged patients to pursue these options of adjunctive therapy. Most doctors
feel that alternative medical practices should be used in cooperation with traditional
medicine and not in place of it. When alternative therapies run amuck, people die.

Alternative Medicine Gone Bad

Some homeopaths still believe Dr. Hahnemann's original theory that diseases
are produced not by bacteria or other injurious biological or chemical agents
but by "miasmas"-deranged vital sources that affect both the body and mind.

Homeopaths treat diseases by administering extremely diluted medications. At these low concentrations, the alleged cures cannot cause any harm but progression of disease or death may occur when these ineffective remedies are chosen over essential prescription medications or appropriate surgery. Some homeopathic practitioners have been arrested and indicted for manslaughter and murder for allowing patients to ignore sound medical advice and opt for non-scientific, imaginative forms of treatment.

Mitra Javanmardi, a 50-year-old Naturopath from Montreal has recently been accused but not convicted of criminal negligence and manslaughter in the death of a 64 year-old patient who died of a heart attack after getting an intravenous injection of a "mineral" treatment. In 2004, Dr. Marisa Viegas, a homeopathic doctor, emailed instructions to a patient of hers not to take any of the medications prescribed to her by another physician for a severe heart condition. Shortly thereafter the patient expired – the cause of death was determined to be: "acute heart failure due to treatment discontinuation." Viegas had her license to practice medicine revoked for professional misconduct as a result of this incident. In another tragedy, Mr. Russell Jenkins sustained a foot injury in December 2006. The wound later became ulcerated and the infection spread to his leg but the 52 year-old shunned conventional treatment saying his 'inner being' told him not to go to hospital. He allegedly sought advice from a homeopath, Susan Finn, who suggested he treat his wound with Manuka honey. Not surprisingly, despite this state-of-the-art (for 200 B.C., maybe) treatment the patient continued to deteriorate rapidly and he became bed-ridden. When Finn visited him the following day, she saw blood on the bed sheets and described a foul smell in Mr. Jenkins's bedroom. His foot was swollen and one of his toes was discolored – the honey wasn't working. He developed gangrene and died in the early hours of April 17. His mother Eileen Jenkins reportedly stated during a Coroner's inquest: "To lose my son is devastating, absolutely. But the way he died, I just can't come to terms with it, when I know all it needed was a phone call for a doctor or ambulance to be called, for antibiotics, and my son would be here today." Susan Finn later stated that despite her best efforts, Jenkins refused to go to a hospital – and she honored his wishes.

In early 2004, a 44 year-old woman was diagnosed with breast cancer by her family physician. She was scheduled for surgery to remove two malignant tumors, one under her right arm and the other in her right breast. The patient refused surgery, however, and chose instead to be treated by a holistic medicine provider, David Eugene Pontius. The treatments began in May 2004 and continued until the patient's death on October 20, 2004. His therapeutic modalities included body "scanning" using a device he called the "Body Scan 2010" and treatments with a Rife Machine and an Oscillator (don't worry, we don't know what they are either).

In June 2004, a CAT scan showed that the cancer had spread and that various organs in her body were now affected. Mr. Pontius also examined her during this month and diagnosed that the pain in the patient's arms was due to a "rib head" being out of alignment. He then performed chiropractic services and "manipulated" the rib in order to relieve the pain. The manipulation relieved the discomfort for approximately 1 hour and then it returned with a vengeance. Mr. Pontius then examined her mouth and told the patient that she had gangrene under two of her teeth and mercury poisoning beneath two others. He then confidently informed her that the infected gums and teeth were the basis of her cancer. Examination by a dentist failed to confirm his diagnoses. Furthermore, cancer is caused by genetic mutations some of which are inborn and others which develop from external factors (our educational tip for the chapter).

Weeks after the dental fiasco Dr. Wendy Breyer, an oncologist and breast cancer specialist, told the withering woman that if she did not receive medical treatment immediately she would die within months. Dr. Breyer was right on with the prognosis – the patient died that Fall. The State of Utah charged Pontius with the unlicensed practice of medicine or naturopathic medicine, both of which were third degree felonies.

In 2006, the family of Dennis G. McDaniel filed a lawsuit against Gregory Haag, Tosca Haag, and Vivian V. Vetrano charging that their "treatment" had resulted in McDaniel's death. For many years, according to their Website, the trio deceptively represented themselves as "doctors" operating the Rest of Your Life (ROYL) Retreat in La Vernia, Texas. The suit charged that the 55 year-old McDaniel, who was suffering from obesity, hypertension and diabetes, died following "detoxification" that included 2 weeks of complete fasting, followed by two more weeks of a "nut milk" diet, and thereafter a diet of raw fruits, vegetables and nut seeds. After several weeks of this therapy, he became unresponsive, non-communicative, and comatose and had to be hospitalized. Upon admission he was dehydrated, malnourished, and in shock. Heroic efforts to save his life proved to be unsuccessful.

Whereas most alternative medical remedies are harmless, others entail significant risks. Yohimbine extracts prescribed for male impotence have been proven to induce hypertension and spasms in the lungs. Blue-green algae may contain a toxic substance (microcystin) that, in large doses, causes acute liver failure in humans. Chiropractic spinal manipulation can rarely cause vertebral artery damage leading to paralysis, stroke, and death. Nonetheless, adults are free to make their own choices when it comes to medical care (at least for now) and they can opt for either traditional or alternative treatment. Unfortunately, children may die due to no fault of their own when a parent or caretaker makes poor choices on their behalf.

Attachment Therapy

A particularly tragic death caused by unorthodox "medical" treatment involves the case of 10 year-old Candace Newmaker. Candace spent time in five foster homes before she was adopted at age six by a single woman, Jeane Newmaker, a nurse practitioner. As occurs in many adoptions, after an initial "honeymoon" period Jeane began to complain that her new daughter was behaving negatively. After just a few months, Jeane attended a national Attachment Therapy (AT) convention in suburban Washington, DC, where she met Bill Goble. Mr. Goble was a North Carolina Attachment Therapist whom she hoped would help Candace bond with her and cure any (real or imagined) problems the girl may have had. Goble had Newmaker fill out a questionnaire at the convention, from which he was able to say Candace was a "fairly severe" case of Reactive Attachment Disorder (RAD), although she apparently did not meet the established medical criteria for that diagnosis. In April 2000, Candace and Jeane Newmaker traveled to Evergreen, Colorado for a $7,000, 2-week, "intensive" session of Attachment Therapy with Jean Connell Watkins and her associate, Julie Ponder.

Attachment therapy (widely known as "holding therapy," "rebirthing," "rage-reduction," or "dyadic developmental therapy") is a dangerous and entirely unscientific practice that preys on adopted and foster children who already have had tough lives. The "rebirthing" procedure is intended to bring children back to the time of their birth by re-enacting labor and delivery from the perspective of the fetus. Reliving this trauma is supposed to recover deeply repressed memories of the original experience of birth: the pain of contractions, the suffocating passage through the birth canal, and the struggle to enter an entirely new world. Following this "treatment" the child is supposed to be reduced to a helpless, infant desperate for a mother. For example, in this case Candace would undergo attachment therapy, be reduced to a neofetus, and bond with her new mother, Jeane, upon her "birth." Attachment therapy techniques rely on forceful physical coercion and restraint, non-consensual touching, verbal abuse, intimidation, enforced eye contact and punishments which included limiting food, water and air intake. The mainstream psychiatric community considers rebirth therapy as being "harmful pseudoscience" and the procedure is severely restricted or banned in several states. Several cases of attachment therapy have culminated in the deaths of the very children whom the therapists were attempting to "heal."

In the Newmaker case many of the treatment sessions had been videotaped. These recordings showed Candace being subjected to cruel and degrading procedures over a period of 2 weeks. In one 2-hour session Candace had her face grabbed 90 times to ensure eye contact with the therapists. In another session, her head was violently shaken 309 times. Adults within inches of her face screamed at her over 50 times while she was being held in Watkins's lap; another adult sat on her legs to ensure her restraint. Attachment therapists call this a "gentle, nurturing," embrace intended to convey an impression of "safety and love." The bonding continued when Candace's obese, adoptive mother lay on top of her for almost 2 hours while licking her face. On several occasions, Watkins and others required this naturally energetic 10-year-old to sit motionless for 10, 20, and 30 minutes at a time. Candace also had her treasured long hair hacked off into a short, ragged mop.

Candace died during the second week of her treatment during a so-called "rebirthing" procedure. Participating in the fatal videotaped session were Watkins and Julie Ponder along with two assisting "therapy parents", Brita St. Clair and Jack McDaniel. Jeanne Newmaker, witnessed the joyous event, ready to step in at the right time and play "Mommy." Following the script for that day's treatment, Candace was placed in a fetal position on the floor and wrapped in a flannel sheet to simulate a womb. Four adults used their hands, feet, and about a dozen large, thick pillows to push against the 75-pound girl with a combined weight of 673 pounds. Candace attempted to free herself while she pleaded and screamed for help and air to no avail. Candace stated several times during the session that she was dying to which Ponder responded, "You want to die? OK, then die. Go ahead, die right now." Twenty minutes into the session, Candace had vomited and urinated inside of the sheet; she was kept restrained. Forty minutes into the session, Jeane Newmaker asked Candace "Baby, do you want to be born?" Candace faintly responded "no"; this would ultimately be her last word. Ponder then screamed at the dying child, "Quitter, quitter, quitter, quitter! Quit, quit, quit, quit. She's a quitter!" Jeane Newmaker felt rejected by Candace's inability to be reborn and was asked by Watkins to leave the room so that Candace would not "pick up on (Jeane's) sorrow." Soon thereafter, Watkins requested the same of McDaniel and Brita St. Clair, leaving only herself and Ponder in the room with Candace. Fifty minutes into the session, Candace went completely quiet. The therapists sat on top of her for another 20 minutes before unwrapping the sheet. By this time Candace was motionless, not breathing and her lips were blue. Upon seeing this, Watkins declared, "Oh there she is, she's sleeping in her vomit." Jeane Newmaker, who had been watching the stillbirth on a monitor in another room, rushed into the room and began CPR while Watkins called 9-1-1. Paramedics were able to restore the girl's pulse and she was flown by helicopter to a hospital in Denver. She was declared brain dead the next day as a consequence of asphyxia.

After a 3-week trial in which the jury twice viewed the 70-minute videotape of the last therapy session the jurors deliberated about 5 hours before finding Watkins and Ponder guilty of reckless child abuse resulting in death. Each received 16-year prison sentences. Watkins was also convicted of a misdemeanor – the unlawful practice of psychotherapy. Jeane Newmaker pled guilty to neglect and abuse charges and was given a 4-year suspended sentence. During the last week of the trial, Colorado Governor Bill Owens signed "Candace's Law" which banned re-enactment of the birth process when it uses restraint that carries a risk of death or physical injury. Unfortunately, it was too late for one pretty, little girl.

Chapter 19
Contagious Caregivers

All sorts of bodily diseases are produced by half used minds.

– George Bernard Shaw

Many infectious diseases are unwittingly transmitted in different ways from one individual to another. Physicians are particularly prone to carrying microbes around since they come into contact with many people who are infected by a myriad of bacteria and viruses. Although doctors take precautions to avoid spreading disease from patient to patient, sometimes hand washing and surgical masks are not enough. Inadvertent spread of infections between patients is not uncommon; it is no wonder that a hospital is a great place to catch a cold or even a more serious, potentially fatal disease. There is no way for doctors to eliminate entirely the possibility of spreading diseases from one person to another – it just goes with the territory. Willfully exposing patients to serious infections, however, is much more serious and may result in civil litigation and even criminal prosecution.

Transmission of infections from patient to patient most commonly occurs via unwashed hands. In essence, the soiled physician plays the role of the rat passing on the Plague. Prior to the adoption of aseptic techniques (and the use of rubber gloves) thousands of women died of puerperal fever, an infection passed between women following delivery via the bloody, dirty hands of the obstetrician. Similarly, many soldiers wounded during the Civil War died of infections spread throughout hospital tents by the very people who were trying to save them. Visitors to the injured men also frequently fell ill. Once the basic habit of hand washing became engrained in the mind of the physician, iatrogenic infections (those caused by doctors) dropped off dramatically. In modern times, doctors are rarely the source of serious outbreaks in hospitals. Even so, they still are quite capable of transmitting diseases to their patients (even in the absence of inappropriate physical relationships).

A recent study which sampled neckties worn by 42 doctors at the New York Hospital Medical Center of Queens found that half of them were inhabited by dangerous bacteria capable of causing pneumonia and life-threatening infections including *Staphylococcus aureus* ("staph infections"), MRSA (methicillin-resistant *Staphylococcus aureus*), *Klebsiella pneumoniae* and *Pseudomonas aeruginosa*. The odds of a physician wearing a contaminated tie were eight times greater than that of security guards in the same hospital. Doctors may also potentially spread

J.A. Perper and S.J. Cina, *When Doctors Kill: Who, Why, and How*,
DOI 10.1007/978-1-4419-1369-2_19, © Springer Science+Business Media, LLC 2010

infections through their clothing and contaminated scrubs. The frightening, antibiotic-resistant bacterium MRSA, a bug that thrives in the hospital setting, may walk out of the hospital and into the gym or kitchen or movie theater along with its host making new acquaintances along the way. Another study showed that if a hospital worker was in the same room with a patient having a MRSA infection, bacteria contaminated their clothes 70% of the time even if the employee had no physical contact with the patient. That's scary.

Given the frequent interaction of hospital employees with numerous sick people there is a high likelihood that an employee will be carrying around some sort of bacteria. Some countries in Europe have attempted to prevent the spread of infection both within the hospital and in the community by having health care workers wear a set of "hospital" clothes in the facility and their own clothes outside of the hospital. The "hospital" clothes and shoes are provided by the hospital itself, a very nice perk not enjoyed in the United States. Of course, this implies that the hospital administration is the arbiter of fashion (which may be not so bad in France). Most American hospitals also have policies requiring their staff to change out of their scrubs and into their street clothes before leaving the facility. Unfortunately, this policy is not well monitored and enforced and in most localities one may encounter doctors or nurses wearing their scrubs around town. For some reason, these walking Petri dishes seem to frequent supermarkets – how lucky for us!

Doctors harboring infections may unknowingly or knowingly transmit them to their patients. Nobody knows how many medical professionals harbor blood-borne pathogens such as Hepatitis B and C and the Human Immunodeficiency Virus (HIV). Over 23,000 healthcare workers, including 1,792 physicians, 5,378 nurses, and 476 paramedics have contracted AIDS. Out of these at least 57 infections (and possibly 139 more) were acquired from an exposure at work. Generally, HIV-positive staff members are allowed to practice freely as long as they follow standard infection-control techniques and have informed their patients that they are carriers of the virus. Some restrictions may be placed on doctors, dentists, nurses and technicians who perform invasive procedures with sharp instruments since these activities carry the greatest risk of exposure to contaminated blood. Although several civil liberties groups have opposed mandated physician disclosure of infection, current regulations force surgeons and other types of doctors infected with HIV or Hepatitis to inform patients of their condition prior to performing any invasive procedure.

The Sad Story of Kimberly Bergalis

The first well-publicized incident of HIV transmission from a doctor to a patient involved Kimberly Bergalis, a 22 year-old Floridian who allegedly was infected by her dentist, Dr. David Acer. Her case stirred an intense and bitter national debate over AIDS testing. Kimberly, the eldest of three daughters, was born in 1968 in Pennsylvania and moved to Florida in 1978. In 1985, Kimberly enrolled at the

University of Florida majoring in business. While attending college, she had two "significant" boyfriends.

In December 1987, Bergalis had two wisdom teeth removed by Dr. Acer, her dentist. Unbeknownst to her, he had been diagnosed with AIDS in the fall of 1987; he later died of the disease in 1990. When she came home on a vacation from college in March 1989, her mother, a nurse, noticed that her daughter appeared seriously ill. Ten months later Kimberly was diagnosed with AIDS. When she became aware of her diagnosis and related it to Dr. Acer's dental extractions she sued the dentist for reckless malpractice. She also began a campaign to enact legislation aimed at preventing AIDS-infected medical personnel from providing unhindered medical care. To settle her lawsuit, Miss Bergalis collected $1 million from Dr. Acer's estate and an undisclosed sum from his insurance company. She continued unabated on her, "You've Ruined My Life" crusade. Kimberly told reporters and Florida health officials in 1990 that she was a virgin who had never taken IV drugs or received a blood transfusion. Despite state-of-the art treatments, AIDS soon transformed her into a shadow of her former self. Nevertheless, she struggled on and even testified before a Congressional Committee in support of her proposed legislation. Before the committee, Bergalis softly stated from her wheelchair: "AIDS is a terrible disease that we must take seriously. I did not do anything wrong, yet I am being made to suffer like this. My life has been taken away. Please enact legislation so that no other patient or healthcare provider will have to go through the Hell that I have."

Spurred on by the public uproar, the Centers for Disease Control (CDC) proposed barring infected healthcare professionals from procedures in which HIV might be transmitted. Soon thereafter the legislation stalled and the CDC backed off following intense opposition from state and local health officials, several powerful medical societies, and advocates for AIDS patients. Opponents of the proposed regulations effectively argued that the Florida case remained an anomaly, that thousands of patients of other doctors with the HIV infection were tested and found uninfected, and that new rules were not needed. The CDC did conclude, however, that Bergalis as well as five other unrelated patients had contracted the same strain of the HIV from Acer; DNA sequencing showed that there was a high correlation between the subtype of the virus carried by the dentist and his patients. A study conducted by the CDC estimated that out of more than 190,000 cases of AIDS reviewed only 13–128 patients *may* have acquired the disease from healthcare workers. Acer's five patients were the only people confirmed to have been infected by this route.

In a posthumous letter addressed to Florida health officials made public by her parents, Kimberly wrote:

"Do I blame myself? I sure don't. I never used IV drugs, never slept with anyone and never had a blood transfusion. I blame Dr. Acer and every single one of you bastards. Anyone who knew Dr. Acer was infected and had full-blown AIDS and stood by not doing a damn thing about it. You are all just as guilty as he was. You've ruined my life and my family's. If laws are not formed to provide protection, then my suffering and death was in vain." She ended by saying: "I'm dying, guys. Goodbye."

When Kimberly's case was diagnosed, Dr. Acer told health investigators that he did not believe he had infected anyone. But he finally notified his patients anyway, informing them of his illness just before he died on September 3, 1990. Experts still question how the infections occurred. The most common theories hold that Dr. Acer bled from a cut finger into an open surgical incision; or, he used instruments on patients that had accidentally punctured his skin; or, that he used dental drills that had not been sterilized after working on another infected patient. While his co-workers and patients gave conflicting statements regarding the cleanliness of his techniques, proponents on the side of Dr. Acer questioned the veracity of Kimberly Bergalis. Regardless of how the disease was spread in this case, it has resulted in the bad-tasting rubber gloves and masks now used by dentists and dental hygienists throughout the country. And there has not been another documented transmission between a dentist and patient since that time.

Blood Money

In June 2008, ABC News reported a corrupt trade in human blood that resulted in the infection of 119 babies and toddlers with the HIV in Kazakhstan, a former Soviet Republic. Most of the children were from poor families living in remote countryside areas. The youngsters were given blood transfusions by local doctors for a variety of fictitious ailments for which they were charged exorbitant fees. No parental consent was obtained and none of the children were ill (until they received the blood). Prosecutors alleged that the profits from the transfusions were split between the doctors and the local blood bank – which had collected blood from all comers in unsterile conditions. Only after ten children had died and the outbreak had become an international scandal were 21 doctors, nurses and officials arrested. Sixteen were found guilty of criminal medical negligence and sentenced to prison over the outbreak. The night before the verdict was announced the crime claimed one more victim – a 2 year-old boy.

Honesty is the Best Medical Policy

Physicians concealing or lying about their contagious status may face criminal conviction for reckless negligence and fraud. Dr. Umesh Gaud was an Indian-born surgeon practicing in East London who had been infected with the Hepatitis B virus while finishing his training. Between 1990 and 1993 he worked at both the London Chest Hospital and the Royal London Hospital as a cardiothoracic surgeon. He obtained these prestigious positions after falsifying his job history and claiming to have been vaccinated against Hepatitis B. When the hospitals asked him to provide a blood sample for pre-employment screening, he substituted blood taken from an immunized patient. After an outbreak of hepatitis among the patients at one of the hospitals, another blood sample was requested and, again, he submitted a sample taken from a non-infected patient.

His deception was discovered in August 1993, when blood was taken from him under the eyes of several witnesses after another outbreak of hepatitis. At least 19 of his patients contracted the disease – he had exposed hundreds more. It is unclear if Dr. Gaud's recklessness will cost anyone their life-only time will tell. Hepatitis can be a chronic, innocuous disease or it can progress to fulminant liver failure, cirrhosis, and death. When he was convicted for "causing a public nuisance" (how British can you get?) the judge branded the physician's behavior as deceitful and deplorable, adding: "What you did was a terrible thing for a doctor to do." As Dr. Gaud began his 1-year prison sentence, the British Department of Health required all surgeons to be immunized against Hepatitis B.

The Last Word

Doctors don't appear to be killing their patients intentionally by infecting them. There are far better ways to do that. In most cases, infections are spread by practitioners who are cutting corners, putting their financial well-being ahead of the welfare of their patients, or jettisoning common sense. It should go without saying that syringes should not be reused and dialysis filters need to be rinsed between patients. Nobody will get the Nobel Prize for figuring out that blood and harvested organs intended to be used for transplantation should be checked for infections prior to giving them to sick people. You don't need Sherlock Holmes to deduce that you should wear gloves and wash your hands after delivering a baby (having done this we recommend washing them a few times). But, to be fair, we should acknowledge that in some settings the possibility of transmitting infection cannot be completely avoided. Consider that doctors use sharp objects to cut bad things out of people from hard-to-reach places in their bodies and that these instruments can cut both surgeons and patients. When this happens blood may be exchanged between the two of them. If the blood is infected, then someone can get sick due to sheer bad luck. We have focused on patients getting infected from their doctors but, in fact, many more caregivers are infected from their patients than vice versa. We will address this in our sequel, *When Patients Kill*. Just kidding. Well, maybe.

Chapter 20
Fictitious Physicians: Where Has Marcus Welby Gone?

Medicine is my lawful wife and literature my mistress; when I get tired of one, I spend the night with the other.

– Anton Chekhov

Medicine and the fine arts have been intertwined for centuries and more than a few physicians have had great success as writers. Drs. Anton Chekhov and Arthur Conan Doyle weren't too bad. Dr. William Carlos Williams wrote some pretty good poetry. More recently, Drs. Robin Cook and Michael Crichton have brought to life stories such as *Coma* and *Jurassic Park*, respectively. And let's not forget that Crichton also gave us the hit television series *"ER"*, the show that catapulted George Clooney ("Dr. Doug Ross"), Anthony Edwards ("Dr. Mark Greene") and Noah Wyle ("Dr. John Carter") to superstardom (well, at least Clooney became a superstar). Clearly some doctors can write. Going back over the past couple of centuries, however, one finds that doctors are just as likely to be characters flowing out of a plume, pen, or printer as they are to be authors. So why do they make such compelling fictional figures?

The answer may lie in that everyone is familiar with doctors. You may or may not have had the pleasure of utilizing the skills of an attorney. Maybe you have not yet had the opportunity to share intense, personal moments with your friendly, local electrical engineer. But chances are you have seen a physician at some point in your life and you have been left with an impression. In broad terms, doctors belonging to the "Greatest Generation" were held in high-esteem and widely accepted as pillars of the community. Since fiction mirrors reality, is it any wonder that the fictitious physicians of the 1960s and early 1970s such as Marcus Welby, Ben Casey, and James Kildare were essentially flawless? Can you imagine if these doctors suffered from Alzheimer disease, a drug addiction, or displayed homosexual tendencies? Things like that just weren't talked about several decades ago although they surely existed. The fact is that doctors were essentially deified on the screen just as they were idolized in reality for the most part. It would seem that doctors were put on a higher pedestal in the past than they are now; somehow, physicians have become all too human.

J.A. Perper and S.J. Cina, *When Doctors Kill: Who, Why, and How*,
DOI 10.1007/978-1-4419-1369-2_20, © Springer Science+Business Media, LLC 2010

Off the Pedestal

Of course, not all fictitious doctors were perfect prior to the advent of modern fiction. Traditionally when doctors in fictional settings were good they were very, very good and when they were bad they were horrid. This is not so in the modern depiction of physicians. Many doctors are now portrayed like other people, a mixture of good and bad. The medical series *House, M.D.* exemplifies this phenomenon. The lead character, Dr. Greg House, is a brilliant, Hopkins-trained diagnostician. He also walks with a cane, abuses his trainees and fellow staff members, insults patients, and ignores most accepted treatment protocols in lieu of his own intuition. Oh, and he is addicted to Vicodin™ (hydrocodone) and is not above stealing prescriptions from dead patients. Suffice it to say that if he truly existed, Dr. House would not have a long career given the current litigious state of medical practice. Nonetheless, this character is popular with the masses because he gives people something they need – a doctor with imperfections. Doctors are not gods. Anyone who watches the news or reads the newspaper or has access to the Internet or purchases a popular novel about doctors that kill knows that physicians make mistakes. Modern medicine is amazing in the scope of diseases that can be cured and doctors still cure many patients (and occasionally earn our eternal gratitude). But some of these same doctors use drugs, get sued, drive drunk, harass nurses, have sex with patients, get divorced, contract AIDS, go to jail, die young, screw up personal relationships, and lie, cheat, and steal. People don't look to doctors to be the shining example of altruistic purity that they were in the past – they want and need doctors to be like the rest of us. And that is what modern films and television gives them.

The very word "Doctor" adds legitimacy and power to any film, television series, or book that chooses to use it or abuse it. Consider Dr. Zhivago, Dr. Strangelove, Dr. Who, Dr. No, Dr. Demento, and Dr. Caligari. Would these titles have the same impact if they were Councilman Zhivago, Strangelove the Handyman, Rabbi Who, Father No, Mr. Demento, or Judge Caligari? As long as people have contact with physicians, doctors will be featured in fiction as they have been for hundreds of years. We could write a whole book on all of the doctors who have been portrayed in literature or on the screen. The exploits of soap opera physicians alone could fill several hundred pages (this is not a promo for a sequel). But in keeping with the theme of this present work, we are going to focus on physicians in fiction who have displayed characteristics similar to those of the murderous physicians found in these chapters.

The Characters

"Dr." Victor Frankenstein

Mary Shelley's protagonist in *Frankenstein; or, The Modern Prometheus* was actually a highly motivated science student rather than a doctor. Nonetheless, in many subsequent adaptations of her novel Victor Frankenstein has been granted a medical degree. Given the fact that he has an intricate knowledge of anatomy and physiology and the manual dexterity of a neurosurgeon this seems fitting. Let's consider it an honorary degree.

"Dr." Frankenstein fits the profile described in the beginning of this book. He believed it was his destiny to create life from nothingness, to imbue "inanimate clay" with a soul. Truly, this mad scientist/surgeon had delusions of being God. Shelley's choice of the subtitle for her novel tells us a few things about the psyche of Frankenstein. Prometheus, according to Greek mythology, stole fire from the gods and brought it to man in order to make the world a better place. In retaliation for his audacity, Prometheus was punished by having an eagle pluck out his liver every day; it regenerated every night to ensure his endless suffering. Frankenstein also attempted to steal something from God which belonged to Him alone – the power over life and death. He was also punished for his arrogance by having his own creation murder his younger brother, best friend, and bride. In the end, Frankenstein died in the Arctic in pursuit of the monster. Frankenstein's curiosity and obsession led him to deliver a grotesque child into this world. Rather than accepting responsibility for his actions, he chose to abandon his offspring with tragic results. Perhaps if he was really a doctor he would have had more compassion.

Dr. Hannibal "the Cannibal" Lecter

Dr. Hannibal Lecter, the creation of former crime scene reporter Thomas Harris, is perhaps the most well-known fictional serial killer of this generation. The American Film Institute (AFI) ranks him as the #1 movie villain of all time (edging out Norman Bates, Darth Vader and the Wicked Witch of the West). He was a brilliant physician having received training both at Johns Hopkins and in Paris. A psychiatrist by trade, he was also adept enough to perform complex brain surgery on one of his victims without killing him – in fact, he fed him his own frontal lobe. Lecter is an alpha-killer.

Whereas the real doctor-killers described in this book had some academic difficulties, Hannibal was an excellent student. It is unclear why he became a murderer but it may have been related to the murder and consumption of his sister in Lithuania in 1944. This horrific crime may have planted the seed of cannibalism in Lecter's mind; dining on his victims became a hallmark of his own murders. Dr. Lecter tended to kill people that he knew, much like real serial killers. He also murdered people who got in his way or threatened him is some way. His crimes were not of a sexual nature yet he was still a sadist who enjoyed the suffering of his victims and the power he had over them. He was a believable character who could have easily fit into the early chapters of this book, but he is not based on any real serial murderer.

Dr. Lecter exercised the ultimate control over his victims – he literally consumed them. By ingesting his victims, he absorbed them completely and took everything away from them. Yet for some reason he did not kill FBI Agent Clarice Starling though he had the opportunity to do so. He explained this at one point by stating that the world was a much more interesting place with her in it, but perhaps it was more than that. Clarice had some deep-rooted psychological problems from her youth that fascinated the physician buried in the psychopath. His interactions with her reflected basic psychoanalytic technique. Perhaps he was hoping that their exchanges would help her to help herself. Lecter was unquestionably a monster, scarier in many ways than Frankenstein's misanthropic creature, but he remained a skilled psychiatrist when it came to Agent Starling. Or maybe he was saving her for dessert.

Dr. Henry Jekyll

The Strange Case of Dr. Jekyll and Mr. Hyde was written by Robert Louis Stevenson in1886. Just as Mr. Edward Hyde is the personification of evil, Dr. Henry Jekyll represents the pinnacle of respectability. This novel was 100 years ahead of its time in that it showed that everyone, even doctors, has the capacity for both good and evil. Dr. Jekyll felt smothered by the trappings of his profession and societal position and needed to create Hyde as an outlet for his deeply buried urges and innate depravity. Over the course of Stevenson's book, Hyde became progressively more evil and Jekyll began to lose control of his alter-ego. Ultimately, the compassionate, respectable Dr. Jekyll could no longer live with the repulsive Edward Hyde so he chose to poison them both. Dr. Jekyll's final action may best be considered a "mercy killing." Although you could argue that Jekyll won in the end by killing Hyde, you can just as easily conclude that evil won out by leading a good man into eternal damnation, the punishment for suicide.

Mr. Hyde was different from many of the serial killers in this book. When he killed it was not necessarily for gratification or gain – it was simply because he wanted to do something bad. Even the evil scientists described in these pages hid behind a thin façade of medical necessity or, at least, curiosity. There were no pretenses with Hyde. He killed simply to take something pure out of the world. It is no wonder that Hyde's antithesis was a physician; the opposite of pure evil is unadulterated goodness. Given the status of doctors in Victorian England, the tale of Dr. Jekyll's fall from grace must have been shocking.

Dr. Christian Szell

When Sir Laurence Olivier questioned Dustin Hoffman with the assistance of a dental drill in the 1976 movie *Marathon Man* the phrase "Is it safe?" became synonymous with torture. Olivier was nominated for an Oscar for his role as Dr. Christian Szell, an aging but highly lethal Nazi war criminal who had been the

"White Angel of Auschwitz" earlier in his medical career. Szell would fit in quite nicely in our "Nazi Murderers" chapters. Over the course of the movie we learn that he is in the United States to recover a collection of diamonds that he had taken from his Jewish concentration camp victims and he was willing to do anything to get it. In addition to killing two people, he gives Hoffman's character a root canal with no anesthetic. Szell is an insidious character who ranks 34th among all-time movie villains according to the AFI (just behind Count Dracula). Despite his obvious capacity for cruelty and ability to kill without remorse, he would have been just an average guy among the doctors at Auschwitz.

Dr. Josef Mengele

Of course, Dr. Mengele is a real figure who committed many atrocities as an S.S. Agent in the Nazi Party during World War II. He was the real "Angel of Death" of the Auschwitz–Birkenau concentration camp and, as its physician, he was responsible for the human experimentation program as well as for sorting the incoming Jews into lines leading either directly to death or to imprisonment and prolonged torment. He was also fictionalized in the 1978 thriller *The Boys from Brazil* starring Gregory Peck in the lead role. In an extension of his real life role as a Nazi scientist, Mengele attempted to clone Hitler in the movie and subsequently re-establish the Third Reich. Interestingly, the fictional Mengele was pursued by Nazi hunter Yakov Liebermann played by Sir Laurence Olivier (the versatile actor who also played the infamous Nazi Dr. Christian Szell).

Dr. Evil (a.k.a. Dougie Powers)

Granted, Dr. Evil is a character in a comedy but he still shares some features with several characters we have encountered. He is most like the physician-dictators in that he was obsessed with power, money, and world domination. He was a physician as evidenced by his statement: "I didn't spend 6 years in evil medical school to be called Mister, thank you very much." In his youth he was an excellent student but overshadowed by his popular brother Austin. This likely resulted in an inferiority complex which manifested itself as an insatiable need for success. He was also the victim of child abuse at the hands of his adoptive parents (when he was insolent he was "placed in a burlap bag and beaten.") His tumultuous upbringing led to a disdain for the remainder of humankind. He indiscriminately killed his own henchmen and even threatened the life of his son, Scott Evil, on several occasions. This physician-killer was willing to take the lives of millions in pursuit of his diabolical schemes, not unlike Josef Stalin. He chose to focus his prodigious intellect on insidious plots including the formation of a "Death Star," the deployment of the "Alan Parsons Project", and the implementation of "Preparation H" instead of saving lives. What a waste!

Dr. Richard Kimble

The lead character of the 1960s television series and the 1993 movie *The Fugitive* epitomizes the troubles befalling a doctor who is deemed guilty until eventually proven innocent. Allegedly, Dr. Richard Kimble was loosely based on Dr. Sam Sheppard. In the movie version, Dr. Richard Kimble (played by Harrison Ford) is a noted vascular surgeon in the Chicago area who inadvertently becomes aware of a serious defect in a drug being produced by a major pharmaceutical company. In order to silence him, a "hit" is ordered but Kimble's wife inadvertently becomes the victim of "the one-armed man." Kimble is convicted of her death based on a mis-interpreted 911 call and sentenced to be executed by lethal injection. Through a fortunate accident, Kimble manages to escape prior to imprisonment. Despite being a fugitive, Dr. Kimble displays his true colors by saving a prison guard trapped in a bus about to be crushed by a speeding train and by rushing an injured boy to the operating room while posing as a low-level hospital employee. In the film, Dr. Kimble eventually is exonerated after being relentlessly pursued by Deputy U.S. Marshall Sam Gerard. In truth, the real evil physician in this movie was Kimble's friend Dr. Charles Nichols. Nichols was a pathologist who was in bed with the pharmaceutical company and he was willing to kill Kimble to ensure the success of the drug. Obviously this is fiction since pathologists are the most honor-able of all physicians.

Dr. Remy Hadley (a.k.a. "Thirteen")

Dr. Hadley (Olivia Wilde) is a beautiful, bisexual, sometimes self-destructive, occa-sionally drug-abusing physician working for Dr. Gregory House (who we have met earlier in this chapter). Over the course of her training, she inadvertently lets one of her patients die through an error of omission. Dr. Hadley had left pills for a patient infected with *Strongyloides*, a type of worm, but had not watched him swallow them. In fact, the medication had been eaten by his dog (which for some reason was allowed to stay in his hospital room) resulting in the death of both the dog and the patient. Hadley's inattention to this detail could have resulted in a civil suit against both her and the hospital but it likely would not have risen to the level of a criminal act.

In late 2008, Hadley developed a romantic relationship with Dr. Eric Foreman, another House protégé who had graduated from the Johns Hopkins Medical School with a perfect 4.0 average. Foreman had also killed a patient by making an incorrect diagnosis and irradiating her instead of treating her for simple infection. In truth, these types of things happen in real life. Unlike reality, however, Dr. House allows his staff to perform unnecessary, painful, and risky tests on his patients without informed consent. This can only happen on television and in V.A. Hospitals. House bases many of his miraculous cures on hunches – these don't hold up well in court if things turn out badly. It would be fair to say that in every episode, someone commits malpractice. In fact, in many cases the doctors of *House M.D.* could be charged with assault and battery and go to prison. That would be a nice twist when the writers run out of other plotlines. Likely in 2011 at this rate.

Dr. Alice Krippen

This is an obscure reference to say the least. Dr. Krippen was played by the noted actress Emma Thompson in the 2007 film *I Am Legend* based on the 1954 science fiction novel by Richard Matheson. This book centers on Dr. Robert Neville, a military physician who is attempting to cure the mutants who represent the last remnants of humanity after a pandemic plague has killed billions. Dr. Krippen, it turns out, was the physician who ended all life as we know it. Krippen appears at the very beginning of the movie in an interview explaining that she has developed a cure for cancer by manipulating the measles virus at the genetic level. She did not anticipate that the virus would be unstable and capable of infecting and killing most everyone who inhaled it. This fictional doctor was the most contagious of all caregivers. But do you know what's really frightening about this story? Even as we speak, scientists and doctors are manipulating genes and molecules in an effort to help humankind, eradicate cancer, and cure a host of diseases. This is a noble effort but there are many respected scientists, physicians and ethicists who are concerned that these man-made mutations could escape and wreak havoc on us all. In many religions God has exterminated most of mankind on occasion. And you know how fond doctors are of playing God.

Is Reality Really Stranger Than Fiction?

What a ridiculous question! Physicians are not wiping out whole cities by unleashing lethal viruses on an unwitting, helpless population, but they are likely involved in the production and purification of biochemical weapons. Medical murderers are not hidden behind metal masks to keep them from cannibalizing their victims, but they do hide behind paper masks as they dissect living men, women and children. Healers don't really drink potions to unleash the animal that hides within them, but they can live double lives – healing by day and torturing and killing by night. Doctors aren't really pursued across the country by U.S. Marshals, but they are sometimes viciously attacked by lawyers, dictators, the media, and politico-religious groups such as the Pro-Life activists. A physician can't build his own island and attempt to take over the world from a secluded fortress, but he can run an island or country with an iron fist and have his every word and whim treated as Gospel. Come to think of it, maybe reality is as strange as fiction. After reading this book, we are sure Hippocrates would think so.

Chapter 21
Doctors to the Stars

> *And also under the (Obama) healthcare plan, pop stars will*
> *still be able to choose their own creepy personal physicians. So*
> *that'll be good.*
>
> – David Letterman

People have always been fascinated with celebrities – and doctors have always been willing to line up to treat them. Going back to antiquity, kings and pharaohs had their personal physicians and today's political elites are no different. The twentieth and twenty-first centuries have also seen the rise of a new generation of gods walking among us, the "superstars." These darlings of the paparazzi include professional athletes, musicians, artists, actors and actresses, religious icons, as well as some celebrities of dubious talent.

Nowadays, celebrities routinely have their "court physicians." These are the descendents of the doctors of yesteryear who "helped" their patients with leeches, bloodletting, enemas, and emetics; only now they use pills, syringes, and prescription pads to mollify their petulant clients. This Faustian doctor/patient relationship can make the physicians rich and famous – or leave them destitute, discredited or imprisoned.

Dr. Feelgood

Fame, money and influence, are often close companions of fate, prompting dangerous self indulgence. While it is true that alcohol abuse and drug addiction are running rampant in Western society at all socioeconomic levels, many people only seem to notice when one of the "beautiful people" are afflicted with these maladies. Celebrities are often surrounded by an entourage or "posse" of close friends who are only too willing to make sure that the gravy train is kept running. These freeloading valets perform a variety of duties for their bosses including thorough ego stroking, scoring drugs, ordering pizza, and dialing 911 in case of an overdose. However, there comes a time when even the best posse is ill-equipped to handle the complex needs of a celebrity addict.

J.A. Perper and S.J. Cina, *When Doctors Kill: Who, Why, and How*,
DOI 10.1007/978-1-4419-1369-2_21, © Springer Science+Business Media, LLC 2010

Enter the "Concierge Physician," a newly labeled entity that has, in fact, been around for decades. These doctors are paid very well to provide customized, personal care to their well-to-do clients. While some of them do, in fact, provide prompt and high quality medical services, other "doctors to the stars" turn into pushers and dealers of prescription medications, violating the most basic professional and ethical standards. In some cases, in addition to serving as the celebrity's primary caregiver, the retained doctor also becomes a close friend, intimate confidant, and even lover.

Celebrities and Abuse of Prescription Drugs

Many celebrities have died following overdoses of illicit drugs such as cocaine and heroin. Others luminaries have been extinguished in alcohol-related fatalities. By and large, these deaths have little to do with the actions of physicians and, as such, will not be further mentioned. Instead, we will take a look at several high profile fatalities spanning five decades involving prescription drug abuse and questionable medical care. After all, you are reading *When Doctors Kill*, not *When Overindulgent Stars Get High and Wake Up Dead*. We are working on that one-it's going to be big!

In recent decades, the United States has experienced a dramatic increase in the abuse of prescription medications (pain relievers, anesthetics, sleeping aids, tranquilizers, stimulants and sedatives). According to government data, millions of Americans abuse prescription drugs. In 2006, 16.2 million Americans ages 12 and older had taken a prescription pain reliever, tranquilizer, stimulant, or sedative for nonmedical purposes at least once during the previous year. In fact, it is estimated that there are currently more prescription drug abusers than illicit drug abusers. Fatal overdoses from prescription painkillers alone have more than doubled from 3,994 in 2000 to 8,541 in 2005 (the last year for which complete data is available) – this doesn't even address the problems associated with sedatives such as Valium and Xanax™. The Centers for Disease Control and Prevention (CDC) has predicted that prescription drug abuse related deaths will continue to increase at an alarming rate.

We have certainly witnessed this trend in our forensic practice. While we still encounter deaths due to heroin or cocaine use, we see several cases a week involving prescription drug toxicity. The abuser routinely obtains these drugs through one of four main routes: stealing them, buying them illegally, accepting them as offerings from their friends (or disciples in the case of celebrities), or obtaining excessive prescriptions and medications from licensed physicians. As this book is focused on doctors who kill, we will focus on the latter means. In some situations, an honest doctor is duped by a deceptive patient who feigns an illness or symptom to obtain drugs. In fact, the Internet has created a cohort of very savvy patients who know just the right things to say to get what they want. With malpractice litigation running rampant, physicians are essentially forced to do something for most everyone who comes through their door for fear of being sued for "failure to treat." In other cases, however, physicians running "pill mills", shady pain clinics, and other high-profit, cash-only practices are eager to build a clientele who knows they can rely on the good doctor to cure what ails them. These unethical practitioners have cast a shadow on the many physicians who correctly and judiciously prescribe medications for pain, mental illness, or emotional stress. In fact, it is likely that some patients who truly need painkillers are being underprescribed badly needed medications because some doctors are afraid of being accused of creating and enabling addicts.

The Rich and Famous have the financial means to rent a "personal physician" to address their urgent or ongoing care needs. Many celebrities would justify the need for round-the-clock medical attention by reminding us just how stressful their lives can be. To be fair, some world-class athletes and performing artists do have to put up with stressors that most of us do not have to endure including:

- Long and strenuous performance hours interfering with the normal "biological clock"
- Weeks to months of grueling rehearsals
- Months of cross country and international travel
- An ongoing battle against aging resulting in dependency on plastic surgery, toxins, hormones, or other remedies
- Unrelenting scrutiny from the media and fans
- A constant fear of tumbling down from stardom into obscurity
- Probing interviews
- Blackmail attempts or civil suits by employees, acquaintances, or strangers threatening disclosure of some real or imaginary scandal
- Innate sensuality leading to sexual excesses and a propensity toward short-lived marriages often followed by acrimonious divorces and litigation
- A sense of loneliness and isolation while in the midst of tumultuous gatherings of fans and "friends"
- A nagging insecurity that anyone who claims to care for them actually loves their persona and not "the real me," and
- A total loss of privacy due to relentless pursuit by the paparazzi

Couple these stressors with a tendency to party all night, eat very little, and embrace the philosophy of "it's better to burn out than to fade away" and you have a recipe for a celebrity fatality waiting to happen.

Whereas, remarkably, some celebrities are able to create a "normal life" for themselves and their families, others cannot cope with the unbearable stress that comes with success. The triad of insomnia, depression and resulting drug abuse/addiction has been afflicting our brightest stars for decades if not centuries. We may call this psychopathological state the "SIDDA" syndrome (Stress, Insomnia, Depression, Drug Abuse). Obviously members of the general population may suffer from this condition, but members of the entertainment elite seem to be particularly prone to developing this condition. Wolfgang Amadeus Mozart, a former child prodigy turned pop star, may have been an early sufferer of this condition.

SIDDA fatalities are likely closely related to another condition afflicting both celebrities and countless others who party themselves to death, DUMASS (Death Using Multiple Addictive Substance Syndrome).

Doctors who choose to treat celebrities are seeking out an inherently high-risk patient population. It is no wonder that they are handsomely compensated for their efforts. Nonetheless, physicians are responsible for treating their patients in a manner consistent with the accepted standard of care regardless of who they are. It is the sworn duty of these concierge doctors to be providers of relief and appropriate therapy, not enablers of drug addiction or, worse still, creators of addicts. By virtue of their training doctors are more aware of the addictive potential of prescription medications than are their patients (rich or poor, famous or not). "Physicians to the stars" may create addicts by flippantly or indiscriminately prescribing and providing medications to their luminous clients just as doctors staffing "pill mills" may create addicts out of patients just like us who have legitimate medical conditions requiring potent prescription drugs. Once a patient has become hooked on a medication, a phenomenon called "tolerance" may ensue. Over time, in order to get the same beneficial effect from a given medication, higher and higher dosages of the drug are required. A doctor who fails to recognize this complication of therapy and, instead, blindly dishes out bottle upon bottle of drugs is not helping the patient. There are often (though not always) viable alternatives that can be explored.

Why would a reputable physician take on the risks associated with treating a prima donna? Well, for one thing it is likely extremely cool to go to a cocktail party and be able whisper, "I am _____ _____'s personal physician." Undoubtedly, this is much more successful than most pickup lines (particularly those used by forensic pathologists such as "No, it's not rigor mortis-I'm just happy to see you"). Second, doctors are fans too and it may well be like living a dream to treat a person that you idolize. Third, the money is good. Rumor has it that Michael Jackson's physician was offered $150,000 per month to take care of the pop icon. Fourth, a physician working on a "for cash" basis doesn't have to worry about haggling with insurance companies or the implications of any national health care overhaul. Last, celebrities talk to their friends just like other patients do. If you do a good job (whatever that may be) for one celebrity, chances are you may earn some other high profile clients. These perks are enough to lure some physicians to wander beyond the fringes of ethical medical care.

There is a lot of pressure on the physician treating a celebrity to trade in the Hippocratic Oath for the business adage "the customer is always right." Some "doctors to the stars" are simply unable to say NO and instead surrender to their patient's demands for excessive amounts of painkillers, antidepressants, sedatives, and sleeping medications. Not unexpectedly, in some instances these patients die as a result of drug overdoses either under accidental or suicidal circumstances. Although the treating physician obviously did not have the intent of killing the patient (it would be rather unwise to kill the "golden goose") they are, nevertheless, clear facilitators of an otherwise preventable death. In many of these cases, the doctor has committed malpractice and risks civil penalties and loss of medical licensure. In some cases, criminal charges may also be in order. In some states, particularly California, there is an apparent prosecutorial trend to view such improper medical conduct in fatal celebrity overdoses as manslaughter, although the chances of conviction appear to be slim. One would like to hope that such aggressive prosecution is based on the merits of the cases and not motivated by political expediency on the part of the prosecutor. That "tough on crime" slogan, though, does look really good on campaign posters if you are running for Governor.

Somewhere Under the Rainbow

Judy Garland (born Frances Ethel Gumm on June 10, 1922) was a dynamic and versatile actress of the stage and screen as well as an enthralling contralto singer. On June 22, 1969 she was found dead in her London apartment, apparently from a drug overdose. Her tumultuous and turbulent life experiences more than explain her tragic and untimely demise at the age of 47 years. Some of her doctors helped Dorothy do to herself what the Wicked Witch of the West was unable to accomplish.

Little Frances Gumm never knew the taste of a normal childhood. While still a toddler she made appearance on the stage of the New Grand Theater in Grand Rapids, Minnesota singing Jingle Bells, as part of a trio with her two sisters. She was featured in Vaudeville acts with her parents and The Gumm Sisters throughout her childhood. Her mother, Ethel, was the stereotypical domineering and controlling type of stage mother, largely oblivious to the intense physical and mental stress on young Frances. Her father Frank was the only person during Frances's early years that showered her with love and tried to protect her from the exhausting demands of the stage. Unfortunately, he died when Frances was only 12.

By the time she was 13, Frances had adopted the stage name of Judy Garland and was put under contract to Metro Goldwyn Mayer. Her career blossomed and she made more than two dozen films, including nine with Mickey Rooney. In order to keep up with the frantic pace of making one movie after another, Garland, Rooney, and other young performers were given amphetamines to boost their energy followed by barbiturates to take before bedtime to allow them to fall sleep. For Garland, this constant regimen of drugs established a pattern of addiction by age 15 and heralded a lifelong struggle to break free from this disease, a fight which she unfortunately lost. In her later life, she would resent the hectic schedule of her youth and felt that MGM studios had stolen her childhood.

In 1939, at the age of 17, she portrayed Dorothy in *The Wizard of Oz*. Her rendition of "Over the Rainbow" has captivated audiences for 70 years and the film vaulted her to superstardom. Judy found herself caught in a cyclone of publicity and pressure following the film and she was seeing a psychiatrist within a year. It was during this period that she also began to ramp up her use of stimulants and depressants. She wrote about the experience years later: "No wonder I was strange. Imagine whipping out of bed, dashing over to the doctor's office, lying down on a torn leather couch, telling my troubles to an old man who couldn't hear, who answered with an accent I couldn't understand, and then dashing to Metro to make movie love to Mickey Rooney." That could mess someone up.

The studio's abuse of their young stars was astonishing. "They'd give us pep pills," she wrote. "Then they'd take us to the studio hospital and knock us cold with sleeping pills... after four hours they'd wake us up and give us the pep pills again..." This regimen of expert medical care resulted in the production of 21 Garland films between 1939 and 1948, including the musicals *Meet me in St Louis* (1944) and the *Easter Parade*. That's a lot of pills. And a lot of very bad medicine.

In 1947 during filming of *The Pirate*, the 25-year-old Garland suffered a nervous breakdown and was placed in a private sanitarium. She was able to complete filming, but later that year made her first suicide attempt. Her mother taped up the cuts she had slashed in her wrists with a piece of broken glass. The next year Judy was cast by MGM in the musical *The Barkleys of Broadway* alongside Fred Astaire but could not finish it because of her disabling drug addiction. She was taking prescription sleeping medication along with illicitly obtained pills containing morphine. When Garland's doctor advised the studio that she could work only in 4- to 5-day increments with extended rest periods between, MGM executives suspended Garland and replaced her with Ginger Rogers. This was a nice break for Ginger.

By the time she was 27 years-old, Judy was being treated with electroshock therapy for depression. Her relationship with MGM further deteriorated in the 1950s resulting in another suspension after she decompensated during filming of "*Annie Get Your Gun.*" The suspension triggered a suicide attempt in 1950 in which she cut her throat with a shard of a broken glass and was sent to a "dry out" clinic where she was given additional electroshock therapy. When studio head Louis B. Mayer was told that Garland would need months to recuperate, he reportedly stated: "I've got millions tied up in this girl, I need her to work."

After release from the facility Judy was immediately cast in the film *Summer Stock*. After completion of this movie, Garland was called to replace a pregnant June Allyson in the leading role of *Royal Wedding* alongside Fred Astaire. Judy failed to report to the set on multiple occasions and on June 17, 1950 MGM studios terminated her contract, branding her as being "irresponsible, unreliable and unemployable." This did not help her deep seated self esteem issues.

In 1957 and several times thereafter, Judy again tried to commit suicide. Her preferred method was incising her wrists. Each time an attempt was reported in the tabloids, her fans would wear band-aids on their wrists in solidarity. She was especially idolized by the gay community, which saw in her tortured existence a reflection of their own difficulties and lifestyle problems. As the drugs took progressively greater hold of her life, Judy's behavior became increasingly unruly, disruptive and demoralizing. By the late Sixties, she was on an expanding list of psychiatric medications, now including Valium and Ritalin™. Ignoring the potential long-term consequences of prescription psychoactive drug use, her doctors continued to meet all of her medicinal needs and requests. They either were unaware of the dangers of the prolonged use of these medications (in which case they were incompetent) or they were too scared or lazy to confront the actress (in which case they passively facilitated her death). Either way, someone should have pulled their medical licenses.

In November 1959 alcoholism and drug addiction prompted another hospitalization. Upon admission, she was 50 pounds overweight (150% of her normal weight) and her liver was tremendously enlarged and affected by hepatitis. Seven weeks later she was discharged after she had lost 30 pounds. She was apparently drug free but was so weak that she had to use a wheelchair. The therapists told her that she would remain a semi-invalid for life and would never sing again, but they were proven wrong by Judy's resiliency. She successfully returned to both films and television and a concert appearance at Carnegie Hall on April 23, 1961, was called by many the "greatest single night in show business."

After hugely successful television specials and guest appearances in the early 1960s, CBS made a $24 million offer to Garland for a weekly television series of her own, *The Judy Garland Show*, which was deemed by the press to be "the biggest talent deal in TV history." The critics praised her television series but, for a variety of technical reasons, it was cancelled in 1964 after only 26 episodes. The demise of the series was personally and financially devastating for Garland, and she never fully recovered from its failure.

A dejected Garland returned to the stage and made various television appearances over the next few years. Most notably, she performed at the London Palladium with her then 17-year-old daughter, Liza Minnelli, in 1964. The concert, which was also filmed for television, was one of Garland's final appearances at the venue. In 1967 Garland was cast as Helen Lawson in *Valley of the Dolls*, the film version of Jacqueline Susann's bestseller featuring the character Neely O'Hara (played by Patty Duke), who was largely based upon Garland herself. As with previous projects, Garland missed days of work, blew repeated takes, and delayed production by refusing to leave her dressing room. She was finally replaced by Susan Hayward.

By early 1969, both her physical and mental health had deteriorated greatly. Depression and an acute sense of loneliness were omnipresent. Judy is reported to have sadly observed: "If I am a legend, then why am I so lonely?" Her five marriages and several affairs were symptomatic of her intense and constant search for meaningful and loving companionship. She performed in London at the "Talk of the Town" nightclub for a 5-week run and made her last concert appearance in Copenhagen in March 1969. Garland was plagued by financial instability, often owing hundreds of thousands of dollars in back taxes and, at times, going totally broke. She was even incapable of paying for her detoxification episodes.

On late Sunday morning, June 22, 1969, Mickey Deans, her fifth husband, found the 47 year-old Garland lying lifeless on the bathroom floor of their rented Chelsea, London house. There were no injuries and Scotland Yard ruled out foul play. Judy, Deans, and a friend had spent the previous night at home eating and watching television. According to friends the singer was said to be in good spirits prior to her death. At the Coroner's Inquest R. E. K. Pocock, the pathologist who performed the autopsy, testified that he found extremely high levels of secobarbital (Seconal, a fast acting barbiturate sleeping pill) in her blood, the equivalent of taking ten 100 mg capsules. But Pocock emphasized that he found no inflammation of the stomach lining and no trace of barbiturates in the stomach suggesting that the Seconal had been absorbed over a considerable period rather than taken in a single, massive dose. At the Inquest, both Deans and her London doctor, Dr. John Traherne, testified that Judy had habitually used Seconal "for many years." Dr. Traherne stated: "I don't think Miss Garland would have been able to sleep without Seconal." So he kept giving her more of it.

The London coroner, Gavin Thursdon, ruled that the cause of death was "an incautious self-overdosage" of barbiturates. Thursdon stressed that the overdose had been unintentional and that there was no evidence to suggest she had committed suicide. Further, Thursdon said the autopsy showed that Miss Garland had been addicted to sleeping pills for years (although, from a forensic pathologist's standpoint, it is unclear to us what findings these might be). "She took more Seconal than her body could tolerate," Thursdon told a courtroom packed with newsmen and fans of the dead singer in describing the cause of death. He continued, "Whether she did this in a daze from previous doses is unclear. But one thing is certain – there is absolutely no evidence this was intentional." The Coroner opined that most likely she had taken several capsules, woken up, and forgetting how many pills she had taken gulped down a few more, a behavior referred to as "automatism." Interestingly, a number of studies have shown automatism in this type of setting to be fallacious, though it is handy to be able to make this argument for personal, professional or legal reasons to rule a probable suicide as an accident.

The death certificate issued by Coroner Thursdon listed the cause of death as "Barbiturate poisoning (quinalbarbitone), incautious self overdosage, accidental." He may be right. Then again, given Judy's history of chronic depression with occasional flare-ups and recurrent suicide attempts, her financial troubles, her waning career, and her string of failed relationships, a strong argument can be made for suicide or, at the least, an undetermined manner of death.

An estimated 20,000 people lined up for hours at the Frank E. Campbell Funeral Chapel waiting to view the open casket. Judy wore the silver gown that she wore at her most recent wedding and her casket was white metal lined with blue velvet. Her mourners included her daughter Liza Minnelli and many entertainment stars including Ray Bolger (the scarecrow from Oz), June Allyson, Lauren Bacall, Jack Benny, Sammy Davis Jr., Cary Grant, Katharine Hepburn, Burt Lancaster, Dean Martin, Mickey Rooney, Frank Sinatra and Lana Turner. Garland was interred in Ferncliff Cemetery, in Hartsdale, New York. Budd Schulbert, a well-known screen writer, novelist and producer, accurately summarized Judy's life in stating: "Judy Garland somehow survived as a star of the first magnitude – a Lady Lazarus who kept rising from the dead, from countless suicide attempts, and broken marriages and nervous breakdowns and neurotic battles with weight and sleep, to somehow pull her jangled nerves together, take command of the Palladium, Palace or Carnegie Hall and bring down that audience one more time."

Both studio employees and doctors willing to ignore her well publicized addiction provided Judy with drugs to control her weight, increase her productivity, get her up, bring her down, and help her sleep. As a teenage star, Garland had been effectively sentenced to a life marred by depression, insomnia and addiction to both uppers and downers. The singer allegedly spent at least $1 million per year on drugs and doctors' fees or inducements. She could not have been a prescription pill addict without the assistance of many medical professionals. That being said, many physicians also made valiant efforts to rehabilitate her.

When Judy Garland died, none of the suppliers of her prescription drugs or any of the studio executives who pushed Judy into addiction were ever condemned or accused of child abuse or criminal wrongdoing. Only decades later, her daughter, Lorna Loft, angrily commented in a 2009 interview:

> What has saddened, disturbed, angered and frustrated me in the last 40 years is still the unethical and irresponsible way that many doctors in the medical field continue to over-prescribe drugs to celebrities and the rich and famous. It seems that we haven't learned anything over the past four decades. My belief is that the responsibility of the addict is absolutely number one, but we can't forget the enablers who have helped them all on their journey into the abyss – the ones who have "lied" to protect, "deceived" to protect, "loved them" to protect, and most importantly, benefitted from their addiction…

> We are facing a moral and ethical dilemma: shameful doctors who took an oath to save lives have now helped destroy them. These people must be severely prosecuted and given long and healthy prison sentences.

As we shall see in a bit, unfortunately for Anna Nicole Smith's doctors, the District Attorney in Los Angeles must have been listening.

Long Live the King – Or Not

There aren't all that many people who have been on a first name basis with the entire world – Elvis' was one of them. Elvis' Aaron Presley, The King, was born on January 8, 1935 in Tupelo, Mississippi. When he was 13, Elvis' and his parents moved to Memphis, Tennessee, one of the hubs of the Blues. After graduating from Humes High School, Elvis' worked a series of odd jobs while singing locally as "The Hillbilly Cat." He earned a local recording contract and, when he was 20, signed a deal with RCA. His popularity and fame started to blossom at a vertiginous pace.

By his mid-20's, Elvis' had become a walking trademark. His sneer, his gyrations, and his hair were adored and emulated everywhere. Truly, he was one of those guys who "women wanted to be with, and men wanted to be like." Despite being arguably the most popular man in the world, he had his critics, particularly when it came to his acting. Nonetheless, his 33 movies did very well at the box-office earning upwards of $150 million dollars. His mother, to whom Elvis' was very close, enjoyed her son's fame and success but was frightened by the frantic and hysterical reaction of his audiences. Her stress contributed to her alcoholism, which likely contributed to her premature death due to heart failure at the age of 46. Elvis' was heartbroken, "grieving almost constantly" for days. This emotional crisis may or may not have further opened his mind to drug abuse.

Several months after his mother's death he began re-experimenting with amphetamines, a drug introduced to him while he was on active duty in the U.S. Army serving in Germany. This was the beginning of Elvis' long, persistent and ill-fated voyage into the drug world. When his tour of duty in the Army was over, Elvis' settled in Hollywood, starring in movies throughout the 1960s. In 1968, he returned to live performances with a television special, which led to a string of successful tours across America. The famous composer and conductor Leonard Bernstein remarked: Elvis' is the greatest cultural force in the twentieth century. He introduced the beat to everything – music, language, clothes, it's a whole new social revolution... the 60's comes from it." In 1973, Presley staged the first global live concert via satellite (*Aloha from Hawaii*), reaching at least one billion viewers live and an additional 500 million on delay. That was ¼ of the world's population.

Despite having it all, Elvis' life was spinning out of control. He was taking stimulants with increasing frequency and in increasing amounts, partly to control his weight (which occasionally pushed 300 pounds) and partly because he liked them. He needed antidepressants to elevate his mood and downers (barbiturates) to combat insomnia. Eventually his drug addiction caused him to act bizarrely and his artistic performances declined dramatically in quality and consistency. His walk was at times unstable, his speech slurred, and he had to cut short or cancel some of his shows. By 1974, Elvis' was a very sick man due to a combination of lifestyle and a number of medical conditions (a dilated colon, glaucoma, mild hypertension and possible arthritis). It is possible that his bowel problems were related to his drug abuse; people taking excessive painkillers often become constipated. His entourage, known as the Memphis Mafia, and his personal doctors indulged the King's every whim.

On January 28, 1975, 20 days after his fortieth birthday, Elvis' was hospitalized for close to a month. The press was told that the hospitalization was because of an enlarged colon, however the primary reason was drug detoxification. A biopsy taken during that admission showed severe liver damage. By December of that year, Elvis' was in financial straits and had to work through the holidays despite a clause in his contract relieving him of all duties during that time of year. On New Year's Eve, Elvis' performed before 80,000 in the huge Silver Dome in Pontiac, Michigan. Artistically the show was a disaster and midway through it the star's pants embarrassingly split at the seams because of his extra weight. This notwithstanding, the show was a financial success and grossed $800,000, a world record for a single show, with half of the take going to Elvis'. A subsequent tour through the South had mixed reviews. Some shows were good, some were fair and some were miserable. He dropped lyrics, mumbled introductions and very nearly stumbled around the stage. On March 31, a Baton Rouge concert had to be cancelled because of singer's "illness" and he was subsequently hospitalized in a two-room suite on the 16th floor of Baptist Hospital. The press was informed that Elvis' was being treated for "exhaustion." The truth is Elvis' apparently nearly overdosed on a number of occasions during this tour and was found at times unconscious or unable to catch his breath.

This may come as a shock, but Elvis' was described by some close acquaintances as a drug experimenter. Just as he wanted the latest car model, he wanted the latest drug du jour whether it was a painkiller, a stimulant, or an anti-depressant. Some of his favorite cocktails included a mix of Valium, ethinamate, Dilaudid, Demerol™, Percodan, Placidyl, Dexedrine, amphetamine, biphetamine, Amytal, Quaalude, Carbrital, cocaine and Ritalin. Elvis' argued with his friends that the many drugs he took were legitimate prescription medications for pain, insomnia, and dieting – except that no one was really fooled. Everyone knew that Elvis' was really yearning for their euphoric effect – the "high." Dilaudid, a very powerful pain medication that causes a dreamy somnolence, was Elvis' favorite drug. He reportedly told one of his friends "I've tried them all, honey, and believe me, Dilaudid is the best." Initially, the drug prescriptions were supplied by a number of doctors, but in Elvis' last couple of years Dr. George Nichopoulos, known as "Dr. Nick," was his primary caregiver.

On August 16, 1977, the 42 year-old Presley had stayed up all night at his 18 room, limestone mansion, Graceland, in Memphis, Tennessee. He had entertained friends, played the piano, sang, and even played racquetball in the early morning. His 21 year-old fiancée, Ginger Alden, a fledgling actress and model, was staying with him in separate quarters adjacent to his master bedroom. Ginger was the last person to see Elvis' alive. At 9:00 AM, Ginger awoke to find Elvis' reading. He told her he couldn't sleep and was going into the bathroom to "read" some more. Ginger knew that meant he was going to take some of his medications. Elvis' syringes were in the bathroom and so was a good part of his personal pharmacy. "Okay," Ginger said, "just don't fall asleep." With that, she rolled over on the big bed and went back to sleep.

At about 2:00 PM she reawakened and went into the bathroom only to find Elvis' lying on the floor unconscious. Most sources indicate that Elvis' was likely sitting in the toilet area, partially nude, and reading when he collapsed. "I thought at first he might have hit his head because he had fallen out of his black lounging chair and his face was buried in the carpet" said Alden. Ginger called Elvis' to him and when she got no response slapped him a few times in an attempt to wake him. She raised the eyelid of one eye and the eye was "just blood red." She quickly summoned road manager Joe Esposito, bodyguard Al Strada, and Dr. Nick. The doctor unsuccessfully attempted mouth to mouth resuscitation and the medics were called. Presley, with his doctor in attendance, was rushed to Baptist Hospital where he was declared dead after additional resuscitation was attempted (including opening his chest to pump his heart by hand). Dr. Nichopoulos had the onerous task of informing Elvis' father of the death. Police on the scene said that there was no indication of foul play.

Under Tennessee statutes Elvis' death was clearly under the jurisdiction of the Shelby County Medical Examiner, Dr. Jerry Francisco. In the case of the sudden, unexpected death of a celebrity the public has a fervent interest in finding out what exactly happened. This is accompanied by intense media publicity and scrutiny – believe us, we know (Anna Nicole Smith came to our Office). Many of the supporters or fans of the deceased celebrity feel a sense of personal loss and are grieved that the world has lost a very valuable individual. Some simply cannot accept that the star was responsible for their own demise and wonder whether someone else was responsible, at least in part, for the death. Conspiracy theories soon emerge and cover-ups are often alleged. This constellation of factors places even a greater than usual burden on the Medical Examiner and law enforcement officials to conduct an extremely thorough and multifaceted investigation when faced with the death of a celebrity.

The investigation of the Medical Examiner must include a thorough review of the medical history; smoking, drinking, and drug habits; the circumstances leading up to death; a thorough and well documented external and internal examination of the body; and extensive toxicological analysis for drugs and medications. All of the physical, chemical, and investigative findings are then integrated to determine the cause and manner of death to within a reasonable degree of medical certainty.

The Medical Examiner of Shelby County seems to have abdicated portions of his responsibility in this case. To begin with, the autopsy was done at the request of the family rather than under Medical Examiner jurisdiction. Dr. Eric Muirhead, a hospital pathologist, performed the autopsy with the assistance of two pathology residents with Dr. Francisco as a witness. Francisco announced that the cause of death was a cardiac arrhythmia even prior to the completion of the autopsy and before any toxicological studies were performed. This proclamation is meaningless – everyone dies of "cardiac arrhythmia" which only means the heart stops. The actual cause of death is the disease or injury which causes the heart to stop. He also said that, "there was no indication of any drug abuse of any kind." This cannot be determined before the lab has completed their analysis of the blood samples taken at autopsy.

Elvis' autopsy did show evidence of severe heart disease, certainly enough to kill him, but also a host of prescription drugs were detected in his system. Toxicological studies were performed on his blood at no less than three independent laboratories. In a press conference on October 21, 1977, Dr. Francisco stated that four drugs were found in significant quantities in the entertainer's bloodstream: ethinamate, methaqualone (Quaalude), codeine and barbiturates. The first two are sedatives, codeine is a narcotic cough suppressant and painkiller, and barbiturates are "downers." Four other drugs including chlorpheniramine (an antihistamine), meperidine (a painkiller), morphine (likely a byproduct of codeine) and Valium were also found in what were said to be "insignificant amounts." The Associated Press quoted Dr. Francisco as saying that the amount of drugs found in Presley's body, collectively, would not have constituted a drug overdose and that it was unlikely that the drugs' chemical reactions within the body could have contributed to his death. He confidently stated that Presley died of heart disease adding, "had these drugs not been there, he still would have died." There is an interesting corollary to consider: in the absence of heart disease, would combined drug toxicity have been considered sufficient to have caused death in this case? If so, one can make a strong argument that they at least contributed to death and the manner of death should be considered accidental rather than natural.

The Medical Examiner's final report listed the probable cause of death as: "HCVD (hypertensive cardiovascular disease)" with "associated ASHD (arteriosclerotic heart disease)" and the manner of death as "natural." Dr. Francisco's ruling was met with skepticism by the press and with criticism by experienced fellow physicians. In 1991 Dr. Muirhead, the retired pathology chief of Baptist Memorial Hospital who had headed the autopsy team, took the first official shot at Francisco. Muirhead, who had remained quiet for 14 years, stated unequivocally that Elvis' "was a drug addict. We knew he was a drug addict because he had been at Baptist to be treated for that." Further, the autopsy team was shocked that death was attributed to heart disease. "We were appalled that he made that announcement," said Muirhead, "there were eight other doctors there who disagreed with him." Nationally known forensic pathologists Dr. Thomas Noguchi and Dr. Cyril Wecht also disagreed strongly with Francisco, asserting that prescription drugs were a major contributory cause to Elvis' Presley's demise. Other forensic experts such as Dr. Michael Baden were more lenient stating; Elvis' had had an enlarged heart for a long time. That, together with his drug habit, caused his death. But he was difficult to diagnose; it was a judgment call." Dr. Joseph Davis, an esteemed forensic pathologist, also reviewed the case and supported Francisco's opinion. Among forensic pathologists, the controversy is ongoing.

In 1980, 3 years after Elvis' death, Dr. Nick was indicted on 14 counts of overprescribing drugs to Elvis', Jerry Lee Lewis, and a dozen other patients. The jury acquitted Dr. Nick on all counts concluding that he was acting in the best interests of his patients. Later that same year, the Tennessee Board of Medical Examiners suspended his medical license for 3 months for overprescribing medications. Dr. Nick's troubles were not over, however. In 1995, the Tennessee Board of Medical Examiners permanently suspended Dr. Nick's medical license after it was revealed that he had been overprescribing drugs to many patients, including Elvis', for many years. It was reported that the doctor had prescribed more than 19,000 doses of medication to Elvis' over the last 2 years of the King's life. Dr. Nick's appeals in 1995 and 1998 to reinstate his medical license were rejected.

Years after Elvis' died, Dr. Nick claimed he was guilty only of caring too much for his patients. He showed this care in an unusual manner. In the final 7 months of Elvis' life, Dr. Nick prescribed 5,300 uppers, downers and painkillers for Elvis', resulting in an average of 25 pills or injectable vials a day. When questioned about the unusual number of prescriptions he had written for the King, he argued that he issued them in order to monitor the singer's drug use and eventually wean him of his addictions. In fact, during his legal proceedings he even claimed to have manufactured 1,000 doses of placebo for his most famous client. Still, it seems that somehow providing Elvis' with multiple prescriptions for Demerol, Nembutal, Dilaudid, Halcion, Didrex, Valium, Placidyl, Haldol, Nubain, Percodan, Nembutal, Stadol, and oxycodone was not effectively treating his addiction.

Dr. Nichopoulos, then 82 years-old, resurfaced in 2009. In interviews given to ABC, CBS, and CNN he complained of having been subjected to an unjustified "witch hunting" and being the "whipping boy" of the media and medical authorities. Conveniently, in the wake of Michael Jackson's death, Dr. Nick announced the upcoming publication of "The King and Dr. Nick: What Really Happened to Elvis' and Me." Dr. Nick has acknowledged that Elvis' was a challenging patient. "Unfortunately there's not a drug you can give somebody to take care of everything. You need a different drug for every situation." He also clarified that he was not only Elvis' physician but also treated up to 150 people on the road with the star. Nichopoulos relayed to the interviewers that Elvis' insisted that all of the prescriptions to his entire entourage be written in his name in order to keep his father, Vernon Presley, from getting upset by the cost of prescription drugs for so many people. "So it looked like he (Elvis') was taking all these drugs because the prescriptions were in his name." Ahhhhh, now it all makes sense!

Anna Nicole Smith

It was difficult to think of a catchy subtitle for this section. Everyone knows that Judy Garland was Dorothy, that Elvis' was the King, and that Michael Jackson was a uniquely talented dancer, singer, and songwriter. But, despite being intimately familiar with the life and death of Anna Nicole Smith (she happened to die in our jurisdiction and came to reside in our Office), we still are not quite sure what she was famous for. This is what we do know.

Anna Nicole Smith was born Vickie Lynn Hogan on November 28, 1967 near Houston, Texas. She was raised by her mother Virgie, a law enforcement officer, after her father had left the family. She did not excel in academics, failing her freshman year of high school and dropping out entirely as a sophomore. She obtained gainful employment at Jim's Krispy Fried Chicken and soon thereafter met her future first husband, Billy Ray Smith, a cook at the restaurant. When Anna was 17 and Billy was 16 they married and the next year they had a son, Daniel Wayne Smith. The couple separated in 1987 and eventually divorced in 1993. Vickie Lynn moved to Houston and worked sequentially at Wal-Mart and Red Lobster. She then turned to exotic dancing for additional income. So far, the same story could be told of thousands of women.

Vickie's big break came in 1992 when she appeared as the cover girl for the March issue of *Playboy* magazine. Vickie Lynn was a throwback to the days of the "blond bombshell" – she had curves and she was proud of them. In fact, she aspired to be the next Marilyn Monroe and she bore an uncanny resemblance to the dead sex goddess in several of her photo shoots. In 1993 she was chosen the Playmate of the Year, a great honor of the soft pornography industry, and had adopted the stage name of Anna Nicole Smith. She was a highly sought after model and her hourglass figure (36DD-26-38) was seen in ad campaigns in the United States and abroad. These were the salad days for Anna Nicole.

Love had also reentered the young stripper's life. In 1991, she met billionaire J. Howard Marshall while performing at Gigi's in Houston. After her divorce from Billy Smith had been finalized, the 26 year-old model married the 89 year-old oil magnate in 1994, officially becoming Vickie Lynn Marshall. Though the couple never lived together, Anna professed to love him deeply. Calloused cynics, however, began to spread rumors that she had married the elderly gentleman for his $1.6 billion, not accepting the possibility that they were soulmates. Some even believed her grief was feigned when Marshall died 13 months after their marriage. The disbelievers included the billionaire's two sons who fought Anna Nicole bitterly over her claim to half of the dead man's estate. Whether she loved him or not, it is clear that Anna Nicole was not doing well after her husband's death for one reason or another – in 1996 she was admitted to the Betty Ford Clinic.

Anna Nicole Smith's legal battle with the Marshalls went on for more than a decade. While the courts sided with Anna Nicole some of the time, they ruled against her on several occasions and in 1996 she filed for bankruptcy. By 2005 the U.S. Supreme Court even weighed in on her case, asserting that she had the right to pursue a share of the estate in federal court. The next year one of Marshall's two sons died, but the case continued on with his widow representing the estate. The estate issue was not resolved at the time of Anna Nicole's death in 2007 raising the possibility that her daughter would inherit millions. A federal appeals court, however, recently decided that Anna and her estate would see none of the $300 million she was seeking.

Anna Nicole Smith was a full figured girl but, unlike most models, did not appear to be all that bothered by it. Nonetheless, in 2003 she signed a deal with TrimSpa, a diet program that helped her to lose almost 70 pounds. Her weight rapidly moved up and down over the next few years, cycling almost as rapidly as her sobriety. In 2004, Anna Nicole was widely ridiculed after slurring her speech and acting erratically at the American Music Awards. Videos of the model taken over the next few years depict Anna as highly intoxicated and childlike; in a few home movies she was wearing smeared clown makeup. In the years leading up to her death, she had developed a full blown addiction to prescription medications, most notably chloral hydrate (a sleeping aid which had been a favorite of Marilyn Monroe's) and sedatives (specifically a class of drug called benzodiazepines).

Anna Nicole was under severe emotional stress the last year of her life. Her estate lawsuit with the Marshalls had not been resolved. Her tenuous relationship with TrimSpa was closely related to her unstable weight. Her acting and producing career was nonexistent. And she was having issues with her family. On September 7, 2006 she gave birth to a daughter , Dannielynn; 3 days later her 20 year-old son Daniel died of a drug overdose while visiting her in the maternity ward. Smith hired well-known forensic pathologist Dr. Cyril Wecht to perform a second autopsy on his body. Dr. Wecht concluded that Daniel had died of an overdose of Zoloft, Lexapro, and methadone. The presence of the latter drug is significant. This medication is used to wean people off of heroin addiction and as a treatment for chronic pain – Daniel suffered from neither condition. It was never determined where he had obtained this drug or from whom. It is quite possible that Daniel got his drugs the same way thousands of teens get them across the country – from his mom's medicine cabinet. But where was Mom getting them?

Anna Nicole obtained her drugs via several means. Some of her medications were obtained through good, old fashioned prescriptions made out in her name. Other drugs were scored by filling prescriptions made out to pseudonyms and close friends, including her lawyer and lover (what a strange combination!) Howard K. Stern and her close friend and physician, Dr. Khristine Eroshevich. There was never a shortage of pills, alcohol, and elixirs around Anna Nicole Smith. Friends were amazed at how many pills she was taking. When she traveled, a tote bag filled with painkillers, sedatives, and chloral hydrate accompanied her. Although allegations have been made that Stern kept Anna Nicole stuporous in order to control her (she apparently could be very domineering when she was sober), Smith also clearly exercised her own free will by voluntarily swallowing excessive medications. Anna's entourage enabled her addiction, but the drugs would not have been around if she wasn't asking for them constantly.

Anna Nicole Smith's fatal road trip from the Bahamas to Florida began on February 5, 2007. Leading up to the trip, she had been in relatively good spirits, having apparently pulled herself out of the depression that followed the death of her son. She was still abusing prescription medications, including methadone, but was apparently relatively functional. In addition to an assortment of pills, she was taking injections into her buttocks of vitamin B-12, Human Growth Hormone, and immunoglobulins to "rejuvenate" her and assist with weight loss. While flying to Florida from the Bahamas she began to complain of pain at her latest injection site; shortly after landing she complained of chills and spiked a fever to 105°F. She was treated with Tamiflu and antibiotics followed by a cold bath and she began to feel a bit better. She attempted to take some cough medicine prior to bed but could not hold it down. Eventually, Anna took two tablespoons of chloral hydrate and was able to fall asleep.

The next day Miss Smith felt tired but her temperature remained below 100°F. She drank plenty of fluids, watched a lot of TV, and napped. That evening, she asked for more chloral hydrate then slept for 1–2 hours. When she awoke, she watched a little television then asked for and was given Klonopin (a seizure medicine also used to treat panic disorder), Soma (a muscle relaxant), Valium (a sedative used for antianxiety disorder), and Topamax (a drug used to treat seizures and migraines) followed by a chaser of chloral hydrate. She was attended to by Howard K. Stern and Dr. Eroshevich.

By February 7, her third day in Fort Lauderdale, Anna Nicole Smith was still on the mend. Early that afternoon, she was found sitting naked in a dry bathtub, a situation that raises questions about her mental state. That evening Anna was very upset when Dr. Eroshevich left Florida for California. She took another dose of chloral hydrate and went to bed but did not sleep well. It is worth noting that chloral hydrate is a liquid medication. We simply don't know if she actually used a tablespoon to take this drug, poured it into a glass, or swigged it from a bottle. We do know she was taking too much of it.

On the morning of February 8, 2007, Howard K. Stern has stated that he woke up around 10:00 in the morning. Anna was already awake and feeling fairly well except for fatigue. He helped her to the bathroom then put her back in bed prior to leaving the hotel to purchase a boat at her request. According to him, he did not see Anna Nicole take any medications that morning nor did he give her any. Anna was then babysat for several hours; it was assumed she was asleep in bed. When her bodyguard's wife, a registered nurse, checked on her at 1:00 PM she was unresponsive and not breathing. Resuscitative efforts by the nurse, the bodyguard, and paramedics ensued but were unsuccessful. She was pronounced dead at 2:49 PM at Hollywood's Memorial Regional Hospital.

The death scene was secured by the local police who initiated an investigation. Staff from the Medical Examiner's Office also responded, confirming the presence of numerous prescription medications in the room. The body was initially examined at the Broward County Medical Examiner's Office that afternoon and samples were taken for toxicological analysis and for microbiological studies to rule out infection. A complete autopsy was completed the next day. Following the procedure, a press conference was held and it was announced that there were no signs of foul play but that additional studies were required to determine the cause and manner of death. Given the circumstances surrounding this fatality and the fact that most young people who die suddenly and unexpectedly in South Florida have taken drugs, an overdose was suspected.

When the first battery of toxicological studies was completed, there was no obvious cause of death. Though several drugs were identified, including acetaminophen, Topomax, diphenhydramine, Klonopin, Valium, Ativan, Robaxin, and Soma, none were at toxic levels. At that time, although a drug overdose could not be excluded since these drugs can act together to kill you even at "safe" levels, the Medical Examiner team's attention was turned to possible infectious causes of death. An interview with Dr. Eroshevich lead the pathologists to dissect the tissue beneath the injection sites. Large abscesses, scars and needle tracks were identified in her buttocks. Infectious disease specialists were consulted and death due to sepsis from infected injection sites was beginning to appear likely. Molecular analysis for interleukins and cytokines was ordered and several markers were elevated, supporting an acute systemic infection. But additional studies were still pending so the cause of death was not finalized.

Real life is not like CSI – sometimes it takes weeks to months to get the results of complex toxicological tests. One goal of the Medical Examiner is to provide answers to the police, the family, and the public in a timely manner but the primary mission is to get the cause and manner of death correct. Despite significant pressure to rule on this fatality prematurely, the Medical Examiner waited until all of the results were in. Doing so in this case prevented a great deal of egg on the face. On the third week following the autopsy, a referral lab informed the Medical Examiner that there was a toxic level of chloral hydrate in the blood. Despite Anna Nicole's probable tolerance to this medication, this drug taken in combination with the cocktail of prescription medications described above, caused her to fall asleep, stop breathing, and die in her bed in the Hard Rock Hotel.

The cause of death in this case was combined drug toxicity and the manner was ruled as accidental. A probable infection was considered a contributory factor in this fatality in that it likely weakened her and may have predisposed her to take excessive medications to try to feel better or get some rest. With the final press conference, the satellite television trucks finally pulled away from the Medical Examiner's Office.

The drug concentrations in Anna Nicole's blood were clearly sufficient to kill, but they were not in the massive range commonly seen in suicides. Homicide was also considered but ruled out. Although the sheer number of prescription drugs present suggested bad medicine, none of the interviews conducted by either the Medical Examiner or the police suggested that anyone other than Anna Nicole Smith was responsible for taking the medications that killed her. Yes, her medications were prescribed and amassed in excess. Yes, she was likely taking medications prescribed in her name as well as drugs prescribed to fake names and friends. And yes, she was being prescribed medications that could easily be abused and, by all accounts, her physicians knew or should have known that she was an addict and that they were providing her with substances that had the potential to kill her. But, unless someone poured the chloral hydrate down her throat or shoved a handful of pills into her mouth the morning of her death, nobody committed homicide in our estimation. The Attorney General of California, however, plans on holding someone accountable.

On November 1, 2009 the Associated Press reported that Stern and two of Anna's physicians, Drs. Khristine Eroshevich and Sandeep Kapoor, have been ordered to stand trial for conspiring to provide controlled substances to the dead celebrity. During the hearing, Gina Shelley, a friend of Anna Nicole, said that she had seen Stern placing pills in Anna's mouth on occasion – "He poured them in her mouth like you would a bird" – though this was not witnessed on the day of her death. The physicians have been accused of providing excessive medications to a known pill addict. During the preliminary hearing in Los Angeles, a pharmacist swore under oath that he had told Eroshevich that "Unless you want your picture on the cover of the National Enquirer, I wouldn't give her (chloral hydrate) because it is a powerful respiratory depressant." Good advice! It will also keep you out of nonfiction bestsellers such as *When Doctors Kill*.

While the behavior of the physicians in this case is certainly questionable from an ethical standpoint and it is likely that their medical licenses are endangered, it will be interesting to see if a jury finds them guilty of any crime other than poor judgment (which is not necessarily illegal). Stern has no medical training, so it will be more problematic establishing criminal fault in his case. Consider that if every friend or family member who gave an addict a pill or an alcoholic a drink was forced to stand trial, the courts would be overwhelmed. More likely than not, in the absence of a smoking gun, Stern will not be found guilty of playing a part in Anna Nicole Smith's death. But you never know. If additional evidence or a shocking eyewitness account of her death surfaces over the course of the trial, we would be happy to consider reclassifying the manner of death in this case. For example, if someone injected her with a powerful anesthetic (such as propofol) to help her sleep we may consider ruling the death as a homicide; of course, if there was no intent to kill we may still deem the death accidental. Barring the unforeseen, the death of Anna Nicole Smith will remain an accidental overdose and the case will remain closed. And her doctors will stand trial in a precedent setting case.

Moonwalk

Michael Jackson sold more than 750 million records and CDs before his untimely death on June 25, 2009 at age 50. By the time you read this, he may have sold over a billion. He was the undisputed "King of Pop" and there will never be another artist like him. He was quite a character.

Michael Joseph Jackson was born the seventh of nine children on August 29, 1958 in Gary, Indiana, an industrial suburb of Chicago. His mother, Katherine, a devout Jehovah Witness, brought music into the home. His father, Joe, also was involved in the upbringing of the kids; allegations of his physical and emotional abuse followed the Jacksons for decades. Joe never lived out his dream of being a professional musician but he did have talented children. He organized his older sons (Tito, Jermaine and Jackie) into a singing group, to which later a fourth son, Marlon, was added. When little Michael joined them in 1964, the Jackson 5 was born.

The group started out working in Gary but then began to tour the Midwest, often opening stripteases and other adult acts in a string of black nightclubs known as the "chitlin circuit." Joe was constantly "motivating" the children to perform their best. In 1968, Berry Gordy, the founder of the legendary Motown recording company, signed them to a contract which lasted until 1975. After that, the Jackson 5 then contracted with CBS records and changed their name back to The Jacksons. They soon embarked on a blazing trail of shows with Michael Jackson serving as their lead song writer and singer. Their appeal crossed over many racial barriers – Michael was a star, but not yet a superstar.

In 1978 Jackson dabbled in the movies, playing the Scarecrow in *The Wiz*, an African American version of *The Wizard of Oz*. Michael's close relationship with Diana Ross, who played Dorothy, lasted up until his death. In many ways she served as a big sister/mother to him, especially in the more troubled moments of his life – eventually, he even began to physically resemble her. Although his performance in *The Wiz* was cute, he was to attain immortality through singing and dancing rather than acting.

Jackson's first solo album, *Off the Wall* in 1979, eventually sold more than 20 million copies worldwide. It was a synthesis of funk songs, disco, soul, soft rock, jazz and pop. And it was very danceable (or so I am told by those who can dance). The "King of Pop" earned his crown in 1982 with *Thriller*, the most commercially successful album of all time with well over a 100 million copies sold. The hit MTV music video was an ingeniously choreographed horror/pop/mini-movie with Michael morphing from an innocent, young man into a monster, leading a cast of zombies through a mesmerizing, ritualistic dance. Even if you weren't a Jackson fan at the time (trust me, I know because I wasn't one) when you saw the video you had to acknowledge his genius. Within a few short years, the planet was filled with Jackson wannabes, emulating his every robotic movement and signature Moonwalk (a dance move based on one of Marcel Marceau's mime routines).

For the next two decades, Jackson became one of the most recognized figures in the world. He amassed hundred of millions of dollars in profits and, although he was a profligate spender, he also was a benevolent philanthropist, raising and donating many millions of dollars to charitable organizations. He also became increasingly weird, both in appearance and behavior. By the present decade, he had earned the sobriquet "Wacko Jacko."

Let's begin by analyzing his increasingly alien appearance. During a 1993 television interview with Oprah Winfrey he admitted that he had taken skin bleaching medications because he had been diagnosed with vitiligo in 1986, a disorder associated with the presence of irregular, patchy, whitish discolorations of the skin caused by a loss of melanin (the normal skin pigment). He had two treatment options, one which would darken the pale areas and the other that would lighten the surrounding skin. Jackson chose the latter alternative, and ended up with a pale, ghostly and ghastly appearance. This choice led some to accuse Michael of trying to become more "white", in a sense disavowing his black heritage. Then there were the surgeries. A lot of them.

In 1979, Jackson had his first facial surgery after breaking his nose during a complex dance routine. However, the surgery was not a complete success, with lingering breathing difficulties leading to a second rhinoplasty ("nose job") in 1980. In 1984 Michael had his nose slightly narrowed and his eyebrows arched. Over the next decade permanent eyeliner was tattooed around his eyes and he underwent additional plastic surgery procedures on his nose, cheeks, lips and chin. His last plastic surgery was done by a German surgeon who took cartilage from Michael's ear to repair his nose, which had been damaged by the prior surgeries. In the end, Jackson was transformed from a handsome, African American man into a sexually ambiguous, sort-of-white, sort-of-person. Dr. Deepak Chopra, a friend of Jackson's for 20 years, said: "What became his compulsion with cosmetic surgery was an expression of self-mutilation, a total lack of respect for himself." Other medical professionals believe that Jackson also had "body dysmorphic disorder," a psychological condition which would cause him to never be satisfied by his own appearance and have no concept of how he is perceived by others. Despite their beauty and many gifts, many celebrities are afflicted with this mental condition. As a matter of fact, so are many everyday folks who believe that they are too fat, too thin, too short, or too tall despite looking just fine.

In addition to mental anguish, Jackson was not a stranger to physical pain or to pain medications. In 1984 he was filming a Pepsi commercial when a pyrotechnic explosion resulted in a shower of sparks landing on Michael's head, setting his hair on fire and causing severe scalp burns. The injuries left him in severe pain requiring treatment with pain medicine and laser therapy. During the 1990s, Jackson became increasingly dependent on prescription drugs, mainly painkillers and strong sedatives, and his health deteriorated dramatically. In 1993, with the help of Elizabeth Taylor and Elton John, Michael entered a rehabilitation clinic but his addiction persisted. And there were doctors willing to provide the King of Pop everything he needed to keep going.

Jackson's emotional pain probably ran deeper than his physical discomfort. Michael was obsessed with clinging to childhood, likely due to the loss of his own youth which was sacrificed for the good of the Jacksons. This manifested itself by surrounding himself with young children, his love of children's games and his habit of speaking in a soft falsetto voice like a child. Michael himself explained that this behavior was prompted by a deep sense of loneliness and deeply rooted feelings that he had been robbed of his childhood and that he was trying (in vain) to recapture it. Jackson's obsession with youth and children eventually lead to a great deal of trouble for the singer.

In 1988, Jackson purchased land near Santa Inez, California where he built his Neverland Ranch. His guests were almost exclusively young children, including many who were disabled. Unfortunately, this benign attachment to children extended to sleeping with them in the same bed, which is considered unusual for a man in his 30's. In the summer of 1993, Jackson was accused of child sexual abuse by a 13 year-old boy named Jordan Chandler and his father, a dentist. The young boy told a psychiatrist and later police that he and Jackson had engaged in acts of kissing, masturbation and oral sex. The case was eventually settled out of court, allegedly at a cost of about 22 million dollars. Jackson was never charged, and the state closed its criminal investigation, citing lack of evidence.

Two short-lived marriages followed in short succession; many believed these were only efforts at shoring up Michael's public image. The first marriage in May 1994 to Lisa Marie Presley, the daughter of Elvis' Presley, ended in divorce in January 1996. The second marriage in late 1996 to his dermatologist's nurse, Debbie Rowe, ended 3 years later. This marriage resulted in two children, Paris Katherine and Prince Michael I. Jackson's third child, Prince Michael Jackson II (nicknamed "Blanket") was born in 2002. In November of that year, Jackson brought his newborn son onto the balcony of his room at the Hotel Adlon in Berlin, as fans stood below. Jackson briefly extended the baby over the railing of the balcony, four stories above ground level, holding him only by his little arm. This thoughtless and immature act (though innocent in Michael's mind) triggered allegations of child endangerment. Jackson later apologized for the incident, calling it "a terrible mistake." He is lucky he didn't dangle a puppy instead – PETA would have been all over him.

Jackson's reputation took another hit in 2003 when he was charged with molestation of a minor, four counts of intoxicating a minor, one count of abduction, and one count of conspiring to hold a boy and his family captive at Neverland Ranch. Jackson denied all counts and asserted that he himself was the victim of a failed extortion attempt. On June 13, 2005, the jury found Jackson not guilty on all charges. The physical and emotional stress associated with exhausting, relentless tours as well as his growing personal problems took their toll, resulting in depression and severe insomnia. He was a classic case of SIDDA. He was also in constant physical pain from years of dancing.

In the waning years of the first decade of this century, Jackson had become a living legend. In fact, in some ways his professional career had died several years before and only the walking freakshow remained. But Michael was ready to change all of that. In July 2009, Jackson was booked to perform a series of major comeback concerts in London entitled *This Is It*, which he suggested was going to be his "final curtain call." Although initially planned for 10 dates, it was increased to 50 concerts after record-breaking ticket sales to more than a million people. However, the shows had to be cancelled because of Michael's unfortunate and premature biological curtain call, at age 50, on June 25, 2009. That was it.

By most accounts, at least one doctor allegedly contributed to Michael Jackson's demise. On the day of his death, Los Angeles Fire Department paramedics responded to a 911 call from the home he was renting at about noon. The unidentified caller stated that Michael Jackson was not breathing and unresponsive with resuscitation being performed by his doctor (ineffectively on a bed, it turns out). When they arrived, within no more than 2 minutes, they were met by Dr. Conrad Murray who identified himself as being Michael Jackson's personal physician. The paramedics placed Jackson on the floor and performed CPR and then took Jackson to UCLA Medical Center, about a 6-minute drive from his home. By the time they arrived at the hospital Jackson was in full cardiac arrest. Dr Murray declined to sign the death certificate and left the hospital shortly after accompanying Jackson to the facility.

The hospital notified the Los Angeles County Coroner of the death and they accepted jurisdiction of the body and planned an autopsy. Meanwhile, the Los Angeles Police Department's (LAPD) Homicide Division started an investigation into the circumstances surrounding the fatality. The next day the forensic pathologists of the Coroner's Office conducted a 3 hour autopsy on the body of Michael Joseph Jackson. Initially, the cause and manner of death were left "pending" citing that the "anatomical findings showed no evidence of trauma to the body or evidence of foul play" and that toxicological and tissue studies were required before the case could be finalized. The LAPD conducted an in-depth investigation, interviewing dozens of individuals, including Jackson's multiple doctors and serving many search warrants both locally and out-of-state. The LAPD also had the assistance of federal, state and local agencies including the United States Department of Justice, Drug Enforcement Administration (DEA), California Department of Justice, Bureau of Narcotics Enforcement (BNE), the Houston Police Department and the Las Vegas Metropolitan Police Department. Within days of the death, Michael's father Joseph was alleging "foul play" while family friends and lawyers were working the talk show circuits and spewing out "drug overdose." One of Michael's closest friends (it is amazing how many "closest friends" a celebrity has after they have died) said he had even warned the family that Michael was going to end up like Anna Nicole Smith. He was right.

The depth and breadth of the LAPD's and Coroner's investigations are not unusual given the high-profile nature of this case. Imaginative plots and wild scenarios pop up frequently after the death of a superstar and many avenues of inquiry must be traveled prior to dismissing them. Both the quality of the police investigation and the thoroughness of the autopsy will be painstakingly scrutinized and often unfairly criticized by the public media.

The investigational fog started to dissipate with the August 2009 unsealing of a batch of documents in Houston, specifically police affidavits that had been submitted in order to permit review of medical records and facilitate search and seizure of evidence from different medical offices. The investigation of treating physicians and their medical records was prompted by the fact that Dr. Sathyavagiswaran, the Los Angeles County Chief Medical Examiner and Coroner, informed the police that Michael Jackson had lethal levels of a short acting anesthetic (propofol) in his blood. The affidavits made it clear that the goal was to secure evidence from Jackson's other doctors that might substantiate whether Dr. Conrad Murray, Michael Jackson's personal physician, had committed manslaughter. Under California law, manslaughter may be considered voluntary or involuntary. In the Jackson case, if any charges are filed, involuntary manslaughter appears to be more likely.

Prior to becoming Michael's personal physician, Dr. Murray was a cardiologist with 20 years of experience with offices in Houston and Las Vegas. In several interviews he indicated that he had been Jackson's doctor for 6 weeks prior to his death and that he had on occasion administered a medication by the name of propofol (Diprivan) diluted with lidocaine to Michael for insomnia. Propofol is a short acting anesthetic that is used for induction of general anesthesia. It causes loss of consciousness very rapidly and it is eliminated from the body in several minutes. Because of the strength of the drug and its fast-acting nature, it is necessary to monitor the patient's heart rate and breathing closely after its administration. As propofol can suppress breathing to the point where a patient's heart stops, it is almost exclusively used under the guidance of an anesthesiologist or other medical professional where resuscitation equipment is available. It is not a sleeping pill nor is it routinely used by cardiologists in the rental homes of celebrities.

Because the medication has to be given intravenously and since it is not usually available in general pharmacies or on the street, addiction to propofol is rather rare amongst the general population. Some physicians have abused it, however, for its ability to block out the world temporarily, allowing them to escape their daily stressors or the demons dwelling in their minds. The problem is that because of the short acting nature of the drug, addicts have to take the drug repeatedly at frequent intervals. Furthermore, the drug is very dangerous because the window of safety between the therapeutic level and the toxic level is very narrow and abusers of this prescription drug may cease to breath. Michael Jackson was afflicted with severe insomnia and he turned to propofol to find a few moments of relief from life – these moments became an eternity.

Dr. Murray related that Michael was very familiar with propofol, which he called his "milk" (the propofol solution has a milky appearance). Jackson had told Murray that he had been prescribed propofol by a number of doctors in the past, including two German physicians during a recent European trip. While serving as Jackson's personal physician, Murray also observed multiple injection marks on the hands and feet of Jackson. When he asked about them, he was told by Jackson that he had been given a "cocktail." If the accusations being leveled at Dr. Murray are substantiated in a court of law, then he was serving as Michael's bartender.

The most potentially damning evidence against Dr. Murray is the timeline of medications that he gave Jackson over the days leading up to the icon's death. By his own admission, on June 22, in order to help Michael sleep, he gave him 25 mg of propofol instead of the usual 50 mg (he was beginning to think the singer was addicted to this drug!) along with lorazepam (Ativan) and midazolam (Versed). On June 23 he gave Jackson only lorazepam and midazolam without propofol and Jackson went successfully to sleep. According to Murray's account, Jackson was again having trouble sleeping the night of June 24. Murray resisted the use of propofol, but this time Jackson wore him down. Starting in the early morning of June 25, he gave Jackson enough drugs to put a class of teenage boys on a field trip to the Playboy Mansion to sleep:

- At 1:30 AM. he injected Jackson with 10 mg of lorazepam
- At 2:00 AM Jackson was still awake and was injected with 2 mg of lorazepam
- At 3:00 AM Jackson was still awake and was given 2 mg of midazolam intravenously, again with no effect, and
- At 7:30 AM Jackson was still awake and Dr. Murray injected him with another 2 mg of midazolam. He also began monitor the singer's blood oxygenation at that time, though it is unclear if Jackson was having trouble breathing

Within a few hours of receiving this last sedative, Michael began to "beg" Murray repeatedly to give him "his milk."

Sometime in the late morning on June 25, the physician finally gave in and allegedly injected his patient with 25 mg of propofol diluted with lidocaine. Jackson finally fell asleep. Murray stated that he monitored Jackson for about 10 minutes and then went to the bathroom for no more than 2 minutes. When he returned he found Jackson comatose and not breathing. Dr. Murray said that he immediately started resuscitation and after a few minutes called for assistance from a security person and Prince, Jackson's eldest son. He continued his efforts until the paramedics arrived and the rest is history. The period during which resuscitation was given by Dr. Murray is apparently in doubt, however, because the police found that Dr. Murray was on the telephone from 11:18 AM to 12:05 PM. It is tough to chat when you are performing CPR. Dr. Murray traveled with the patient to the hospital and told Dr. Cooper, the Emergency Room physician, that he gave Jackson only 2 mg of lorazepam during the night and an antidote; he apparently did not mention any other drugs, including propofol.

On Friday August 28, 2009, the Los Angeles County Coroner's office officially ruled Michael Jackson's death a homicide, stating that it was primarily caused by acute propofol intoxication. The Coroner's report also listed benzodiazepines (sedatives including lorazepam and midazolam) as contributing to the singer's death. "The drugs propofol and lorazepam (Ativan) were found to be the primary drugs responsible for Mr. Jackson's death," the news release read; other drugs detected included midazolam (Versed), diazepam (Valium), and lidocaine. The manner of death was determined to be homicide since the cause of death, an overdose, was said to have been caused by "injection by another." Dr. Conrad Murray would have to be the "another."

The autopsy report and the detailed toxicology reports were temporarily sealed at the request of the LAPD and Los Angeles County District Attorney on grounds that the death is still under investigation and charges may be filed. As of today, criminal charges of manslaughter had not yet been pressed against Dr. Murray though they appeared to be imminent several months ago. But it seems to be just a matter of time and timing (there will be a Governor's race coming up in California and the Attorney General is a candidate) before such criminal charges will be proffered. In theory, Jackson's doctor could go on trial around the same time as Anna Nicole Smith's physicians.

If manslaughter charges are leveled at Dr. Murray they most likely will be based on his administration of drugs to a known addict, the inappropriate administration of a drug (propofol) not recommended for use as a sleeping aid, failure to take appropriate measures to combat possible serious drug side effects, inappropriate resuscitation measures, and a delay in seeking emergency assistance. While such charges may be more than sufficient for a determination of gross medical negligence and malpractice in a civil trial and there may be enough evidence to revoke Dr. Murray's medical license, it is much less clear that the District Attorney could secure a conviction on a criminal charge such as involuntary manslaughter, much less murder. The defense in a criminal trial is likely to argue that:

- There was a clear lack of "mens rea" ("evil intent") to kill Michael Jackson
- Dr. Murray tried his utmost to keep this patient alive and wean him of his addictions
- Michael Jackson was apparently addicted to propofol while in Germany, well before Dr. Murray treated him
- Dr. Murray advised Jackson of the propofol risks and side effect, so adequate informed consent was obtained
- Michael Jackson was addicted to a number of prescription drugs, some obtained from other physicians, as the postmortem toxicology revealed the presence of several drugs which had not been prescribed or given to Jackson by Dr. Murray, and of which Dr. Murray had no knowledge
- Propofol is not an illegal drug
- While it is true that the manufacturer recommends propofol as an anesthetic drug and not as a sleeping aid, physicians use many drugs for conditions not recommended by official sources and in some cases they are quite effective
- Some medical publications have indicated that propofol significantly improves the recovery from insomnia-related symptoms and it may have been an effective therapy in Jackson's case
- In the entire United States there have been very few (only 48) deaths due to propofol toxicity, and
- If a combination of drugs killed Jackson, rather than propofol alone, and Jackson was taking several of these drugs without Murray's knowledge, it will be difficult to determine beyond a reasonable doubt that Murray's actions alone resulted in death. Michael's own actions may have pushed him over the edge

To sum up this defense strategy, "drugs kill addicts, not the doctors who administer or prescribe them."

On the other hand, a conviction of involuntary manslaughter might be sustained against Dr. Murray if the jury can be convinced that Dr. Murray was recklessly negligent and caused the death of Michael Jackson on the grounds that Dr. Murray:

- Knowingly prescribed improper and excessive medications to an obvious addict
- As a cardiologist, was neither qualified nor sufficiently knowledgeable to safely administer and monitor propofol, an anesthetic

- Lacked the skilled or the training for attempting to cure Jackson of his drug addiction
- Administered excessive amounts of propofol via injections to Michael Jackson and that the singer did not inject himself
- Did not have the necessary resuscitation skills, equipment and personnel required to treat Jackson should he stop breathing (a common complication of propofol toxicity)
- Made no efforts to consult with drug treatment experts as to the diagnosis and treatment of Jackson's drug addiction, and
- Inappropriately monitored and treated the Jackson's terminal collapse by performing inadequate CPR on a bed rather than on a firm surface and delayed notifying emergency medical personnel for mysterious reasons

In other words, "drugs don't kill people, bad doctors who give addicts drugs do."

As juries are well known to be unpredictable, one can only guess as to what their decision would be should this case go to trial. It is worth remembering that the burden of proof for any criminal trial will rest with the District Attorney – they have the hard job. In a civil trial, such as a malpractice suit, the burden will be on Dr. Murray to successfully defend himself.

We have not yet discussed one other facet of this case. Whether Dr. Murray's acts were criminal or not, whether he should be allowed to practice medicine or not, or whether he should or should not have been providing Jackson this dangerous drug, we cannot deny that Michael Jackson had free will. Michael Jackson was addicted to sedatives and pain pills and he repeatedly asked for the drugs that eventually killed him. One of the people who knew him stated emphatically: "Michael knew what he was doing." "He knew that the drugs he was taking – that the amount that he was taking – could kill him at any moment. And many people tried to stop him and discourage him, and it's very, very sad and tragic that he lived with so much pain that he couldn't stop." Jackson was in physical pain from years of physical abuse related to dancing and the rigors of performing and in mental and emotional agony from the loss of his childhood and his yearning to one day find it. But in the end, his choices killed him. The courts will only be deciding if Dr. Murray helped and, if so, how much.

Jackson never gave a farewell concert. Nonetheless, a movie ("*This Is It*") depicting the rehearsals for a final tour that never materialized earned $150 million within weeks of its release. His memorial service on July 7, 2009 was broadcast live around the world, attracting a global audience of up to one billion people. Now Little Michael finally has a chance to play and be whoever he wants to be.

Shooting Stars

The actions of physicians in combination with the personal choices made by the celebrities resulted in the deaths of the stars described above. Many other celebrities have died of overdoses related to prescription drug abuse and others have struggled with addictions to sedatives and painkillers. In some cases, there is little doubt that doctors provided these addicts with medications and turned a blind eye to overt substance abuse. In others, practitioners may have been duped into providing drugs to famous patients with fictitious illnesses or prescribing medications to groupies hoping to ingratiate themselves with a celebrity by providing them with a few pills. This is nothing new-groupies have been helping their idols to die for years. Other celebrities, however, have proven to be quite capable of helping themselves into the grave by abusing prescription medications with little assistance from fans or physicians.

Nearly 50 years ago, Marilyn Monroe died of an apparent suicidal overdose of barbiturates. Her drugs were prescribed by physicians, yet by all accounts at least one doctor was trying to wean her of her drug dependence. In 1965 Dorothy Dandridge, the first African American to be nominated for an Academy Award for Best Actress, was found dead by her manager. Her death was ruled to be due to an accidental overdose of imipramine, an antidepressant, that she took for a bipolar disorder. Jimi Hendrix, the famous American guitarist, was found dead in his girl-friend's London hotel room (although some have claimed that he died in the ambulance on the way to the hospital). The cause of death noted on the coroner's report was "inhalation of vomit" after "barbiturate intoxication (quinalbar-bitone)", the same prescription medication that had killed Monroe. In 1996 Margaux Hemmingway, a 42-year-old model and actress and granddaughter of Ernest Hemingway, was found dead in her apartment in Santa Monica, California. She died of a suicidal overdose of phenobarbital. Heath Ledger won a posthumous Oscar for his role as the Joker following his accidental drug overdose in early 2008. Although two doctors were investigated by the DEA following his death, no charges were filed and the U.S. Attorney in New York decided there were no "viable targets" for criminal prosecution. None of the above were following "doctor's orders" when they died.

Can It Be Stopped?

The short answer is "no." It is simply impossible (and probably unconstitutional) to make people stop acting in their own worst interests. That being said, steps can be taken to make it more difficult to obtain, abuse, and overdose on prescription medications. The first step is to recognize that there is a national prescription drug abuse epidemic that affects both the rich and famous as well as the masses. Doctors overprescribe pain medications and sedatives to Grammy Winners, Academy Award nominees, truck drivers, plumbers, and housewives. In many states, especially Florida, there has been an unfortunate blooming of "pill mills" where cash is exchanged for pills to treat ubiquitous lower back pain, migraines, and fibromyalgia. In fact, the authors have recently been informed that there are more pain clinics in their county than McDonald's restaurants. Just down the street from the Medical Examiner's Office, one can glance in the parking lot of the local pain clinic and study our newest South Florida tourists, the so-called "pillbillies," who obtain oxycodone and alprazolam for their "illnesses" and transport them back to Kentucky and West Virginia for distribution.

A few states have passed legislation requiring the creation of mandatory and confidential pharmacy databases. In theory, these information warehouses will facilitate the tracking of doctors who are giving out pills upon request. Unfortunately, though this sounds good, such measures have met with only limited success. Until stiffer penalties for both the prescribing physicians and abusing patients are enacted and enforced, people will continue to kill themselves, their friends, and their idols with prescription medications. And there will be physicians willing to inadvertently assist them.

Doctors have killed people, no doubt about it. But the death toll from medical murder, malfeasance, experimentation, terrorism, euthanasia, and tyranny is dwarfed by the carnage that patients have inflicted on themselves and those around them, including the ones they profess to love, by drug abuse. But who wants to read about that.

Suggested Reading

Chapters 1 and 2: In the Beginning; Perfect Intentions, Imperfect People

J Addison. The Healing Gods of Ancient Civilizations. University Books, New York, 1962.

I al-Jawziyya. Natural Healing with the Medicine of the Prophet. Pearl Publishing House, 1993–2008.

T Blanchard. Joining Heaven and Earth; Maimonides and the Laws of Bikkur Cholim (Visiting the Sick). National Center for Jewish Healing, New York, 1994.

N de S Cameron. The New Medicine: Life and Death After Hippocrates. Chicago Bioethics Press, 2002.

S Davies. Jesus the Healer. SCM Press, 1995.

Y Donden. Health Through Balance: An Introduction to Tibetan Medicine. Snow Lion Publications, 1986.

P Fenton. Tibetan Healing: The Modern Legacy of Medicine Buddha. Quest Books/Theosophical Publishing House, 1999.

A Greenbaum. The Wings of the Sun: Traditional Jewish Healing in Theory and Practice. Breslov Research Institute, Jerusalem, Israel/Monsey, NY, 1990.

T Grimsud. God's Healing Strategy: An Introduction to the Bible's Main Themes. Pandora Press U.S., 2000.

G Hart, M Forrest. Asclepius: The God of Medicine. RSM Press, 2000.

J Larchet. The Theology of Illness. Oakwood Publications, 2002.

C Morgan. Medicine of the Gods; Basic Principles of Ayurvedic Medicine. Charles T. Banford Company, 1994.

R Orr, N Pang. The Use of the Hippocratic Oath: A Review of 20th Century Practice and a Content Analysis of Oaths Administered in Medical Schools in the United States and Canada in 1993. The Journal of Clinical Ethics 8(4): 377–388, 1997. http://www.llu.edu/llu/bioethics/update/u141b.htm.

H Radest. From Clinic to Classroom: Medical Ethics and Moral Education. Praeger Publishers, 2000.

Chapter 3: The Alpha Killers: Three Prolific Murderous Doctors

A Esmail. Physician as serial killer – the Shipman case. The New England Journal of Medicine 2005; 352:1843–1844.

Harold Shipman's clinical practice 1974–1997. A clinical audit commissioned by the Chief Medical Officer of Britain Health Ministry. London, UK: Department of Health, 2001.

R Kaplan. The clinicide phenomenon: an exploration of medical murder. Australasian Psychiatry 2007; 15(4):299–304.

H Kinnell. Serial homicide by doctors: Shipman in perspective. British Medical Journal 2000; 321:1594–1597.

F Martin. The crimes, detection and death of Jack the Ripper. Barnes and Noble Books, 1987.

A McLaren. A prescription for murder – the Victorian serial killings of Dr. Thomas Neil. Chicago University Press, 1995.

M Newton. The encyclopedia of serial killers, 2nd ed. Checkmark Books, 2006.

A Rule. Bitter Harvest: A woman's fury, a mother's sacrifice. Simon & Shuster, 1998.

M Sitford. Addicted to murder. The true story of Dr Harold Shipman. London: Virgin Press, 2004.

P Sugden. Complete history of Jack the Ripper. Carrol and Graaf Publishers, 2002.

B Whittle, J Ritchie. Prescription for murder. The true story of mass murderer Dr. Harold Frederick Shipman. Time Warner Paperbacks, 2004.

C Wilson. The mammoth book of history of murder – the history of how and why mankind is driven to kill. Carrol and Graaf, 2000.

C Wilson, D Wilson. Written in blood: a history of forensic detection. Carroll and Graf, 2003.

Chapter 4: America's Contribution to Medical Mayhem

W Clarkson. The Good Doctor. St. Martin's Paperbacks, 2007.

C Evans. Killer Doctors: The Shocking True Crimes of Medical Deviates Who Practiced in Murder. Penguin Group, 2007.

K Iserson. Demon Doctors: Physicians as Serial Killers. Galen Press, 2002.

H Kinnell. Serial homicide by doctors: Shipman in perspective. British Medical Journal 2000; 23(321): 1594–1597.

G Olsen. Starvation Heights: A True Story of Murder and Malice in the Woods of the Pacific Northwest. Warner Books, 1997.

A Rule. Bitter Harvest. Pocket Books, 1999.

A Rule. Last Dance Last Chance – Ann Rule's Files. Pocket Books, 2003.

H Schechter. The Serial Killer Files. Ballantine Books, 2003.

G Scott. Homicide by the Rich and Famous – A Century of Prominent Killers. Westport Publishers, 2005.

J Stewart. Blind Eye: The Terrifying Story of a Doctor That Got Away with Murder. Simon and Schuster, 2000.

Chapter 5: International Men of Mystery: Other Serial Killers

E Carrere. L'adversaire; ed Gallimard – Collection, La Bibliotheque Gallimard, 2003.

Internet People's Daily January 16, 2001 at http://english.peopledaily.com.cn.

Killer's beliefs in omens, spirits led to attack on toddler. South Africa's Herald on-line (Port Elizabeth), October 28, 2008.

C Mack, D Mack. A Field Guide to Demons, Fairies, Fallen Angels, and Other Subversive Spirits. Holt Paperbacks, Owl Books edition, 1999.

Maxim Petrov. Wikipedia at http://en.wikipedia.org/wiki/Maxim_Petrov.

S Okie. Dr. Pou and the Hurricane – Implications for Patient Care During Disasters. The New England Journal of Medicine 2008; 358:1–5.

M Pistorius. Strangers on the Street: Serial Homicide in South Africa. Penguin Global, 2005.

A Pou. Hurricane Katrina and Disaster Responsiveness. The New England Journal of Medicine 2008; 358:1524.

D Schmidt. Natural Born Celebrities: Serial Killers in American Culture. University of Chicago Press, 2005.

J Shephard. Land of the Tikoloshe. Longman Green and Company, 1955.

Ticoloshe's friend. Time Magazine, February 20, 1956.

P Vronski. Serial Killers: The Method and Madness of Monsters. Berkley Trade, 2004.

Chapter 6: To Catch a Killer: Investing Serial Murder

S Egger. Serial Murders – An Elusive Phenomenon. Praeger Press, 1990.

C Ferguson, D White, S Cherry, M Lorenz, Z Bhimani. Defining and classifying serial murder in the context of perpetrator motivation. Journal of Criminal Justice 2003; 31(3): 287–292.

J Fox, J Levin. Extreme Killing: Understanding Serial and Mass Murder. Sage Publications, 2005.

S Giannangelo. The Psychopathology of Serial Murder – A Theory of Violence. Greenwood Press, 1996.

R Holmes, Stephen Holmes. Profiling Violent Crime: An Investigative Tool, 3rd ed. Sage Publications, 2002.

K Iserson. Demon Doctors: Physicians as Serial Killers. Galen Press, 2002.

R Kaplan. The clinicide phenomenon: an exploration of medical murder. Australasian Psychiatry 2007; 15(4): 299–304.

H Kinnell. Serial homicide by doctors: Shipman in perspective. British Medical Journal 2000; 23(321): 1594–1597.

A McLaren. A Prescription for Murder: The Victorian Serial Killing of Dr. Thomas Neill Cream. University of Chicago Press, 1995.

L Miller. Practical Police Psychology – Stress Management and Crisis Intervention for Law Enforcement. Charles C. Thomas, 2006.

H Morrison, Harold Goldberg. Inside the Minds of the World's Most Notorious Murderers. Harper Collins, 2004.

W Petherick. The Science of Criminal Profiling: All Killers Have Their Own Modus Operandi. Barnes & Noble, 2005.

P Vronski. Serial Killers: The Method and Madness of Monsters. Berkley Trade, 2004.

B Yorker, K Kizer, P Lampe, A Forrest, J Lannan, D Russell. Serial murders by healthcare professionals. Journal of Forensic Sciences 2006; 51(6): 1362–1371.

Chapter 7: The Nazi Murders

M Burleigh. The Third Reich – A New History. Hill and Wang, 2001.

F Dikotter. Race Culture: Recent Perspectives on the History of Eugenics. The American Historical Review 1998; 103: 467–468.

R Evans. The Third Reich in Power, 1933–1939. Penguin Books, 2005.

H Gallagher. By Trust Betrayed: Patients, Physicians, and the License to Kill in the Third Reich. Henry Holt and Co., 1990.

D Kevles. In the Name of Eugenics: Genetics and the Uses of Human Heredity. Harvard University Press, 1995.

C Koonz. Ethical Dilemmas and Nazi Eugenics: Single-Issue Dissent in Religious Contexts. The Journal of Modern History 1992; 64 (Supplement: Resistance Against the Third Reich; pp. S8–S31).

A LeBor, R Boyes. Seduced by Hitler – The Choices of a Nation and the Ethics of Survival. Barnes & Noble Books, 2000.

R Lifton. The Nazi Doctors Medical Killing and the Psychology of Genocide. Basic Books, 2000.

P Mehta. Human Eugenics: Whose Perception of Perfection? The History Teacher (Long Beach, California) 2000; 33: 222–240.

S Milgram. Obedience to Authority: An Experimental View. Harper Perennial Modern Classics, 2004.

R Proctor. Racial Hygiene: Medicine Under the Nazis. Harvard University Press, 1988.

R Proctor. The Nazi War on Cancer. Princeton University Press, 1999.

L Weber. The Holocaust Chronicles. Publications International Ltd., 2003.

P Weindling. Health, Race and German Politics Between National Unification and Nazism, 1870–1945. Cambridge University Press, 1989.

P Weingart. German Eugenics Between Science and Politics. The University of Chicago Press, 1989.

S Weiss. The Race Hygiene Movement in Germany. Osiris, University of Chicago Press, 1987; 3:193–236.

Chapter 8: Hitler's "Scientists"

G Annas, M Godin eds. The Nazi doctors and the Nurenberg code: Human rights in human experimentation. Oxford University Press, 1992.

N Baumslag. Nazi doctors, human experimentation and typhus. Praeger Publishers, 2005.

D Bogod. The Nazi hypothermia experiment. Anaesthesia 2004; 59(12):115.

A Caplan. When medicine went mad: Bioethics and the holocaust. Humana Press, 1992.

R Lifton. The Nazi doctor, medical killings and the psychology of genocide. Basic Books, 2000.

L Matalon. Children of the flames: Dr. Mengele and the untold story of the twins of Auschwitz. New York: William Morrow, 1991.

Nurenberg trial proceedings v. 4 20 Dec. 1945, Nurenberg Trials Page by Yale Law School. http://www.yale.edu/lawweb/Avalon/init/proc12-20-45.htm.

J Preuss, B Madea. Gerhart Panning (1900–1944): a German forensic pathologist and his involvement in Nazi crimes during Second World War. American Journal of Forensic Medicine and Pathology 2009; 30(1):14–17.

N Schaefer. The legacy of Nazi medicine. The New Atlantis 2004; 5:54–60. http://www.thenewatlantis.com/publications/the-legacy-of-nazi-medicine.

V Spitz. Doctors from hell; The horrific account of Nazi experiments on humans. Sentient Publications, 2005.

P Weindling. Nazi medicine and the Nurenberg trials: From medical war crimes to informed consent. Palgrave Mc Millan, 2005.

Chapter 9: Made in Japan: Unethical Experiments

D Barenblatt. A Plague upon Humanity: the Secret Genocide of Axis Japan's Germ Warfare Operation. Harper Collins, 2004.

W Barnaby. The Plague Makers: The Secret World of Biological Warfare. Frog Ltd, 1999.

S Endicott, E Hagerman. The United States and Biological Warfare: Secrets from the Early Cold War and Korea. Indiana University Press, 1999.

H Gold. Unit 731 Testimony. Charles E Tuttle Co., 1996.

S Handelman, K Alibek. Biohazard: The Chilling True Story of the Largest Covert Biological Weapons Program in the World – Told from Inside by the Man Who Ran It. Random House, 1999.

S Harris. Factories of Death: Japanese Biological Warfare 1932–45 and the American Cover-Up. Routledge Press, 1994.

R Harris, J Paxman. A Higher Form of Killing: The Secret History of Chemical and Biological Warfare. Random House, 2002.

N Kristof. Confronting Gruesome War Atrocity. New York Times, March 17, 1995.

T Tsuchiya. In the Shadow of the Past Atrocities: Research Ethics with Human Subjects in Contemporary Japan. Eubios Journal of Asian and International Bioethics 2003; 13:100–102.

P Williams. Unit 731: Japan's Secret Biological Warfare in World War II. Free Press, 1989.

Chapter 10: Good Old Fashioned American Ingenuity-and Evil

S Baker, O Bradley, L Marks. Effects of untreated syphilis in the Negro male, 1932 to 1972: A closure comes to the Tuskegee study. Urology 2004; 65(6):1259–1262.

D Black. Acid: A New Secret History of LSD, 2nd ed. Vision, 2003.

W Bowart. Operation Mind Control: Our Secret Government's War Against Its Own People. Dell, 1978.

F Camper. The MK/Ultra Secret. Christopher Scott (CS) Publishing, 1997.

A Collins. In the Sleep Room: The Story of CIA Brainwashing Experiments in Canada. Key Porter Books, 1998.

R Delagado, H Leskovac. Informed Consent in Human Experimentation: Bridging the Gap Between Ethical Thought and Current Practice. UCLA Law Review 1986; 34(1):67–160.

A Goliszek. In the Name of Science: A History of Secret Programs, Medical Research, and Human Experimentation. St. Martin Press, 2003.

A Hornblum. Acres of Skin: Human Experiments at Holmesburg Prison. Routledge Press, 1999.

J Jones. Bad Blood: The Tuskegee Syphilis Experiment. Free Press, 1993.

M Lee, B Shlain. Acid Dreams: The Complete Social History of LSD: The CIA, the Sixties, and Beyond. Grove Press, 1994.

J Marks. The Search for the Manchurian Candidate; The CIA and Mind Control. W.W. Norton & Co., 1991.

A McCoy. A Question of Torture: CIA Interrogation, from the Cold War to the War on Terror. Metropolitan Books, 2006.

J Moreno. Undue Risk: Secret State Experiments on Humans. Routledge Press, 2000.

J Moreno. Mind Wars: Brain Research and National Defense. Dana Press, 2006.

J Ranelagh. The Agency: The Rise and Decline of the CIA. Touchstone Books, 1987.

R Singer. Consent of the Unfree: Medical Experimentation and Behavior Modification in the Closed Institution. Law and Human Behavior 1977; 1(1):1–43.

J Stevens. Storming Heaven: LSD and the American Dream. Grove Press, 1998.

G Thomas. Journey into Madness: The True Story of Secret CIA Mind Control and Medical Abuse. Bantam Press, 1989.

U.S. Congress: The Select Committee to Study Governmental Operations with Respect to Intelligence Activities, Foreign and Military Intelligence (Church Committee Report). Report no. 94-755, 94th Cong., 2nd Session, Washington, DC: GPO, 1976.

U.S. Senate: Joint Hearing Before the Select Committee on Intelligence and The Subcommittee on Health and Scientific Research of the Committee on Human Resources; 95th Cong., 1st Session, August 3, 1977.

J Vankin, J Whalin. Eighty Greatest Conspiracies of All Time. Citadel Press, 2004.
H Washington. Medical Apartheid: The Dark History of Medical Experimentation on Black Americans from Colonial Times to the Present. Doubleday, 2007.
E Welsome. The Plutonium Files: America's Secret Medical Experiments in the Cold War. The Dial Press, 1999.

Chapter 11: Physician Kill Thyself

L Altman. Who goes first: The story of self experimentation in medicine. Random House, NY, 1987.
L Andrew. Physicians' suicide. E-Medicine WEB MD Emedicinemedscape.com/article/806779. overview.
L Dendi, M Boring. The story of self experimentation. Random House, NY, 1987.
L Dyrbe, M. Thomas, F Nassie, et al. Burnout and suicidal ideation amongst U.S. medical students. Annals of Internal Medicine 2008; 149(5): 334–341.
A Fiks. Self experimentation: Sources of study. Edited by W Bullow. Praeger, Westport and London, 2003.
C Fontenot, W O'Leary. Dr. Forssman's self-experimentation. American Surgeon 1996; 62(6): 514–515.
J Franklin, J Sutherland. Guinea pig doctors: The drama of medical research through self experimentation. Morow Press, NY, 1984.
E Harris. Eight scientists who became their own guinea pigs. New Scientist Health. http://www.newscientist.com/article/dn16735-eight-scientists-who-became-their-own-guineapigs.html?full =true.
I Kerridge. Altruism or reckless curiosity? A brief history of self experimentation in medicine. Internal Medicine Journal 2003; 33: 203–207.
A Martinelli, A Czelusta, S Peterson. Self-experimenters in medicine: heroes or fools? Part I. Pathogens. Clinics in Dermatology 2008; 26(5): 570–573.
M Myers, C Fine. Suicide in physicians, towards prevention. Medscape General Medicine. http://www.medscape.com/view article/462612.
K Rose, I Rosow. Physicians who kill themselves. Archives of General Psychiatry 1973; 29(6): 800–805.
E Schernhammer. Taking their own lives – the high rate of physicians' suicide. The New England Journal of Medicine 2005; 352 (24): 2473–2476.
E Schernhammer, G Colditz. Suicide rate amongst physicians: a quantitative and gender assessment. American Journal of Psychiatry 2004; 161: 2295–2302.

Chapter 12: Libel Plots Against Physicians

J Brent and V Naumov: Stalin's Last Crime. The Plot Against the Jewish Doctors 1948–1953. Harper Collins Publishers, 2003.
J Brooks. Thank You, Comrade Stalin!: Soviet Public Culture from Revolution to Cold War. Princeton University Press, 2000.
M Clarfield. The Soviet "Doctors' Plot" 50 years on. British Medical Journal 2002; 325: 1487.
N Cohn. Warrant for Genocide: Myth of the Jewish World-Conspiracy and the Protocols of the Elders of Zion, 3rd ed., Serif, 1996.
V Hatchinski. Stalin's last years: delusions or dementia. European Journal of Neurology 1999; 6(2): 129–132.

S Montefiori. Stalin: The Court of the Red Tsar. Vintage, 2005.

L Rapoport. Stalin's war against the Jews: the Doctors' Plot and the Soviet solution. Toronto: Free Press, 1990.

Y Rapoport. The doctors plot of 1953. Translated by N.A. Perova and R.S. Bobrova. Cambridge University Press, 1991.

Vicious spies and killers under the Mask of Academic Physicians. Pravda, January 13, 1953 as translated by Wikipedia, http://en.wikipedia.org/wiki/Doctors'_plot.

World Medical Association. Charges against Russian doctors. British Medical Journal 1953; i(suppl): 136.

Chapter 13: Judge, Jury, Executioner, and Doctor

E Abbott. The Duvalier and Their Legacy. Touchstone Publishing, 1991.

J Anderson. Che Guevara: A Revolutionary Life. Grove Press, 1997.

B Anzulovic. Heavenly Serbia: From Myth To Genocide. New York University Press, 1999.

L Benson. Yugoslavia; A Concise history; Revised and updated edition, 2nd ed. Palgrave-MacMillan, 2004.

P Constable. Haiti's Shattered Hopes; Journal of Democracy. Johns Hopkins University Press, 1992.

B Diederich, Al Burt. Papa Doc and the Tontones Macoutes. Marcus Wiener Publishing, 2005.

J Ferguson. Papa Doc, Baby Doc: Haiti and the Duvaliers. Blackwell Publishers, 1988.

A Finlan. The Collapse of Yugoslavia 1991–1999. Osprey Publishing, 2004.

G Greene. The Comedians. Penguin Classics, 1991.

E Guevara. The Motorcycle Diaries: A Journey Around South America. London: Verso, 1996.

E Guevara. Latin America: Awakening of a Continent. Ocean Press, 2008.

E Guevara and H Villegas. Guerrilla Warfare. Authorized Edition, Ocean Press, 2006.

R Harris. Death of a Revolutionary, Che Guevara's Lost Mission. W.W. Norton & Co, 2007.

J Hart. Che: The Life, Death, and Afterlife of a Revolutionary. Basic Books, 2004.

N Hawton. The Quest for Radovan Karadzik. Hutchinson Press, 2009.

T Judah. The Serbs; History, Myth and the Destruction of Yugoslavia, 2nd ed. Yale University Press, 2000.

T Judah. Kosovo: War and Revenge, 2nd ed. Yale University Press, 2002.

R Kaplan. Balkan Ghosts: A Journey Through History. Picador Press, 2005.

J Kees van Donge. Kamuzu's legacy: the democratization of Malawi. African Affairs1995; 94(375): 227–257. http://afraf.oxfordjournals.org/cgi/content/citation/94/375/227.

R Mahmutcehajic. The Denial of Bosnia (Post-Communist Cultural Studies). Pennsylvania State University Press, 2000.

J Mertus. Kosovo: How Myths and Truth Started a War. University of California Press, 1999.

G Mwakikagile. Africa After Independence: Realities of Nationhood. Continental Press, 2006.

H Pierre. Haiti, Rising Flames from Burning Ashes. University Press of America, 2006.

M Plimmer. Bryan King. Beyond Coincidence. Icon Books, 2005.

A Segal, B Weinstein. Haiti: The Failure of Politics. Praeger Publishers; 1992.

P Short. Banda. Routledge, Kegan and Paul Publishers, 1974.

C Stewart. Hunting the Tiger: The Fast Life and Violent Death of the Balkans Most Dangerous Man. Thomas Dunne Books, 2008.

C Strader. The Muslim-Croat Civil War in Central Bosnia 1992–1994. University Press, 2003.

T Williams. Malawi, the Politics of Despair. Cornell University Press, 1978.

Chapter 14: Trading Treatment for Terror

Y Aboul-Enein. Ayman al-Zawahiri's Knights Under the Prophet's Banner: The al-Qaeda Manifesto. Book Review. U.S. Army SCSC; Military Review, 2005.

G Davis. Religion of Peace? Islam's War Against the World. World Ahead Publishing, 2006.

M el-Zayed. The Road to al-Qaeda: The Story of Bin Laden's Right Hand Man. Critical Studies on Islam. Pluto Press, 2004.

S Emerson. Jihad Incorporated: A Guide to Militant Islam in US. Prometheus Books, 2006.

M Levitt. Hamas: Politics, Charity and Terrorism in the Service of Jihad. Yale University Press, 2007.

A Nussea. Muslim Palestine: The Ideology of Hamas. Routledge, 1998.

M Rosaler. Hamas: Palestinian Terrorists (Inside the World Most Infamous Terrorist Organization). Rosen Publishing Books, 2002.

B Rubin, J Colp Rubin. Anti-American Terrorism and the Middle East: A Documentary Reader. Oxford University Press, 2002.

P Williams. The Al Qaeda Connection. Prometheus Books, 2005.

Chapter 15: Guilty Until Proven Innocent

E Anderson. House panel OKs bill sparked by Dr. Anna Pou case. The Times-Picayune, May 14, 2008. http://www.nola.com/news/index.ssf/2008/05/baton_rouge_legislation_that.html.

J Bohannon. Science in Libya: evidence overruled: medics on death row. Science 2005; 308:184–185.

Courage amid Katrina chaos. ABC News, December 16, 2005. http://abcnews.go.com/2020/HurricaneKatrina/story?id=1410279&page=1.

Doctors Call for Release of Medical Workers Accused of Infecting Libyan Children with HIV. Medical News Today, October 30, 2006.

G Filosa. Investigation of physician in Katrina case protested – care for patients at hospital praised. The Times-Picayune, July 18, 2007.

D Griffin, K Johnson. Medical experts never testified in Katrina Hospital deaths. August 27, 2007, CNN.com, http://www.cnn.com/2007/US/08/26/hospital.grandjury/index.html.

HIV trial in Libya. Wikipedia, http://en.wikipedia.org/wiki/HIV_trial_in_Libya.

T Hundley. Libya frees nurses, doctor accused of infecting children. Chicago Tribune, July 24, 2007. http://www.highbeam.com/doc/1G1-166761657.html.

C Kollas, B Boyer-Kollas, J Kollas. Criminal prosecution of physicians providing palliative or end-of-life care. Journal of Palliative Medicine 2008; 11(2): 233–241.

C Kromm, S Sturgis. Hurricane Katrina and the guiding principles on internal displacement. The Institute for Southern Studies – Southern Exposure 2008; 36(1).

E Langston. AMA: Justice served for Dr. Pou. Position Statement of American Medical Association, July 24, 2007.

M Neil. Katrina hospital death charges dropped. ABA Journal; Law News Now, July 5, 2007. http://www.abajournal.com/news/katrina_hospital_death_charges_dropped/.

New Orleans MD charges dropped. Internal Medicine News, August 15, 2007.

S Okie. Dr. Pou and the Hurricane – implications for patient care during disasters. The New England Journal of Medicine 2008; 358(1):1–5.

Physicians for Human Rights (PHR) press releases on the accused nurses and doctor in Libya. PHR Library, 2007. http://physiciansforhumanrights.org/library/press-releases-libya-nurses.html

J Simon. Death sentence for medics in Libyan HIV case. The Guardian, May 6, 2004. http://yaleglobal.yale.edu/display.article?id=3819

Chapter 16: Euthanasia and Assisted Suicide: What Would Hippocrates Do?

M Betzold. Appointment with Doctor Death. Momentum Books LLC, 1993.

I Byock. Kevorkian: Right Problem, Wrong Solution [Letter to the Editor], The Washington Post, January 1994, p. A23.

Doctor death. Dr. Jack Kevorkian is back on his crusade. Is he an angel of mercy or a murderer? Time Magazine, May 31, 1993.

G Dworkin, R Frey, S Bok. Euthanasia and Physician-Assisted Suicide. Cambridge University Press, 1998.

C Dyer. Withdrawal of food supplement judged as misconduct. British Medical Journal 1999; 318: 895.

Findlaw's compilation. http://news.findlaw.com/legalnews/lit/schiavo/.

R Fine. From Quinlan to Schiavo: medical, ethical, and legal issues in severe brain injury. Proceedings of Baylor University Medical Center 2005; 18(4): 303–310.

H Groenewoud, P van der Maas, G van der Wal, et al. Physician-assisted death in psychiatric practice in the Netherlands. The New England Journal of Medicine 1997; 336: 1795–1801.

G Harris, B Tamas, N Lind. Dynamics of Social Welfare Policy: Right Versus Left. Rowman and Littlefield, 2008.

H Hendin. Seduced by Death: Doctors, Patients and Assisted Suicide. W.W. Norton & Company, 1998.

D Hillyard, J Dombrink. Dying Right: The Death with Dignity Movement. Routledge, 2001.

J Hoefler. Managing Death. Basic Books, 1997.

D Humphry. Final Exit: The Practicalities of Self Deliverance and Assisted Suicide for the Dying. Bantam Books, 2002.

B Jennett. The Vegetative State: Medical Facts, Ethical and Legal Dilemmas. Cambridge University Press, 2002.

J Kevorkian. Prescription Medicine. The Goodness of Planned Death. Prometheus Books, 1993.

A Mclean. Briefcase on Medical Law. Routledge Cavendish, 2003.

S McLean, A Britton. The Case for Physician Assisted Suicide. Pandora Press, 1997.

T Moore, M Cohen, C Furberg. Serious adverse drug events reported to the Food and Drug Administration 1998–2005. Archives of Internal Medicine 2007; 167(16): 1752–1759.

J Moreno. Arguing Euthanasia: The Controversy over Mercy Killing, Assisted Suicide, and the "Right to Die." Touchstone, 1995.

A Murray. Suicide in the Middle Ages. Oxford University Press, 2000.

M Otlowski. Voluntary Euthanasia and the Common Law. Oxford University Press, 1997.

Pope John Paul II. Care for patients in a "permanent vegetative state. Origins 2004; 33(43): 737, 739–740. http://www.vatican.va/holy_father/john_paul_ii/speeches/2004/march/documents/hf_jp-ii_spe_20040320_congress-fiamc_en.html.

T Quill. Death and Dignity: Making Choices and Taking Charge. W.W. Norton & Company, 1994.

S Rosenblatt. Murder of Mercy: Euthanasia on Trial. Prometheus Books, 1992

T Rutter. US Supreme Court decides physician assisted suicide is unconstitutional. British Medical Journal 1997; 315: 9.

M Seguin. A Gentle Death. Key Porter Books, 1994.

D Short. Should Doctors Support the Living Will? Chapter 4 in "Euthanasia: an edited collection of articles from the Journal of the Christian Medical Fellowship." CMF, London, 1994. http://www.cmf.org.uk/ethics/content.asp?context=article&id=1366.

W Smith. Forced Exit: The Slippery Slope from Assisted Suicide to Legalized Murder. Spence Publishing Company, 2003.

P van der Maas, G van der Wal, I Haverkate, et al. Euthanasia, physician assisted suicide, and other medical practices involving the end of life in the Netherlands, 1990–1995. The New England Journal of Medicine 1996; 335: 1699–1705.

H White, J Jalsevac. Kevorkian denounces "Tyrant". Pushes for euthanasia in Florida speech. St. Petersburg News, January 16, 2008.
J Wise. Australian euthanasia law throws up many difficulties. British Medical Journal 1998; 317: 969.

Chapter 17: Malpractice or Murder?

T Albert. Malpractice or murder? American Medical News, October 22/29, 2001.
G Annas. Medicine, death and the criminal law. The New England Journal of Medicine 1995; 333:527–530.
D Baker, M Wolf, J Feinglass, et al. Health literacy and mortality among elderly persons. Archives of Internal Medicine 2007;167(14):1503–1509.
L Berlin. Consequences of being accused of malpractice. American Journal of Radiology 1997; 169:1219–1223.
L Berlin, J Spies, B Silver, J Brenner. Malpractice issues in radiology. Maer Roentgen Ray Society, 1993.
D Brahams. Doctors and manslaughter. Lancet 1993; 341:1404.
M Crane. Practice medicine, land in jail. Wall Street Journal, February 21, 1995; A24.
E Duncanson, V Richards, K Luce, J Gill. Medical homicide and extreme negligence. American Journal of Forensic Medicine and Pathology 2009; 30(1):18–22.
R Eisenberg, L Berlin. When does malpractice become manslaughter? American Journal of Radiology 2002; 179:331–335.
I Loudon. Maternal mortality in the past and its relevance to developing countries today. American Journal of Clinical Nutrition 2000; 72(1):241S–246S. http://www.ajcn.org/cgi/content/full/72/1/241S.
E Monico, R Kulkarni, A Calise, J Calabro. The criminal prosecution of medical negligence. The Internet Journal of Law, Healthcare and Ethics 2007; 5(1). http://www.ispub.com/ostia/index.php?xmlFilePath=journals/ijlhe/vol5n1/criminal.xml.
Navy Heart Surgeon imprisoned in 1984 is practicing again. New York Times, December 24, 2008.
Physician charged with manslaughter after OR death. American Medical News, November 4, 1996; 34.
A Sadetzki, A Chetrit, A Lubina, M Stovall. Risk of thyroid cancer after childhood exposure to ionizing radiation for Tinea Capitis. Journal of Clinical Endocrinology and Metabolism 2006; 91(12):4798–4804.
The People v Einaugler; 618 NYS2d 414 (NY App 1994).

Chapter 18: It's All Natural

G Colata. On fringes of health care, untested therapies thrive. The New York Times, December 11, 2008.
G Costa. Attachment therapy on trial: The torture and death of Candace Newmaker. In Child Psychology and Mental Health by Jean Mercer, Laary Sarner, Linda Rosa. Praeger, 2003.
J Crellin, F Ania. Professionalism and Ethics in Complementary and Alternative Medicine. Routledge, 2001.
E Ernst. Healing, Hype, or Harm? A Critical Analysis of Complementary or Alternative Medicine. Imprint Academic, 2008.

N Faas. Integrating Complementary Medicine into Health Systems. Aspen Publication, 2001.

J Klastersky, S Schimpff, H Senn. Complementary Medicine by in Supportive Care in Cancer: A Handbook for Oncologists, Chapter 30. Informa Health Care, 1999.

S Saper, S Kales, J Paquin, et al. Heavy metal content of ayurvedic herbal medicine products. Journal of the American Medical Association 2004; 292:2868–2873.

A Shang, K Huwiler-Müntener, L Nartey, P Juni, S Dorig, J Sterne, et al. Are the clinical effects of homoeopathy placebo effects? Comparative study of placebo-controlled trials of homeopathy and allopathy. Lancet 2005; 366:726–732.

S Singh, E Ernst. Trick or Treatment: The Undeniable Facts About Alternative Medicine. W.W. Norton & Company, 2008.

D Studdert, D Eisenberg, F Miller, D Curto, T Kaptchuk, T Brennan. Medical malpractice implications of alternative medicine. Journal of the American Medical Association 1998; 280:1610–1615.

M Weintraub, D Studdert, T Brennan. Legal implications of practicing alternative medicine. Journal of the American Medical Association 1999; 281: 1698–1699.

Chapter 19: Contagious Caregivers

R Angler. Scientists linked to Heimlich investigates – Experiment infects AIDS patient in China with malaria. The Cincinnati Enquirer, February 16, 2003.

Corrupt doctors infect 100 Kazakh children with HIV. ABC News, June 28, 2007.

Deliberately infecting AIDS patients with malaria. Reuters, April 14, 2003.

C Dyer. Surgeon jailed for infecting patient. British Medical Journal 1994; 309:896.

Egypt-justice-AIDS: Egyptian doctors, nurses jailed for infecting patients with AIDS. Agence France-Presse, September 24, 2002.

Feds say doctor exposed patients to infection. Posted by Chronicle News Service, November 14, 2007; 22:02.

L Gostin. HIV-infected physicians and the practice of seriously invasive procedures. The Hastings Center Report, 1989; 19.

J Jones. Public Health crisis due to negligence at endoscopy center. Health Line. http://www. healthline.com/blogs/healthline_connects/labels/unsafe%20practice.html.

B Lambert. Kimberly Bergalis is dead at 23: Symbol of debate over AIDS tests. New York Times, December 9, 1991.

B Lambert. Infected doctor told to get patients' consent. New York Times, April 19, 2002.

J Manier. Four organ patients get HIV donor's infection is 1st such case in U.S. in 22 years. Chicago Tribune, November 13, 2007.

H Minich, J Moreno, R Nichols, et al. Infected physicians and invasive procedures; safe practice management. Clinical Infectious Diseases 2005; 40:1665–1672.

S Nuland; The doctors' plague: Germs, childbed fever, and the strange story of Ignac Semmelweis. W.W. Norton & Company, 2004.

A Reitsma, M Closen, M Cunningham, et al. Infective physicians and invasive procedures. Clinical Infectious Diseases 2005; 40:1665–1672.

D Shelton. Patient sues over getting HIV, hepatitis from infected kidney donor. Chicago Tribune, November 18, 2008.

J Smith, L Berlin. Malpractice issues in radiology: the infected or substance abuse impaired radiologist. American Journal of Radiology 2002; 178:567–571.

D Spurgeon. Doctors and officials should not have been charged over infected blood, lawyers say. British Medical Journal 2007; 335:743.

P Terekerz, R Pearson, J Jagger. Infected physicians and invasive procedures: National policy and legal reality. Milkbank Quarterly 1999; 77(4):511–529.

A Toufexis, L Griggs, D Thompson. When the doctor gets infected. Time, January 14, 1991.

P Vitttello. Hepatitis found again among doctor's patients Nassau County. New York Times, November 20, 2007.
I Wilson. When doctors become patients. Oxford University Press, 2007.

Chapter 20: Fictitious Physicians: Where Has Marcus Welby Gone?

Dubner S. When Doctors Write. Posted March 28, 2007, http://freakonomics.blogs.nytimes.com/2007/03/28/when-doctors-write/, researched January 19, 2009.
http://en.wikipedia.org/wiki/I_Am_Legend_(film), last modified January 24, 2009; accessed January 25, 2009.
http://www.nationmaster.com/encyclopedia/Dr._Christian_Szell, Nationmaster.com, 2003-5; accessed January 25, 2009.
http://en.wikipedia.org/wiki/The_Boys_from_Brazil_(film), last modified January 28, 2009; accessed January 29, 2009.
http://www.nlm.nih.gov/hmd/frankenstein/frank_modern_1.html, last modified February 13, 2002; accessed January 25, 2009.
http://en.wikipedia.org/wiki/Hannibal_Lecter, last modified January 27, 2009; accessed January 28, 2009.
http://www.cliffsnotes.com/WileyCDA/LitNote/Dr-Jekyll-and-Mr-Hyde-About-the-Novel-A-Brief-Synopsis.id-88,pageNum-2.html, John Wiley and Sons; accessed January 25, 2009.
http://en.wikipedia.org/wiki/AFI%27s_100_Years..._100_Heroes_and_Villains, page last modified January 29, 2009; accessed January 29, 2009.
http://en.wikipedia.org/wiki/Dr._Evil, page last modified January 21, 2009; accessed January 29, 2009.
http://iamlegend.warnerbros.com/, 2008; accessed January 29, 2009.

Chapter 21: Doctors to the Stars

Ambulance report on Marilyn's death. http://www.angelfire.com/stars/mmgoddess/AMBULANCE.html.
K Anger. Hollywood Babylon. Dell Publishing, 1975.
Anna Nicole Smith. http://en.wikipedia.org/wiki/Anna_Nicole_Smith.
M Baden, J Hennessee. Unnatural Death: Confessions of a Medical Examiner. Random House, New York, 1992.
S Boteach. The Michael Jackson Tapes: A Tragic Icon Reveals His Soul in Intimate Conversation. Vanguard Press, 2009.
M Boyer. The Hollywood Culture: What You Don't Know Can Hurt You. XLibris Corporation, 2008.
Broward County Medical Examiner's Office Investigative Report. 2/8/07. http://www.broward.org/medical/investigative_report.pdf.
P Brown, P Broeske. Down at the End of a Lonely Street: The Life and Death of Elvis' Presley. Signet Press, 1998.
Celebrities using heroin. http://www.heroinhelper.com/bored/celebrities/index.shtml, 2004.
G Clarke. Get Happy; The life of Judy Garland. Dell Publishing, 2000.
L Deutsch. Pharmacist says he warned against drug for Smith. Associated Press 10/20/09. http://abcnews.go.com/Entertainment/wireStory?id=8868438.

L Deutsch. Three held for trial in Anna Nicole death. Associated Press 11/1/09. http://www.fancast. com/blogs/celebrities/three-held-for-trial-in-anna-nicole-death/.

D Eby. Actors and addiction. Talent Development Resources. http://talentdevelop.com/articles/ AAA.html.

Elvis' Presley. Rolling Stone, 2009. http://www.rollingstone.com/artists/elvispresley/biography.

S Giancana, C Giancana, B Giancana; Double Cross: the Explosive, Inside Story of the Mobster Who Controlled America. Grand Central Publishing, 1993.

A Goldman. Elvis': The Last 24 Hours. 1990.

F Guiles. Legend: The Life and Death of Marilyn Monroe. Scarborough House, 1992.

P Guralnick. The Last Train to Memphis. Little, Brown & Co., 1994.

P Guralnick. Careless Love: The Unmaking of Elvis' Presley. Little, Brown & Co., 1999.

J Halpering. Unmasked: The Final Years of Michael Jackson. Simon Spotlight Entertainment, 2009.

A Higginbotham. Doctor Feelgood. The Observer, August 11, 2002.

J Hopkins. Elvis': The Biography. Plexus, 2007.

M Jackson. Moonwalk. Doubleday, 1998.

T Jordan. Norma Jean: My Secret Life with Marilyn Monroe. William Morris & Co., New York, 1989.

Judy Garland, 47, Found Dead. The New York Times, June 23, 1969. http://www.nytimes.com/ books/00/04/09/specials/garland-obit.html.

M Kusinitz. Celebrity Drug Use; Encyclopedia of Psychoactive Drugs, Series 2. Chelsea House Publications, December1987.

CK Lawford. Moments of Clarity: Voices from the Front Lines of Addiction and Recovery. William Morrow, December 2008.

B Leaming. Marilyn Monroe. Crown Publishers, New York, 1998.

L Loft Interview. Live Journal, 2009. http://community.livejournal.com/ohnotheydidnt/37815902.html.

N Mailer. Marilyn Monroe: A Biography. Grosset & Dunlap, 1973.

D Marsh. Elvis'. Smithmark Publishing, 1997.

B Mason. Elvis' Presley. Penguin Group, 2007.

A Nash, B Smith, M Lacker, L Fike. Elvis' and the Memphis Mafia. Aurum Press, 2005.

T Noguchi, J Dimona. Coroner. Simon and Schuster, 1983.

D Pinsky, S Young. The Mirror Effect: How Celebrity Narcissism is Seducing America. Harper Collins Publishers, March 2009.

Police affidavits in Michael Jackson's case. http://www.examiner.com/x-19141-Hollywood- Concerts-Examiner~y2009m8d25-Michael-Jackson-search-warrant-in-its-entirety-minus- redactions-by-law-enforcement.

G Posner. Elvis' Doctors Speaks. The Daily Beast, 2009. http://www.thedailybeast.com/blogs- and-stories/2009-08-14/elviss-doctor-speaks/1/.

P Presley. Elvis' and Me. Putnam, 1985.

D Shipman. Judy Garland: The Secret Life of an American Legend. Hyperion Books, 1993.

R Simone. The Mysterious Death of Michael Jackson – The REAL Story. Headroom Kindle Books, 2009.

D Spoto. Marilyn Monroe: The Biography. Cooper Square Press, 2001.

Statistics of abuse of prescription medications. Source: National Survey on Drug Use and Health. http://www.samhsa.gov/.

G Stromberg, J Merrill. The Harder They Fall; Celebrities Tell Their Real Life Stories of Addiction and Recovery. Hazelden, April 2005.

A Summers. Goddess: The Secret Lives of Marilyn Monroe. MacMillan, New York, 1985.

JR Taraborrelli. Michael Jackson: The Magic, the Madness, the Whole Story, 1958–2009. Hachette Book Group, 2009.

R Veach. The case for Michael Jackson's Doctor. Oup Blog, Oxford University Press, September 14, 2009. http://blog.oup.com/2009/09/michael-jackson-doctor/.

D Wolfe. The Last Days of Marilyn Monroe. William Morrow, New York, 1998.

B Woodward. Wired: The Short Life and Fast Times of John Belushi. Pocket Publisher, 1985.

Index